Concise Textbook of Equine Clinical Practice Book 3

This concise, practical text covers the essential information veterinary students and nurses, new graduates, and practitioners need to succeed in equine medicine, focussing on respiratory and gastrointestinal diseases. Written for an international readership, the book conveys the core information in an easily digestible, precise form with extensive use of bullet points, lists, diagrams, protocols, and extensive illustrations (over 300 full-colour, high-quality photographs).

Part of a five-book series that extracts and updates key information from Munroe's *Equine Surgery, Reproduction and Medicine,* Second Edition, the book distils best practice in a logical straightforward clinically based approach. It details relevant clinical anatomy, physical clinical examination techniques and findings, normal parameters, aetiology/pathophysiology, differential diagnoses, diagnostic techniques, management and treatment, and prognosis. The emphasis is on information tailored to general equine clinicians with just enough on advanced techniques to make the practitioner aware of what is available elsewhere.

- The respiratory system is split into sections on surgical and medical conditions of the upper and lower respiratory tract.
- The gastrointestinal system is divided into the upper tract, including the oral cavity and dentistry, and the lower tract and peritoneal cavity.

Ideal for veterinary students and nurses on clinical placements with horses as well as practitioners needing a quick reference 'on the ground'.

Concise Textbook of Equine Clinical Practice Book 3

Respiratory and Gastrointestinal Diseases

Tim Barnett
Laura H. Javsicas
Graham Munroe

Edited By

Graham Munroe

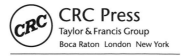

CRC Press
Taylor & Francis Group
Boca Raton London New York

CRC Press is an imprint of the
Taylor & Francis Group, an **informa** business

First edition published 2024
by CRC Press
2385 NW Executive Center Drive, Suite 320, Boca Raton, FL 33431

and by CRC Press
4 Park Square, Milton Park, Abingdon, Oxon, OX14 4RN

ISBN: 9781032548388 (hbk)
ISBN: 9781032066165 (pbk)
ISBN: 9781003427711 (ebk)

DOI: 10.1201/9781003427711

Typeset in Sabon
by Evolution Design & Digital Ltd (Kent)

Printed in the UK by Severn, Gloucester on responsibly sourced paper

 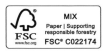

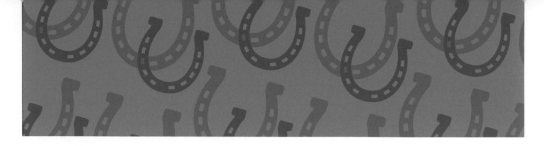

Table of Contents

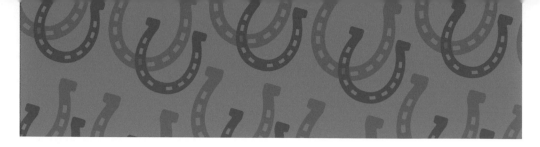

Preface

A vast array of clinical equine veterinary information is available for the under- and post-graduate veterinarian and veterinary nurse to peruse. This is contained in textbooks, both general and specialised, and increasingly online at websites of varying quality and trustworthiness. It is easy for the veterinary student or nurse, recent graduate, and busy general or equine practitioner to become overwhelmed and confused by this diverse range of information. Often what is required, particularly in the clinical situation, is a distillation of the essential knowledge and best practice required to treat the horse in the most suitable way. This concise, practical text is designed to provide the essential information needed to understand and treat clinical cases in equine practice.

This book focuses on medical and surgical conditions of the respiratory and gastrointestinal tracts. It is part of a five-book series, which between them will cover all the areas of equine clinical practice. The information is extracted and updated from *Equine Clinical Medicine, Surgery and Reproduction* (Second Edition) that was published in 2020. It is written for an international readership and is designed to convey the core, best-practice information in an easily digested, quick reference form using bullet points, lists, tables, flowcharts, diagrams, protocols, and extensive illustrations and photographs.

The respiratory system is split into sections on surgical and medical conditions of the upper and lower respiratory tract. The gastrointestinal system is divided into the upper tract, including the oral cavity and dentistry, and the lower tract and peritoneal cavity. All the material in the two clinical systems is approached in the same logical straightforward clinically based way. There are details of relevant clinical anatomy, physical clinical examination techniques, normal parameters, aetiology/pathophysiology, clinical examination findings, differential diagnosis, diagnostic techniques, management and treatment, and prognosis. The emphasis is on information tailored to general equine clinicians with just enough on advanced techniques to make the practitioner aware of what is available elsewhere.

The intention of this series of books is for them to be used on a day-to-day basis in clinical practice by student and graduate veterinarians, and nurses. The spiral binding format allows them to lie open on a surface near to the patient, readily available to the veterinary student or practitioner whilst looking at, or treating, a clinical case.

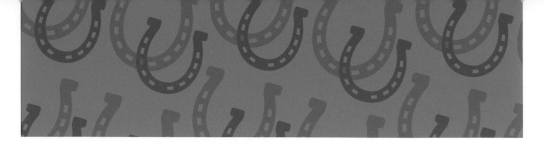

About the Authors

Tim Barnett qualified from the University of Edinburgh in 2005. After a period in general practice, he joined Rossdales in Newmarket, working as an orthopaedic assistant and then completing an 18-month internship in the hospital and diagnostic centre. He undertook a surgical residency at the University of Edinburgh before re-joining Rossdales in 2014. He worked in general practice and then as part of the horses-in-training team before moving into the surgical and dental referral group. He became clinical director of Rossdales in 2021. He was awarded an MSc with Distinction from the University of Edinburgh 2014 for his work on postoperative findings in horses undergoing laryngoplasty and attained the RCVS Certificate in Advanced Veterinary Practice and became a Diplomate of the European College of Veterinary Surgeons (EVCS) in 2015. He became a Diplomate of the European Veterinary Dental College (EVDC) in 2018. He holds RCVS specialist status in both equine surgery and dentistry.

Laura H. Javsicas is board certified by the American College of Veterinary Internal Medicine in Large Animal Medicine and has special interests in neonatology, ultrasonography, cardiology, gastrointestinal diseases and emergency/critical care medicine. She graduated from the University of Pennsylvania before completing an internship at the Hagyard Equine Medical Institute in Lexington, KY. She then completed an equine internal medicine residency at the University of Florida following which she became a member of the faculty.

She joined Rhinebeck Equine, a full-service ambulatory and referral hospital, in 2013 where she provides emergency and elective internal medicine services within the hospital and out in the field.

Graham Munroe qualified from the University of Bristol with honours in 1979. He spent 9 years in equine practice in Wendover, Newmarket, Arundel, and Oxfordshire, and a stud season in New Zealand. He gained a Certificate in Equine Orthopaedics and a Diploma in Equine Stud Medicine from the RCVS while in practice. He joined Glasgow University Veterinary School in 1988 as a lecturer and then moved to Edinburgh Veterinary School as a senior lecturer in large animal surgery from 1994 to 1997. He obtained the FRCVS in 1994 and DipECVS in 1997 by examination. He was awarded a PhD in 1994 for a study in neonatal ophthalmology. He has been visiting equine surgeon at the University of Cambridge Veterinary School, the University of Bristol Veterinary School and Helsingborg Hospital, Sweden. He was team veterinary surgeon for British Driving Teams from 1994–2001, the British Dressage Team from 2001–2002 and the British Vaulting Team in 2002. He was a FEI veterinary delegate at Athens 2004 Olympics. He currently works in private referral surgical practice, mainly in orthopaedics. He has published over 60 papers and book chapters.

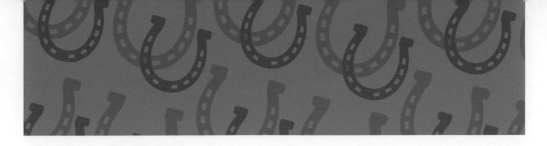

Abbreviations

4-BAD	Fourth branchial arch defects
ADAF	Axial or medial deviation of the aryepiglottic folds
AHS	African horse sickness
BAL	Bronchoalveolar lavage
CAD	*Cricoarytenoideus dorsalis*
CAL	*Cricoarytenoideus lateralis*
CDI	*Clostridium difficile* infection
CFT	Complement fixation titre
CK	Creatine kinase
CNS	Central nervous system
CO	Cardiac output
COPD	Chronic obstructive pulmonary disease
CPE	*Clostridium perfringens* enterotoxin
CRI	Constant rate infusion
CRT	Capillary refill time
CSF	Cerebrospinal fluid
CT	Computed tomography
DDSP	Dorsal displacement of the soft palate
DIC	Disseminated intravascular coagulation
DMSO	Dimethyl sulphoxide
DPJ	Duodenitis/proximal jejunitis
DSS	Dioctyl sodium succinate
ECG	Electrocardiography
EcoV	Equine coronavirus
EE	Eosinophilic enterocolitis
EGGD	Equine glandular gastric disease
EGS	Equine grass sickness
EGUS	Equine gastric ulcer syndrome
EHM	Equine herpesvirus myeloencephalopathy
EHV	Equine herpesvirus
EIP	Equine interstitial pneumonia
EIPH	Exercise-induced pulmonary haemorrhage
EIV	Equine influenza virus
ELISA	Enzyme-linked immunosorbant assay (iELISA = indirect ELISA)
EMPF	Equine multinodular pulmonary fibrosis
EOTRH	Equine odontoclastic tooth resorption and hypercementosis
EPM	Equine protozoal meningitis
ERAV	Equine rhinitis A virus
ERBV1	Equine rhinitis B virus type 1
ERBV2	Equine rhinitis B virus type 2
ESGD	Equine squamous gastric disease
ETR	Excessive transverse ridges
EVA	Equine viral arteritis
FB	Foreign body
FEI	Fédération Equestre Internationale

GA	General anaesthesia
GI	Gastrointestinal
HA/H	Haemagglutinin
HAI	Haemagglutination inhibition
i/m	Intramuscular
i/v	Intravenous
IAD	Inflammatory airway disease
IMHA	Immune-mediated haemolytic anaemia
IMTP	Immune-mediated thrombocytopenia
IRU	Increased radiopharmaceutical uptake
IU	International units
LCV	Large colon volvulus
LRT	Lower respiratory tract
MDI	Metered dose inhaler
MEED	Multisystemic eosinophilic epitheliotropic disease
MLST	Multilocus sequence typing
N	Neuraminidase
NG	Nasogastric
NPC	Nasopharyngeal collapse
NSAID	Non-steroidal anti-inflammatory drug
OIE	Office International des Epizooties
p/o	Per os
PCR	Polymerase chain reaction
PCV	Packed cell volume
PEH	Progressive ethmoidal haematoma
PHF	Potomac horse fever
qPCR	Quantitative ('real-time') polymerase chain reaction
RAO	Recurrent airway obstruction
RDPPA	Rostral displacement of palatopharyngeal arch
RL	Right limb
RLN	Recurrent laryngeal neuropathy
RNA	Ribonucleic acid
SAA	Serum amyloid A
SCC	Squamous cell carcinoma
SCID	Severe combined immunodeficiency
SG	Specific gravity
SI	Small intestine
SRH	Single radial haemolysis
TL	Tracheal lavage
URT	Upper respiratory tract
UV	Ultraviolet
VapA	Virulence-associated protein A
WBC	White blood cells

"Veterinary students will love this! I have seen the success of similar books in small animal medicine and how useful they can be on rotations when a quick reference is needed. I think it would equally be of benefit to residents and practitioners needing quick refreshers."
Carla Lusi, University of Melbourne, Australia, author of *Fascial Anatomy of the Equine Forelimb* (CRC Press)

"I think this Equine textbook will be exceptionally well received. Although the original book *Equine Clinical Medicine, Surgery and Reproduction* really helped me personally through university, I could only ever use it at my desk or at the library. More concise books allow students and new grads to have them at hand all the time, especially during rotations for quick reference. Leave the 1500-page book at home and take just what they need for the day! Each disease or syndrome has the same layout, allowing a very quick reference, and the images are amazing. They are good quality and allow very immersive learning."
Sophie Neasham, veterinary surgeon, UK

"While the volume *Equine Clinical Medicine, Surgery and Reproduction*, Second Edition is a great resource for reference, say, when wanting to research differential diagnoses for a case or brush up on a disease, it is not practical to be used out in the field. This smaller, more focused reference guide is more amenable to practical day-to-day veterinary use. For example, when out on a call and you need a quick reference on how to treat a specific presentation, having a resource which is concise and targeted is more user friendly than a large volume."
Rachael Harmer, veterinary medicine student at the University of Surrey (2016–2021), UK

Respiratory System

INTRODUCTION

- horses are athletic animals:
  - use a small proportion of their respiratory capacity at rest.
  - subtle respiratory disease can significantly decrease exercise capacity in athletes.
  - usually present for respiratory disease investigation earlier than other species.

Clinical examination of the respiratory tract

Aims

- aim of clinical examination is to reach one of four initial preliminary diagnoses:
  - infectious upper respiratory tract (URT) disease.
  - non-infectious URT disease.
  - infectious LRT disease.
  - non-infectious LRT disease.
- clinical examination must include assessment of tract from the nares to lungs:
  - further investigations then required to establish precise aetiology and diagnosis:
    - microbiology, endoscopy, and cytology.
    - radiography and ultrasonography.
    - specialist investigations, including respiratory function testing, in some cases:
      - assist diagnosis and assess response to treatment.
- examination of the respiratory tract at rest can be insensitive in detecting signs:
  - nasal discharge, epistaxis, or pronounced coughing cases are exceptions.
  - disease detectable at rest, particularly of the lower tract (LRT):

- likely to be of moderate or severe intensity.
- horses with significant respiratory disease (causing poor performance) may appear normal when examined at rest.

Features of different disease classifications

- each of the four groups of diseases has a typical set of presenting signs:
  - not every individual case will present with every clinical sign on the list.
- **Infectious URT disease:**
  - several animals in a group affected.
  - younger animals.
  - pyrexia   ○ depression.
  - mucopurulent or purulent nasal discharge.
  - lymphadenopathy.
  - cough.
- **Non-infectious URT disease:**
  - single animal affected   ○ any age.
  - no pyrexia no depression.
  - mucopurulent or purulent haemorrhagic nasal discharge.
  - variable lymphadenopathy.
  - facial distortion   ○ respiratory noise.
  - possible coughing/dysphagia.
- **Infectious LRT disease:**
  - individuals or groups   ○ any age.
  - pyrexia   ○ severe depression.
  - mucopurulent or purulent haemorrhagic nasal discharge.
  - often no lymphadenopathy.
  - coughing ○ tachypnoea ○ dyspnoea.
  - may be rapidly fatal.
- **Non-infectious LRT disease:**
  - usually individual individuals.
  - older horses.
  - no pyrexia   ○ no depression.

DOI: 10.1201/9781003427711-1

- o exercise intolerance and/or poor performance.
- o mucopurulent or purulent nasal discharge.
- o coughing o tachypnoea o dyspnoea.

Clinical examination

- important to follow the same rigorous procedure for all clinical examinations:
  - o take a detailed clinical history.
  - o observation from a distance.
  - o close observation.
  - o hands-on physical examination.

History and signalment

- Age:
  - o young horses more likely to have infectious or congenital diseases.
  - o older horses more often have non-infectious diseases.
  - o both types of disease can occur in any age group.
- Use:
  - o athletes with a history of poor performance:
    - ♦ more likely to have subtle disease on clinical examination at rest.
- Transport or other stress:
  - o pleuropneumonia may be more likely.
- Mixing with other age groups and through markets/dealer yards:
  - o predisposition to URT infections.
- Several in the group:
  - o   infectious disease more likely.
- Abnormal respiratory noise at exercise:
  - o non-infectious URT disease likely.
- Attitude:
  - o depression is more common with infectious diseases or with severe dyspnoea.
- Coughing:
  - o equine airway is insensitive compared with other species.
  - o **coughing is therefore not a sensitive indicator of respiratory disease:**
    - ♦ specific indicator of respiratory disease.
    - ♦ character of the cough is not informative:
      - – productive coughing in horses is unusual.
      - – frequent, dry, hacking cough in some equine influenza cases

in naïve horses, although most cases do not present in this way.
- Nasal discharge:
  - o nature and volume:
    - ♦ unilateral or bilateral may help to indicate the source of the discharge:
      - – LRT discharges are usually bilateral.
  - o after exercise or transport may indicate an LRT origin.
  - o copious discharge when the head is lowered:
    - ♦ may indicate a guttural pouch origin.
    - ♦ after prolonged transport if horses not been able to lower their heads.
- Vaccination history.
- Worming history.

Observation from a distance

- general demeanour should be assessed.
- respiratory rate prior to stimulating the horse:
  - o normal resting rate: 8–14 breaths per minute.
- respiratory effort:
  - o normal inspiratory effort: mainly thoracic with some abdominal component.
  - o normal expiratory effort: mostly elastic thoracic recoil with barely detectable abdominal (rectus abdominis) movement.
  - o respiratory effort easily detectable at rest: horse is likely to have dyspnoea.

Close observation

- nostril flare at rest indicates moderate to severe dyspnoea.
- nasal discharge should be characterised:
  - o unilateral/bilateral.
  - o serous/mucoid/mucopurulent/purulent.
  - o haemorrhagic o epistaxis.
- facial symmetry should be assessed, with close attention paid to the maxillary area.

Abnormal noises

- normally little or no noise during inspiration at rest and light exercise.
- may be noise on expiration related to vibration of the false nostril.
- fat or unfit horses may make a respiratory noise:
  - o disappears as fitness improves.

- breathing and stride patterns are intimately linked:
  - at the canter, expiration occurs as the forelimbs strike the ground.
- abnormal noises are related to airway obstruction either by:
  - dynamic collapse of the airway:
    - usually most apparent during exercise due to increased negative pressures.
    - causes inspiratory noise e.g. nasopharyngeal or laryngeal origin.
  - physical airway compression:
    - fixed obstructions cause both inspiratory and expiratory noise.
    - nasal or tracheal problems may present in this way:
      - thickening of the airway lining.
      - mass within the airway.

Physical examination of the respiratory tract

Nares

- assess patency by testing for airflow from both nostrils using a small piece of cotton wool.
- presence of swelling or injury.
- dilation at rest (indicates marked dyspnoea).
- discharge:
  - mucopurulent discharge occurs with all causes of airway inflammation.
  - does not automatically indicate infection.

Nasal cavity and paranasal sinuses

- external rostral facial symmetry and presence of swelling (especially over maxillary bone).
- percussion over sinuses or nasal cavity:
  - dullness and/or pain.
  - holding the tongue out of the mouth while percussing may augment dullness.
- detailed oral examination is required if sinus disease is suspected:
  - majority of cases of sinusitis are secondary to dental disease.

Lymph nodes

Submandibular lymph nodes

- located between the horizontal rami of the mandible.
- palpable in normal horses as a group of small, loosely associated lymphoid nodules.
- drainage from rostral nasal cavity and nasopharynx.
- enlarged in cases of URT infection and some dental disease cases.

Retropharyngeal lymph nodes

- located dorsal to the oesophageal pharynx.
- ventral to the floor of the medial pouch of the guttural pouch:
  - nodes are clearly visible through the guttural pouch floor on endoscopy.
- not palpable in normal horses.
- all drainage of lymph from the head passes through these nodes:
  - enlarged in response to infection.
  - must be grossly enlarged before they are palpable.

Parotid lymph node

- drains the orbit and ear region.
- sometimes abscessates in *Streptococcus equi* infection.

Guttural pouches

- palpate retropharyngeal area for swelling or pain:
  - not a sensitive indicator of guttural pouch disease.
- obvious distension usually indicates tympany:
  - occasionally, may also occur in severe cases of empyema.

Larynx

- palpate the dorsal surface of the larynx for:
  - symmetry of left and right dorsal cricoarytenoid muscles and laryngeal cartilages.
- **Slap test:**
  - slap just caudal to the withers induces a brief contralateral adduction of the arytenoid cartilage.
  - palpated as a flick of the cricoarytenoid muscle or visualised endoscopically.

- recent research has cast doubt on its relevance to the respiratory examination.
- induction of a cough by squeezing the larynx (laryngeal sensitivity?):
  - highly subjective procedure that has limited clinical value.
- auscultation of the larynx may provide some information about the larynx:
  - laryngeal noise may be audible on lung auscultation and can be confusing.

Trachea

- palpation of the trachea can help detect:
  - physical deformity.
  - squeezing the trachea to induce a cough is carried out by some clinicians:
    - highly subjective and has limited value.
- auscultation of the trachea is worthwhile:
  - tracheal noise radiates to the lung field.
  - airway discharges pool at the thoracic inlet and may indicate distal airway and lung pathology.

Lung field auscultation (Fig. 1.1)

- auscultation area of the lung field is triangular in shape:
  - cranial boundary:
    - caudal edge of triceps muscle between caudal border of scapula and olecranon.
  - dorsal boundary:
    - horizontal line from caudal border of scapula to tuber coxae.

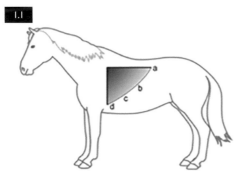

FIG. 1.1 Normal area of auscultation of the horse's lungs. (a) Level with the tuber coxae at the 18th rib. (b) Mid-thorax at the 13th rib. (c) Level with the shoulder at the 11th rib. (d) Point of the elbow. (Adapted from https://veteriankey.com/lower-respiratory-tract-2/)

- caudal boundary:
  - slopes cranioventrally from 16th or 17th intercostal space to olecranon.
- normal adult horses have little audible noise in any part of the lung field:
  - foals and thin adults have more obvious noise on auscultation.
  - hilar region, immediately dorsal to the heart base:
    - contains the major divisions of the bronchial tree.
    - air movement noise (bronchial sounds) heard on inspiration, with quiet bronchial sounds on expiration.
  - peripheral lung field is quiet:
    - barely perceptible air movement sounds on inspiration or expiration.
  - audible lung field may be:
    - expanded in horses with severe recurrent airway obstruction.
    - decreased ventrally with pleural effusion or pulmonary consolidation.
- auscultation at rest is not a sensitive means of assessing the lung fields:
  - slow breathing rate and small tidal volume compared to exercise.
  - sensitivity improved by auscultation during and immediately after rebreathing.
- rebreathing exam performed as follows:
  - use a large-volume plastic bin liner and fold free edges over to give better control.
  - introduce the bag over the horse's muzzle:
    - gather the free bag to form a good seal between the bag and the muzzle.
    - hold the bag in position under the noseband of the head collar.
    - horse rebreathes the air from the bag and carbon dioxide increases.
    - breathing rate and effort increases accentuating abnormal sounds.
  - keep the bag in place for as long as the horse will tolerate it.
  - auscultation of the thorax:
    - with the bag in place.
    - after the bag is removed, horse continues to take deep rapid breaths for 1–2 mins.

- better than occluding the nostrils which is usually not well tolerated.
- surprisingly small range of abnormal sounds heard in horse lungs:
  - **Wheezes:**
    - musical, sighing sounds generated by air moving through airways narrowed by bronchoconstriction and/or discharges.
    - less marked airway constriction generates bronchial sounds that are harsher and more audible than normal, rather than wheezes.
  - **Crackles:**
    - short, harsh sounds like bubble wrap packaging.
    - generated by collapsed small airways or alveoli:
      - surface tension effects of discharge.
      - snapping open at the end of inspiration and during expiration.
    - fluid or bubbling sounds are very unusual in horses.
    - crackles are usually not due to emphysema (rare pathology in horses).
- **Friction rubs:**
  - high-pitched, squeaky sounds generated by inflamed pleural surfaces rubbing together.
  - indicates pleuritis or pleuropneumonia.

Lung field percussion

- valuable information on presence of pleural effusion and, possibly, extent of the inflated lung field.
- carried out either by:
  - placing the first two fingers of one hand over an intercostal space and tapping these fingers firmly with the tips of the first two fingers of the other hand.
  - more effectively, by using a plexor and pleximeter.
- cranial to caudal, with each intercostal space percussed from dorsal to ventral:
  - identify areas of hyporesonance.
  - indicates absence of air-filled lung (i.e. pleural fluid and/or consolidated lung).
- remarkably accurate for identifying pleural fluid lines.

- occasionally, hyperresonance may occur in severe equine asthma cases due to lung hyperinflation.

Diagnostic tests

Respiratory endoscopy

- simple, well tolerated and extremely informative investigation for both URT and LRT.
- direct examination of most of the tract and collection of lavage and biopsy samples.
- 8–12 mm diameter fibreoptic or digital video endoscopes are standard equipment in equine practices:
  - 1.0–1.5 metres long suitable for examination of the URT and proximal trachea:
    - not beyond the carina.
  - 2.4–3.5-metre video endoscopes required for examination of the bronchial tree and collection of bronchoalveolar lavage (BAL) samples.
- sedation (combination of alpha-2 agonist and butorphanol) usually indicated:
  - reduce coughing, increase patient compliance, and reduce risk of damage to patient and instrument.
  - **meaningful assessment of pharyngeal and laryngeal function:**
    - **only possible in unsedated horses.**
    - sedation causes relaxation of nasopharynx, flaccidity of the soft palate, and decreased arytenoid abduction.
- examination should include:
  - both sides of the nasal cavity including the ventral and middle meati:
    - check for discharge from the region of the nasomaxillary openings.
  - Nasopharynx and soft palate (Fig. 1.2).
  - Guttural pouches:
    - entry requires an implement, either:
      - closed biopsy forceps [Fig. 1.3].
      - or a solid, semi-rigid plastic introducing device.
      - inserted via the endoscope's biopsy channel to lever open the nasopharyngeal ostium of the pouch and allow entry of the endoscope.

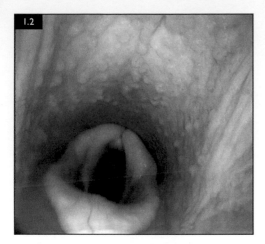

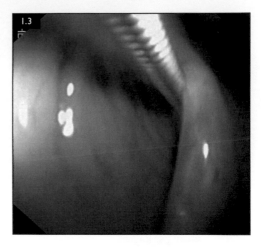

FIG. 1.2 Endoscopic view of a pharynx with pharyngeal folliculitis. This inflammatory reaction can be encountered in a number of situations including with viral infections of the URT. (Photo courtesy Gaby van Galen)

FIG. 1.3 A closed biopsy instrument is inserted into the pouch and, as the endoscope is rotated, the pouch opening elevates to facilitate entry of the endoscope.

- ○ Larynx:
  - ◆ resting position, movement, and symmetry of the epiglottis, aryepiglottic folds, arytenoids, vestibular folds, vocal folds, and lateral ventricle should be assessed.
  - ◆ observe during and after swallowing for:
    - – transient positional abnormalities (e.g. epiglottic entrapment).
    - – difficult-to-visualise abnormalities (e.g. subepiglottic cysts).
  - ◆ **Note endoscopically induced dorsal displacement of the soft palate is common and does not necessarily indicate this abnormality occurs during exercise.**
- ○ Trachea:
  - ◆ proximal trachea is relatively insensitive (examined with little coughing).
  - ◆ discharge from the lung pools at the thoracic inlet.
- ○ Carina and bronchial tree:
  - ◆ trachea becomes progressively more sensitive along its length.
  - ◆ beyond the carina the airway should be desensitised with 1% lidocaine.

Respiratory tract radiography

- • URT:
  - ○ radiography can provide valuable diagnostic information about:
    - ◆ dental disease.
    - ◆ sinus disease.
    - ◆ dorsal nasal cavity.
    - ◆ bone and cartilage skeleton:
      - – skull, maxillary and ethmoid turbinates, nasal septum, sinus walls.
- • LRT:
  - ○ thoracic radiography can provide information on:
    - ◆ chronic unresponsive equine asthma (pulmonary fibrosis).
    - ◆ exercise-induced pulmonary haemorrhage (EIPH) (focal consolidation).
    - ◆ pleuropneumonia/ bronchopneumonia:
      - – pulmonary abscess, pulmonary consolidation, mediastinal masses, and thoracic trauma (pneumothorax).
- • **Equipment:**
  - ○ URT:
    - ◆ all views of the head and cranial neck regions of the URT can be obtained with standard general practice X-ray machines.

- considerable superimposition of different structures in the head:
  - lateral, dorsoventral, and lateral oblique views help interpretation.
- CT imaging of the head has greater diagnostic sensitivity and specificity:
  - may require referral with cost implications.
- LRT:
  - thoracic radiography requires high-powered equipment:
    - not possible with small portable practice machines.
  - multiple overlapping lateral projections are required to image the lung field.
- **Interpretation:**
  - thoracic radiographs require recognition of the four major pulmonary patterns:
    - **Bronchial:** increased visibility of bronchial tree due to chronic airway disease and mineralisation of the airway wall.
    - **Interstitial:** increased density of lung interstitium due to inflammation or fibrosis:
      - common, but non-specific, pulmonary radiographic abnormality.
    - **Alveolar:** air-filled bronchi (tubular lucencies) silhouetted against fluid-filled alveoli (radio-opaque lung field):
      - 'air bronchograms', which are associated with pulmonary oedema.
    - **Vascular:** increased visibility of the pulmonary vasculature:
      - congenital conditions producing left-to-right shunts:
        - ◊ e.g. ventricular septal defect.
  - **these patterns indicate pathological changes and not specific diseases.**

Thoracic ultrasonography

- very useful for identifying:
  - pleural fluid.
  - peripheral pulmonary disease where there is:
    - decreased air in the peripheral lung.
    - lung lesions extend into the pleural space.

- adhesions between parietal and visceral pleura.
- provides a valuable guide for both thoracocentesis and lung biopsy.
- **Equipment:**
  - superficial pathology:
    - 7.5 to 15.0 MHz tendon transducer at depth setting of 5 to 6 cm.
    - 6.0 to 10.0 MHz microconvex transducer at depth setting of 6 to 10 cm.
  - deep pathology:
    - 5.0, 3.5 or 2.5 MHz transducer and/or increased depth (25 to 30 cm).
    - adults with severe pleural or pulmonary disease, or the horse is obese.
- **Interpretation:**
  - normal lung is air-filled and reflects the ultrasound beam:
    - creates bright white line at the air interface of the pulmonary surface.
    - no lung detail revealed.
  - visceral pleural surface creates reverberation artefacts known as 'comet tails'.
  - pleural fluid is readily visible:
    - information about the nature of the fluid (cellularity and fibrin content).
    - location within the pleural space and whether there is pocketing.

Paranasal sinus percutaneous centesis and sinuscopy

- boundaries of the maxillary sinus are defined as follows:
  - **Dorsally:** line drawn from medial canthus of the eye to nasoincisive notch.
  - **Rostrally:** the rostral limit of the facial crest.
  - **Ventrally:** the facial crest.
  - **Caudally:** line drawn from the middle of the orbit to the facial crest.
- boundaries of the frontal sinus are as follows:
  - **Caudally:** line drawn from the temporomandibular joint to the midline.
  - **Rostrally:** midpoint of a line drawn from the medial canthus of the eye to the nasoincisive notch joined to the midline.

○ **Laterally**: medial canthus of the eye.

Percutaneous sinus centesis

- simple way of obtaining a lavage sample from the sinuses in a standing, sedated horse.
- local anaesthetic infiltrated subcutaneously, and a small incision made.
- 3–4 mm Steinmann pin in a chuck used to drill through the bone into the sinus.
- catheter then introduced and a saline lavage taken.
- **Caudal maxillary sinus entry site:**
  ○ approximately 3–4 cm dorsal to facial crest and 3–4 cm rostral to medial canthus.
- **Rostral maxillary sinus entry site:**
  ○ approximately 3–4 cm rostral to caudal site.
- **Frontal sinus entry site:**
  ○ midpoint of a line drawn from the medial canthus to the midline.

Sinuscopy

- entry points and preparation for sinuscopy (Fig. 1.4) are the same as for centesis except that a larger pin size or trephine hole is required to provide access for the endoscope.
- trephine hole into the frontal sinus provides access to:
  ○ caudal maxillary sinus via the frontomaxillary opening.
  ○ ventral conchal sinus if forceps are used to create an opening into this space.

Tracheal (TL) and bronchoalveolar (BAL) lavage

- TL and BAL are essential in all cases of LRT disease:
  ○ samples are suitable for cytology, bacteriology/virology, and parasitology.
- TL samples are representative of both lungs as discharges pool in the trachea:
  ○ preferred sample for bacteriology/virology in infectious lower airway disease.
  ○ generally, provide poor samples for cytology (cells are degenerate).
  ○ may not accurately reflect current events in the lung.

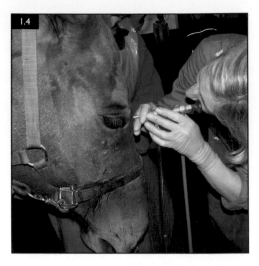

FIG. 1.4 Sinuscopy of the frontal sinus carried out under standing sedation. The portal used for this and the one visible beneath the right eye can also be used to collect material from the sinuses (sinocentesis).

- BAL samples provide an accurate, current reflection of events in the lung:
  ○ not representative of the whole lung as only one segment of lung is sampled.
  ○ samples are suitable for generalised lung diseases (e.g. equine asthma).
  ○ preferred sample for cytology but may miss focal abnormalities.

Tracheal lavage

- TL can be performed transendoscopically or transtracheally:
  ○ small risk of bacterial contamination of transendoscopic samples from nasal cavity and nasopharynx.
- endoscope is advanced to the mid-cervical trachea or beyond the thoracic inlet:
  ○ sterile catheter inserted through the biopsy port.
  ○ using a catheter with a sterile plug reduces the risk of bacterial contamination.
  ○ 20–30 ml of sterile saline is injected into the trachea and runs:
    ♦ caudally from a cervically positioned endoscope.
    ♦ cranially from a heart base-positioned endoscope.
- catheter is advanced into the saline pool and a sample aspirated.

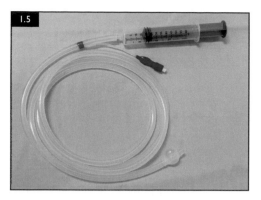

FIG. 1.5 Flexible nasotracheal catheter with an inflatable cuff used for performing BAL in horses. The tube is passed blindly into the caudodorsal region of either the right or the left lung for lavage.

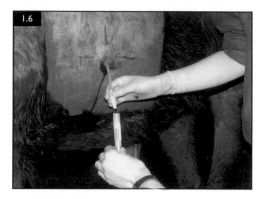

FIG. 1.6 A chest drain has been inserted on the left side under aseptic conditions, with local anaesthetic infiltration. Note the marks on the skin (made at the point of maximum collection of pleural exudate as determined by previous ultrasonography).

- TL collected percutaneously using either a commercial kit or an intravenous catheter:
  - cases where it is important to collect the sample using a sterile collection method.

Bronchoalveolar lavage

- BAL requires a 2.4–3 m endoscope or a commercial 2.4 m BAL catheter (Fig. 1.5).
- endoscopic collection carried out by wedging the endoscope in the cranial lung lobe.
- catheter collection passes the tube blindly into the LRT where it becomes wedged:
  - cuff is then inflated.
- 300–500 ml of prewarmed sterile saline should be infused:
  - 50–250 ml gently aspirated.
  - fluid should have a frothy appearance (presence of surfactant).

Thoracocentesis

- used to confirm the presence of pleural fluid, obtain samples for cytology and bacteriology, and to drain pleural fluid.
- **should be guided by ultrasound examination:**
  - identifies fluid pocketing and adhesions which may make drainage difficult.
- **ventral entry site:**
  - about a hand's breadth above the olecranon at approximately the 8th intercostal space on the left (i.e. caudal to the heart).

  - 7th intercostal space on the right, depending on the precise location of the fluid.
  - immediately cranial to border of the rib at the desired intercostal space:
    - avoids the intercostal artery, vein, and nerve.
    - take care to avoid the lateral thoracic vein.
- **procedure:**
  - skin close clipped/shaved and sterilised.
  - local anaesthetic infiltrated subcutaneously and into the intercostal space.
  - large-bore (24–30 French) chest drain and trochar are inserted directly into the pleural space through a stab incision (Fig. 1.6).
  - following entry, trochar is withdrawn and the drain inserted further:
    - should provide fluid drainage.
  - large volumes of fluid:
    - leave drain in place with a one-way valve to prevent air aspiration.

Lung biopsy

- rarely undertaken because of complications including:
  - epistaxis, pneumothorax, and sudden death.
- reserved for cases where all other investigations have failed to achieve a diagnosis.

- do not carry out if pulmonary infection is suspected.
- refer when this procedure is required.

Pulmonary function tests

- Pulmonary function testing:
  - difficult because of lack of patient compliance and need for specialised equipment.
  - sometimes useful in assessing severity of disease or response to treatment, but not generally required or available in practice.
- Blood gas analysis:
  - simple to perform, but not abnormal at rest unless moderate to severe pulmonary or cardiovascular disease is present.
  - arterial blood samples collected into a heparinised syringe from the transverse facial artery for immediate analysis.
  - hypoxia (PaO_2 <80 mmHg) and hypercapnia ($PaCO_2$ >45 mmHg) result from ventilation–perfusion mismatching in the lung.
  - treadmill and field exercise testing allow more rigorous assessment of the respiratory (and cardiac, locomotor,

and metabolic) systems than examination at rest.
- Treadmill testing combined with simultaneous endoscopy:
  - used to identify dynamic abnormalities in the nasopharynx (dorsal displacement of the soft palate and dynamic collapse of the larynx and pharynx).
  - superseded by overground (dynamic) endoscopy:
    - ◆ URT visualised while the horse is performing its normal exercise programme.

Thoracoscopy

- allows direct inspection and assessment of:
  - thoracic cavity.
  - mediastinum and its contents.
  - lung surface.
- increased accuracy of diagnosis/prognosis for pleural and some pulmonary diseases.
- performed in sedated, standing horses using local analgesia and a rigid endoscope.
- procedure is well tolerated, but some horses may develop a transient pneumothorax.

Surgical conditions of the respiratory tract

NOSTRIL

Alar fold disease (redundant/hypertrophy/ collapse/stenosis)

Definition/overview

- Alar fold forms the ventral aspect of the nasal diverticulum (false nostril):
  - divides it from the rostral nasal passage.
- extends from the alar cartilage caudally to the rostral aspect of the ventral nasal concha.
- elevated during exercise and closes off false nostril.

- failure of function or abnormalities can lead to abnormal inspiratory noise at exercise.

Aetiology/pathophysiology

- cause varies between individual cases, but possibilities include:
  - increased size or thickening of the alar folds.
  - abnormal function of the transversus nasi muscle (elevator of alar cartilages).
- individuals with abnormally narrowed nostrils may suffer from similar problems.

- American Saddlebred horse and Standardbreds may be more commonly affected:
  - possible genetic conformation abnormalities of the nostril region.

Clinical presentation

- loud vibratory noise from nostril region at exercise – especially at faster gaits:
  - worse on expiration.
  - rarely noise at rest.
- variable effects on exercise tolerance but often none.
- occasionally still collapsed into the nostril at end of work.
- nostril and false nostril conformation may/may not be abnormal.

Differential diagnosis

- 'High blowing' is used to describe where the folds vibrate during expiration only:
  - normal situation.
  - causes no clinical effects.
  - noise usually louder at the beginning of work and decreases with exercise.
- other causes of abnormal respiratory noise and nostril traumatic damage and deviation.

Diagnosis

- temporary mattress suture through the dorsal nostril and false nostril, passing over the bridge of the nares and through the other side (Fig. 1.7):
  - placed under local anaesthesia.
  - tied on top of a swab in the midline.
  - examined before/after suture placement to assess difference in noise/performance.

Management

- none required unless exercise intolerance or the noise is very loud.
- bilateral resection of the alar folds under GA has been described:
  - returned to exercise after suture removal at 2 weeks postoperatively.

Prognosis

- fair for noise reduction and return to normal exercise levels.

Atheroma

Definition/overview

- congenital epidermal inclusion cyst of the false nostril.
- oval-shaped cyst (Fig. 1.8).
- may have some effect on performance, but it is principally a cosmetic disease.
- treatment is removal with an excellent prognosis.

Aetiology/pathophysiology

- congenital abnormality which develops during the first 1–2 years of life.

Clinical presentation

- visible and palpable soft fluctuant swelling is present on the muzzle:
  - 2–5 cm in diameter and approximately 5 cm caudal to the nostril.
- easily palpated via the false nostril and non-painful.
- rarely causes any respiratory obstruction.

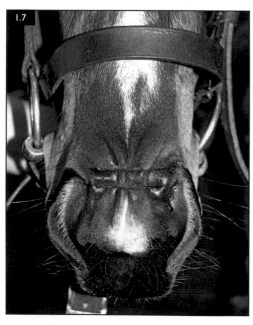

FIG. 1.7 A temporary mattress suture opening the false nostril used as an aid to the diagnosis of alar fold collapse.

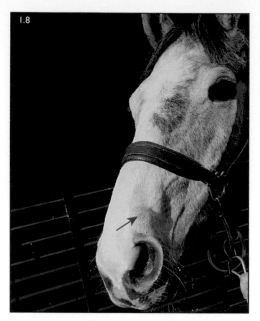

FIG. 1.8 Typical atheroma (arrow) in the false nostril of a young Thoroughbred racehorse.

Diagnosis

- clinical findings and centesis aspiration of grey, greasy contents (Fig. 1.9).

Management

- injection with 10% formalin in the standing, sedated horse:

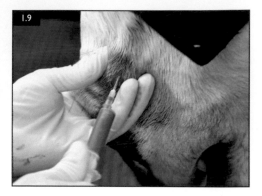

FIG. 1.9 Aspiration of grey greasy sebaceous material from the cyst prior to injection of formalin.

- o contents are aspirated and similar volume of formalin–saline is injected (5 ml).
  - o swelling for 24 hours and cyst gradually regresses over 7 days.
- stab incision made under local anaesthesia, via the false nostril into the cyst:
  - o cyst lining reamed out, using a laryngeal or ventricular 'Hobday' burr.
- surgical removal is seldom necessary.

Prognosis

- excellent and recurrence is very rare.

NASAL PASSAGES AND PARANASAL SINUSES

Wry nose

Definition/overview

- complex congenital deformity of the nose:
  - o shortening/deviation of maxilla, premaxilla, nasal bone, vomer bone, and nasal septum.
  - o occasionally milder mandibular deformity and/or dorsoventral deviation.

Aetiology/pathophysiology

- unknown aetiology but may be genetic.
- may be more frequent in Arabian and draught breeds, and possibly primiparous mares.

- true incidence is not known.
- some cases associated with contracted foal syndrome and seen following dystocia.

Clinical presentation

- visible deviation of the maxilla.
- respiratory stridor at rest.
- more severely affected animals may not be able to suckle.

Differential diagnosis

- clinical presentation is typical.

Diagnosis

- clinical signs.

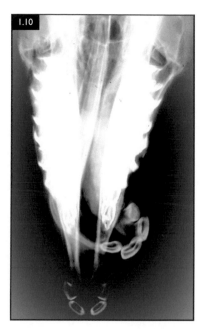

FIG. 1.10 Dorsoventral radiograph of a wry nose in a foal. Note the markedly deviated upper jaw.

- radiography of upper and lower jaws in lateral and dorsoventral projections (Fig. 1.10).

Management

- mildly affected foals can be managed conservatively:
  - spontaneous improvement has been reported.
- surgical correction or euthanasia in more severe cases.

Prognosis

- good results have been reported post-surgery.

Deformity of the nasal septum

Definition/overview

- variety of rare congenital and acquired conditions:
  - cause deviation and/or thickening of the nasal septum.
- usually cause abnormal respiratory airflows and noises.

- diagnosed on digital palpation, endoscopy, dorsoventral head radiographs and CT.
- some animals can cope with these problems without treatment, but surgical removal of the septum may be necessary.

Aetiology/pathophysiology

- multiple conditions reported to result in thickening and deviation of the nasal septum:
  - thickening:
    - haemartoma
    - congenital cystic degeneration.
    - neoplasia ◆ amyloidosis.
    - post-traumatic injury.
    - severe bacterial/mycotic infection of the septum following URT disease.
  - deviation:
    - congenital malformations such as wry nose.
    - expanding masses in nasal cavity or paranasal sinuses (neoplasia, cysts).

Clinical presentation

- variable nasal passage and respiratory obstruction.
- respiratory stertor at rest and exercise intolerance.
- facial swelling and/or asymmetry.

Differential diagnosis

- reduced airflow in one nostril with marked stertor – associated conchal swelling:
  - expansile mass within the paranasal sinuses:
    - sinus cyst.
    - severe primary sinusitis.
    - large progressive ethmoidal haematoma (PEH).

Diagnosis

- digital palpation via nares:
  - may reveal abnormalities of rostral septum and abnormal airflow.
- endoscopy of nasal passages:
  - unrewarding due to the severity and narrowness of meati.
- radiography:
  - dorsoventral head radiographs may reveal bony and septal deformities.
- CT or MRI.

Management

- mild deformities or thickening may not require treatment if the horse performs limited exercise.
- severe cases, or where return to athletic ability is desired:
  - surgical removal of the septum is necessary.

Prognosis

- good results have been reported.
- surgery in these cases can have multiple complications.

Choanal atresia/stenosis

Definition/overview

- rare congenital condition involving failure of the development, or narrowing, of a hole (the choana) between the nasal passages and the nasopharynx.
- occasionally, congenital narrowing or stenosis of the airway at this level that presents later in life as a respiratory noise and/or exercise intolerance.

Aetiology/pathophysiology

- Bucconasal membrane separating the nasal cavities from the pharyngeal cavity thins progressively and perforates before parturition.
- cause of failure of membrane to rupture is unknown.

Clinical presentation

- bilateral cases are almost invariably fatal at birth due to severe respiratory distress.
- unilateral cases present at a young age with:
  - respiratory noise, reduced airflow from one nostril and reduced exercise tolerance.
  - other abnormalities may be present.
  - poor athletic potential.

Differential diagnosis

- bilateral:
  - all causes of respiratory obstruction and distress in the newborn foal.
- unilateral:
  - other causes of respiratory distress in the young horse including:

- permanent dorsal displacement of the soft palate.
- expansile mass within the paranasal sinuses, including sinus cysts.

Diagnosis

- endoscopic examination is definitive (Fig. 1.11):
  - can be difficult to interpret as cannot pass through to the pharynx.
  - examination via the contralateral nares in a unilateral case.
  - one or both entrances from nasal passages to nasopharynx may appear narrowed in stenosis cases.

Management

- bilateral – emergency orotracheal intubation and/or tracheotomy.
- endoscopic laser surgery if membranous obstruction.
- surgical removal using a frontonasal bone flap or laryngotomy.

Prognosis

- good for survival of unilateral cases.
- return to normal exercise tolerance is often poor.

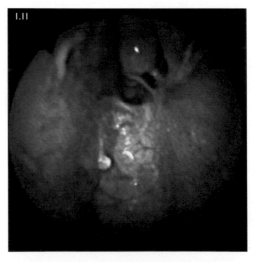

FIG. 1.11 Endoscopic view of a unilateral (left side) choanal atresia. Left side is the caudal nasal septum, upper aspect is the ethmoturbinates, right side is the caudal ventral turbinate, and the lower aspect is the abnormal membrane covering the upper part of the ventral meatus.

- concurrent congenital abnormalities affect the prognosis.

Fungal rhinitis

Definition/overview

- frequent complication of other nasal or sinus disease, or their treatment:
  - predisposed by treatment with antibiotics or antiseptics.
- primary fungal infections of the URT caused by specific fungal species are rare:
  - tend to occur in specific regions of the world.
  - cryptococcosis, rhinosporidiosis, phycomycosis, and coccidioidomycosis.

Aetiology/pathophysiology

- most isolated fungus is *Aspergillus fumigatus* but *Pseudoallescheria boydii* has been cultured.
- mainly secondary invaders of tissue damaged by:
  - trauma   ○ sinonasal surgery.
  - nasal or sinus masses such as PEH.
  - persistent nasal discharge, either from disease of paranasal sinuses or the lungs.
- primary fungal rhinitis is very rare, particularly in temperate climates.

Clinical presentation

- chronic, unilateral, nasal discharge:
  - blood-stained, mucopurulent or purulent.
  - often malodorous.
- submandibular lymph node enlargement.
- worsening or persistence of nasal discharge post-surgery.

Differential diagnosis

- other causes of chronic nasal discharge and epistaxis including:
  - PEH, guttural pouch disease and other paranasal sinus diseases.
  - complication, rather than differential diagnosis, of most causes of nasal discharge.

Diagnosis

- endoscopy is diagnostic (Fig. 1.12):
  - fungal plaque is often yellowish/greenish white and covered in thick exudate.
  - one or more plaques on dorsal/ventral conchae in nasal passages.
  - samples should be taken for cytology, culture and sensitivity.

Management

- removal of the plaque(s) using endoscopy.
- topical antifungal agents:
  - enilconazole, miconazole, ketoconazole, and natamycin solutions.
  - nystatin powder for difficult to lavage lesions.
- correction of any predisposing cause:
  - antibiotic and/or antiseptic treatments may have to be withdrawn.

Prognosis

- very good.
- recurrence or persistence of lesions is rare:
  - **fungal infection is a result of an underlying disease that requires treatment.**
- limiting the use of antibiotics helps to prevent the development of this disease.

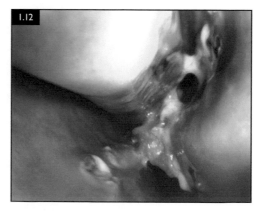

FIG. 1.12 Large mycotic plaque in the middle meatus. The horse had a history of intermittent epistaxis.

Primary sinusitis

Definition/overview

- frequent condition, particularly of animals with a history of URT disease.
- anatomy of the paranasal sinus compartments is complex.
- clinically the sinus compartments (Fig. 1.13) can be divided into two:
  - rostral maxillary/ventral conchal:
    - ◆ lateral and medial to the teeth and infraorbital canal.
    - ◆ own separate drainage ostia in the middle meatus.
  - all the others, including the frontal, conchofrontal and caudal maxillary:
    - ◆ these all communicate with each other through large openings.
    - ◆ drain via single slit-like opening in caudal middle meatus.

Aetiology/pathophysiology

- URT infection leads to:
  - increased mucus production and compromised mucociliary clearance.
  - stagnation of the mucus in the dependent sinuses.

- relatively small and poorly sited drainage ostia are further compromised by surrounding mucosal inflammation (hyperplastic with chronicity).
- secondary bacterial infection (mixed growth) is common:
  - increased production of fluid (purulent).
  - empyema and inspissation of the exudate can occur with chronicity.
- drainage even more restricted in rostral maxillary and ventral conchal sinuses:
  - once empyema established successful drainage is hard to achieve.
  - increasing exudate may cause expansion of the conchal walls of the paranasal sinuses and increasing obstruction of the airway.

Clinical presentation

- unilateral mucopurulent or purulent nasal discharge which is often copious (Fig. 1.14):
  - increased after exercise or ground feeding.
  - increasingly malodorous with chronicity.

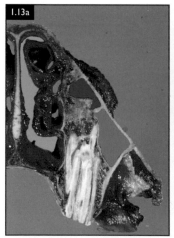 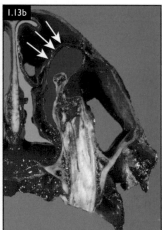 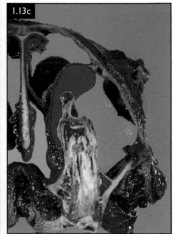

FIG. 1.13 (a) Cross section of the head at the level of tooth 208, showing the nasal meati (bright green) and the rostral maxillary sinus (blue); (b) cross section of the head at the level of tooth 209, showing the nasal meati (bright green) and the rostral maxillary and ventral conchal frontal sinus (blue); (c) cross section of the head at the level of tooth 210, showing the nasal meati (bright green), the rostral maxillary and ventral conchal frontal sinus (blue) and the caudal maxillary sinus (background green). Note the conchal 'bulla' of the rostral maxillary sinus (arrows in b).

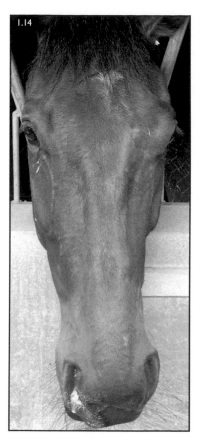

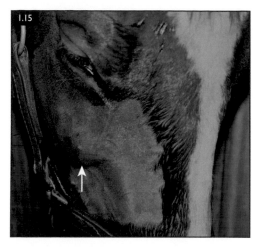

FIG. 1.15 [3.18 in 2E] Facial swelling caudal to the rostral margin of the facial crest, typical of an expansile lesion within the sinus (arrow).

FIG. 1.14 Horse with a right-sided unilateral purulent nasal and ocular discharge typical of sinusitis.

- unilateral submandibular lymphadenopathy.
- conchal swelling, reduced airflow, abnormal respiratory noise and exercise intolerance.
- facial swelling (Fig. 1.15).
- occlusion of nasolacrimal duct – epiphora and/or ocular discharge.

Differential diagnosis

- secondary sinusitis, particularly that due to dental disease.
- other causes of unilateral nasal discharge include:
  - guttural pouch disease, particularly empyema.
  - rhinitis (particularly fungal rhinitis).
  - occasional horses with mucopurulent tracheal discharges preferentially expelled down one nostril.

Diagnosis

- based on the history, clinical signs, endoscopy, sinuscopy, and radiography.
- careful examination of the mouth for any cheek tooth pathology (upper three caudal).
- endoscopy is less valuable in sinusitis than in many other conditions of the URT:
  - conchal swelling.
  - discharge from the caudal maxillary sinus drainage angle.
  - only possible to advance the endoscope into the maxillary sinus if architecture has been damaged by previous surgery or mycotic infection.
  - sinocentesis and/or sinuscopy allow collection of samples for bacteriology, visualisation of the lining and lavage of the paranasal sinuses.
- radiography:
  - most important diagnostic technique for diagnosis of sinusitis (Fig. 1.16).
  - one or more horizontal free gas/fluid interfaces may be noted (Fig. 1.17).
  - more commonly in primary sinusitis, sinus compartments are filled completely:
    - fluid opacity replacing the normal gas density of the sinus (Fig. 1.18).
    - dorsoventral view displacement of nasal septum by gross distension of sinus.

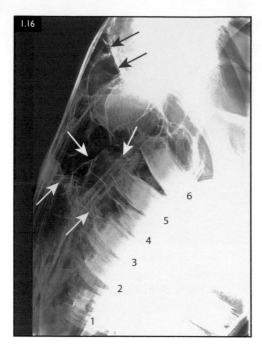

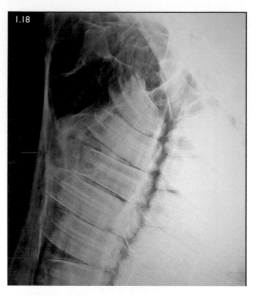

FIG. 1.18 Soft tissue or fluid density within the rostral maxillary sinus only, illustrating the lack of fluid lines in many cases of sinusitis (arrow).

FIG. 1.16 Laterolateral radiograph of a normal horse's head, showing the rostral edge of the maxillary sinuses (yellow arrows), the caudal edge of the frontal sinus (red arrows) and the 'bulla' of the rostral maxillary sinus (white arrows). The teeth are numbered as cheek teeth from 1 rostral (206) to 6 (211). The fourth cheek tooth (209) is easily identified as the shortest tooth.

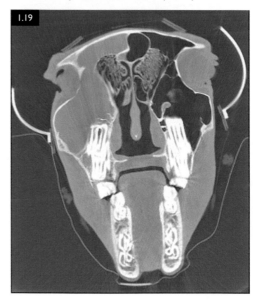

FIG. 1.19 CT scan of a horse with fluid density filling the entire right paranasal sinus compartments.

♦ occasionally material becomes confined to the ventral conchal sinus.
♦ chronic cases, lining of sinuses or their contents may become mineralised.
• standing CT (Fig. 1.19):
   ○ more detailed imaging of head and clearer differentiation of cause.

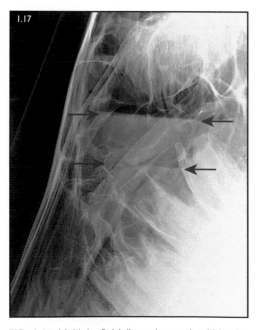

FIG. 1.17 Multiple fluid lines (arrows) within the paranasal sinus compartments.

Management

- depends on its severity.
- simple early case with fluid lines visible in the sinus compartments:
  - systemic antibiotics for 1–3 weeks usually curative.
  - culture/sensitivity of nasal discharge, or fluid obtained from trephined sinus.
  - regular light exercise.
  - grazing and feeding all food from the floor encourages drainage.
- cases that fail to respond to conservative treatment are managed by:
  - sinus lavage (inspissated material may not respond to simple flushing alone):
    - ♦ trephine caudal maxillary sinus or frontal sinus (Fig. 1.20).
    - ♦ sinuscopic examination of the sinuses.
    - ♦ Foley or other self-retaining catheter is placed and sutured to the skin.
    - ♦ irrigated with copious volumes of fluids, preferably under pressure:
      - – tap water, saline or dilute 0.05–0.1% povidone–iodine disinfectant solution q12–24h for 5–7 days.
    - ♦ instillation of an antifungal agent after irrigation may be recommended:
      - – fungal sinusitis is a common complication of sinus lavage.

- failure of treatment for primary sinusitis may be due to ongoing sinusitis of the rostral maxillary and ventral conchal sinus compartment:
  - trephination of the rostral maxillary sinus is more difficult:
    - ♦ sinus is small, particularly in young horses.
    - ♦ large amount of the space is occupied by the root of the teeth 109/209.
  - communication between rostral maxillary and ventral conchal sinuses is poor:
    - ♦ hence the ventral conchal sinus may remain poorly lavaged.
    - ♦ formation of inspissated pus is common.
- management of primary sinusitis that has not responded to conservative therapy and sinus lavage is surgical (Fig. 1.21):
  - this may be possible in the standing sedated horse via a large nasofrontal flap or trephine holes and endoscopic guidance (Figs. 1.22, 1.23).

Prognosis

- good, as many cases respond to conservative treatment, lavage or sinoscopy.
- more guarded where surgical intervention is required, as complications are common.
- reduced in patients with PPID.

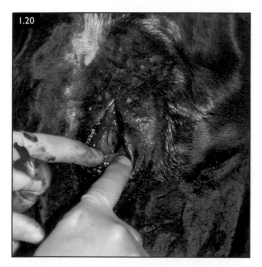

FIG. 1.20 A trephine into the conchofrontal sinus.

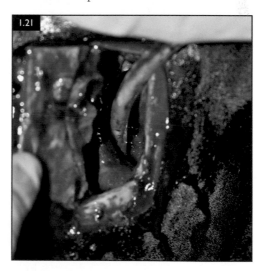

FIG. 1.21 Catheter placed into the rostral maxillary sinus after removal of the bulla of the sinus via a frontonasal flap.

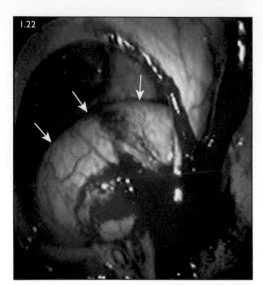

FIG. 1.22 'Bulla' of the rostral maxillary sinus (arrows), distended by purulent contents, is clearly visible endoscopically from a frontal trephine.

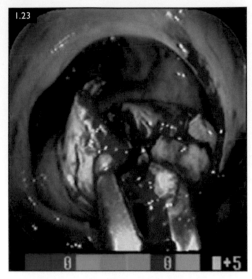

FIG. 1.23 Removal of the roof of the rostral maxillary sinus, using arthroscopy rongeurs.

Secondary sinusitis

Definition/overview

- most commonly a sequela to dental periapical infection.
- other causes include:
  - sinonasal neoplasia.
  - facial fractures or trauma.
  - occlusion of drainage by expansile lesions such as:
    - ♦ PEH or sinus cysts.
  - immunosuppression, especially in Cushingoid older ponies
  - fungal sinusitis.

Aetiology/pathophysiology

- periapical infections of tooth roots can result in sinusitis:
  - teeth 109/209 (most common) and occasionally caudal root of teeth 108/208 usually in the rostral maxillary and ventral conchal sinuses.
  - teeth 110/210 and 111/211 in the caudal maxillary sinuses.
- most common neoplasm of nasal passages is squamous cell carcinoma (SCC) (Fig. 1.24):
  - many other tumours have been reported from the paranasal sinuses:

- ♦ lymphosarcoma, adenocarcinoma or ossifying fibroma.
  - neoplastic-like conditions such as fibrous dysplasia.
- any condition that either forms a focus of necrotic or infected tissue within the sinuses, or occludes the normal drainage channels, can result in secondary sinusitis.

Clinical presentation

- similar to primary sinusitis.
- more often purulent and malodorous nasal discharge with dental sinusitis:

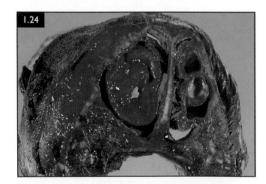

FIG. 1.24 Post-mortem cross section through the head of a horse with a SCC of the maxillary sinuses. The invasive nature of the tumour is clearly visible.

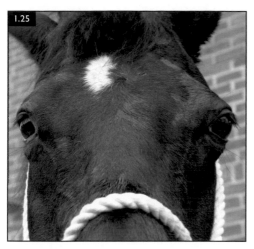

FIG. 1.25 Exophthalmos of the left eye caused by a neuroendocrine tumour.

○ foetid halitosis is common with dental disease.
• space-occupying lesions have less discharge and more likely to have:
  ○ facial swelling.
  ○ nasal obstruction.
  ○ unilateral epiphora.
  ○ exophthalmos (Fig. 1.25).

Differential diagnosis

• primary sinusitis.
• specific diagnosis for secondary sinusitis is essential to make a treatment plan and prognosis:
  ○ smaller amounts of sinus fluid often on radiographs in secondary sinusitis (Fig. 1.26).
  ○ mycotic sinusitis is an important differential diagnosis and can develop following treatment for a primary sinusitis.

Diagnosis

• similar to primary sinusitis.
• radiography of sinuses and teeth:
  ○ specific oblique views of apices of teeth.
  ○ periapical changes of infection are not always clear:
    ♦ lavage of sinuses for several days prior to repeat radiographs.
• detailed oral examination including oral endoscopy (Fig. 1.27):

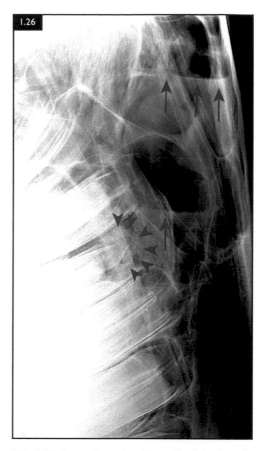

FIG. 1.26 Secondary sinusitis, with fluid lines in the rostral maxillary and conchofrontal sinuses (arrows) and periapical sclerosis of tooth 109 (arrowheads).

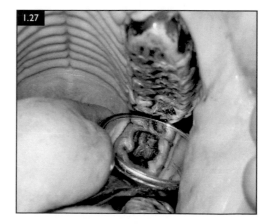

FIG. 1.27 Oral examination with a dental mirror revealing infundibular necrosis of tooth 209.

- essential for complete dental evaluation and identification of orosinus fistulae.
- CT of head in standing horse:
  - useful imaging modality in secondary sinusitis cases.
- sinoscopy:
  - masses and dental lesions may be identified on examination after lavage.

Management

- depends on the underlying disease:
  - dental disease:
    - oral extraction or surgical removal.
  - surgical repair of orosinus fistulae.
  - surgical management of sinus cysts or PEH.
  - surgical treatment of neoplasia usually unrewarding and recurrence common.
- underlying sinusitis usually requires treatment once the inciting cause is removed:
  - systemic medication.
  - sinus lavage.

Prognosis

- good for uncomplicated dental sinusitis following extraction:
  - reduced with post-tooth removal complications:
    - orosinus fistulation.
    - persistent dental or bone fragments.
    - alveolar, maxillary bone or turbinate infection.
  - secondary fungal and/or anaerobic bacterial infections are quite common postoperatively.
- neoplastic sinus disease has a poor prognosis – most are invasive and/or malignant.
- complications can lead to prolonged treatment, considerable costs, and difficult client relations.

Empyema of the conchal bullae

Definition/overview

- less common variation of sinusitis:
  - inspissation occurs in the conchal bullae:
    - centre of the scrolled turbinate bones, rostral to the paranasal sinuses.

Aetiology/pathophysiology

- presumed to be very similar to primary sinusitis.

Clinical presentation

- identical to primary sinusitis with:
  - chronic, often malodorous, unilateral nasal discharge.
  - facial swelling.

Differential diagnosis

- primary sinusitis is the principal differential diagnosis.

Diagnosis

- clinical examination and poor response to treatment of primary sinusitis.
- endoscopy may allow direct visualisation of a draining tract from the conchus overlying the bullae (Fig. 1.28).
- CT provides unequivocal diagnosis.

Management

- treatment of any associated sinusitis and underlying cause.
- surgical drainage and debridement of the affected bullae.

Prognosis

- good if drainage is established and inspissated pus removed.

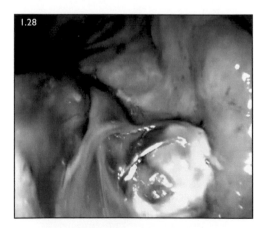

FIG. 1.28 Conchal ulceration as a result of empyema of the conchal bulla.

Fungal sinusitis

Definition/overview

- infrequent condition of the paranasal sinuses.

Aetiology/pathophysiology

- often secondary to another disease process, such as tumours.
- frequent complication of the treatment of sinusitis:
  - common history of treatment for sinusitis with antibiotics and/or antiseptics:
    - original primary sinusitis often resolves but mycotic infection develops during treatment.
    - clinical signs will often not alter, although the disease process changes.
- primary mycotic sinusitis is recognised but rare in temperate climates.
- infections are often erosive and may damage the nasal conchae or infraorbital canal:
  - erosion of nasomaxillary opening may allow an endoscope to be passed directly into the paranasal sinus.

Clinical presentation

- typical of sinusitis with:
  - unilateral, often malodorous, nasal discharge.
  - unilateral submandibular lymph node enlargement.
- chronic history and often previous antibiotic/antiseptic treatment.

Differential diagnosis

- other causes of sinusitis, especially those causing secondary sinusitis.

Diagnosis

- endoscopic examination of the nasal meatus usually reveals:
  - no abnormalities, or possibly scanty discharge from nasomaxillary sinus drainage angle.
- radiography is frequently unrewarding with limited signs:
  - possible fluid lines in the maxillary sinuses, but often no abnormalities.

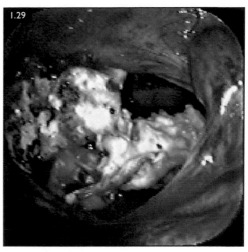

FIG. 1.29 Sinuscopic view of mycotic sinusitis

- Gamma scintigraphy frequently reveals:
  - intense IRU within the affected area of paranasal sinuses similar to tooth abscess.
- definitive diagnosis requires direct sinus endoscopy (sinusoscopy):
  - via a trephine hole, either in the caudal maxillary or the frontal sinuses.
  - mycotic plaques have a typical diphtheritic appearance:
    - microscopic examination of samples identifies fungal hyphae (Fig. 1.29).

Management

- sinoscopic removal of the diphtheritic plaques by arthroscopy rongeurs.
- irrigation with antifungal agents via an indwelling catheter:
  - enilconazole for 2–3 weeks.

Prognosis

- good with resolution after several weeks of topical treatment.

Facial trauma involving the nasal cavity and paranasal sinuses

Definition/overview

- relatively common condition of variable severity.

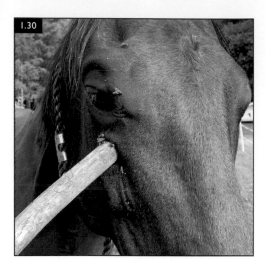

FIG. 1.30 Facial injury. The horse made a complete recovery following removal of the stake. (Photo courtesy Barney Fraser)

- caused by impact with solid objects during falls/collisions or by kicks.
- variable degrees of soft and bony tissue damage can occur:
  - secondarily cause injury to the eye, URT, and cranial vault.
- head lacerations should be primarily repaired where possible:
  - wounds and injuries of the head heal well compared with elsewhere.
  - carry a good prognosis.

Aetiology/pathophysiology

- traumatic (not always confirmed in every case) (Fig. 1.30).
- may or may not be skin lacerations depending on the specific cause.
- degree of bony damage can range from:
  - superficial trauma to non-displaced cracks.
  - depression fractures (may be comminuted).
  - large areas of bone damaged overlying the paranasal sinuses +/− nasal passages in severe cases.

Clinical presentation

- mild to moderate epistaxis on the affected side which may last several days:
  - increasingly mucopurulent with secondary infection of sinuses.
- variable soft tissue swelling:

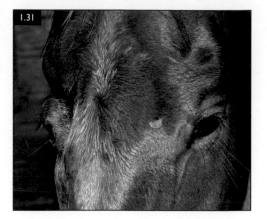

FIG. 1.31 Depression fracture of the right orbit in a National Hunt racehorse, which was kicked by another horse.

  - may hide true extent of any bony deformity.
- variable wounds:
  - small punctures to large flaps of skin or severe lacerations.
- variable bone deformation:
  - degree, site, and extent of damage:
    - depression fractures are common (Fig. 1.31).
- epiphora due to damage to the nasolacrimal duct.
- subcutaneous emphysema suggests penetration of the paranasal sinuses or nasal cavity.

Differential diagnosis

- conditions that cause head deformity, including expansile masses or erosive tumours within the paranasal sinuses.
- eliminate other causes of epistaxis, including guttural pouch mycosis, ethmoidal haematoma and fungal rhinitis.

Diagnosis

- clinical examination:
  - careful palpation may reveal extent and severity of injuries.
- full ophthalmic and neurological examination:
  - damage to the orbit, eye or cranial vault should be considered.
- **radiography** including lesion-specific obliques:
  - presence of fluid in sinuses and fractures.

o often difficult to interpret the results.
- **ultrasonography** to assess bone topography:
  o can be complicated by subcutaneous gas.
- CT is much more reliable, particularly for the detection of blood in the sinuses.

Management

- simple lacerations should be repaired primarily.
- puncture wounds cleaned regularly and lavaged for a few days.
- antibiotics and non-steroidal anti-inflammatory drugs (NSAIDs) are indicated:
  o decrease swelling, pain, and incidence of secondary sinusitis.
- sinus lavage for a few days is indicated in cases with obvious bleeding into the sinuses.
- management of fractures of the facial bones depends on degree of injury:
  o non/minimally displaced fractures can heal well when treated conservatively.
  o more displaced and depressed fractures can also be treated conservatively:
    ♦ cosmetic defects, and in nasal bones, possible respiratory obstruction.
  o loose fragments of bone should be removed, often possible in the standing animal.
  o anatomical restoration of larger/depressed fractured bones within 48 hours under GA.

Prognosis

- good:
  o most fractures and wounds heal without functional problems:
  o cosmetic result varies with original injury and treatment – conservative or surgical.
  o most cases have a firm swelling left after healing has finished.

Nasal amyloidosis

Definition/overview

- rare disease where deposits of amyloid occur in various sites of the URT with or without skin deposits:

- nostrils, alar folds, nasal septum, nasal conchae and, more rarely, nasopharynx and guttural pouches (Fig. 1.32).
- amyloid is formed secondary to a chronic immunological stimulation:
  o often not identified in these cases.
- clinical signs may include:
  o thickened and raised nodular mucosal masses, often with areas of haemorrhage.
  o nasal discharge, often containing small amounts of blood.
  o nasal obstruction and respiratory noise.
  o exercise intolerance.
- other signs associated with primary disease, e.g. weight loss.
- differential diagnosis includes other causes of nasal discharge, epistaxis, and soft tissue formation in the URT.
- diagnosis on clinical examination of nasal lesions and endoscopic examination of the rest of respiratory tract:
  o biopsy and histopathology confirm the diagnosis.

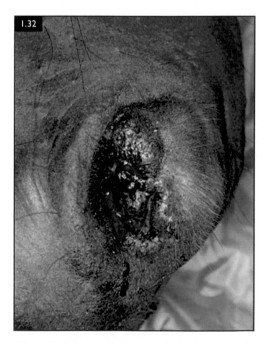

FIG. 1.32 A horse that presented with intermittent bilateral epistaxis and which on examination had firm, ulcerated, multiloculated masses in both nostrils. Biopsy confirmed amyloidosis. There were also masses involving both palpebral conjunctivae.

- identify and treat any underlying primary disease if identified.
- local surgical excision in the nostrils or transendoscopic laser ablation elsewhere.
- local URT lesions can recur and carry a guarded prognosis.
- primary problems can lead to a poor prognosis.

Progressive ethmoidal haematoma

Definition/overview

- develops from nasal or sinus surface of the ethmoidal labyrinth.
- behaves as a tumour, being progressive and expansile:
  - histology does not reveal any neoplastic tissue.
- most affected horses present with a low-grade nasal discharge, often with blood.
- diagnosed by endoscopy and radiography.
- variety of options are available for their treatment.

Aetiology/pathophysiology

- aetiology unknown, but not neoplastic.
- repeated submucosal haemorrhage from the surface of the ethmoidal labyrinth, underneath normal respiratory epithelium, and associated with significant fibrosis.
- mass is a mixture of blood, haemosiderin and fibrous tissue.
- masses can arise within the caudal nasal cavity or the paranasal sinuses.

Clinical presentation

- low-grade, recurrent, unilateral epistaxis or serosanguineous, non-odorous, nasal discharge:
  - old blood and no association with exercise.
- occasional alternative presentations include:
  - airway obstruction.
  - abnormal respiratory sounds at exercise.
  - poor performance.
- larger masses can lead to:
  - facial deformity.
  - spread to pharynx and cause dysphagia.

- spread down nasal passages to appear at the nares.
- rarely, expansion through the cribriform plate may lead to:
  - neurological and headshaking signs.

Differential diagnosis

- principal differential for investigation is epistaxis:
  - guttural pouch mycosis.
  - trauma, mycotic rhinitis, and sinonasal neoplasia.

Diagnosis

- endoscopy (Fig 1.33):
  - identification of nasal lesions and, via sinuscopy, paranasal sinus masses:
    - smooth-walled, reddish green/yellow.
    - paranasal sinus masses are common:
      - bleeding or serosanguinous exudate from sinus drainage angle.
      - nasal conchal swelling.
  - bilateral lesions are common (50%):
    - **always examine both nasal passages and paranasal sinuses.**
- standing lateral/DV radiography of the head for sinus lesions:
  - defined soft tissue mass rostral/dorsal to ethmoidal labyrinth (Fig. 1.34).

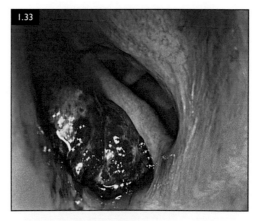

FIG. 1.33 Endoscopic view of an ethmoidal haematoma obscuring part of the view of the ethmoid turbinates. Note the typical appearance and mild haemorrhage from the mass. (Photo courtesy Tim Greet)

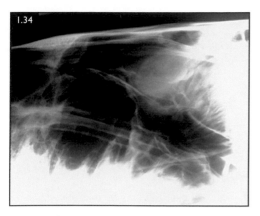

FIG. 1.34 Standing lateral radiograph of the paranasal sinuses in a horse with an ethmoidal haematoma. Note the teardrop-shaped soft tissue mass situated rostral to the ethmoid within the frontal sinus.

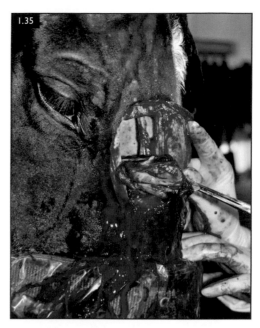

FIG. 1.35 Removal of a PEH via a frontonasal flap in a standing sedated horse.

- ○ fluid lines due to bleeding or secondary infection.
- CT:
  - ○ identification of lesion and anatomical localisation including sphenopalatine sinus.
  - ○ more accurate prognostication and greatly aids in management planning.

Management

- number of treatments available depending on size, position, accessibility, equipment, and finances.
- 10% formalin injection via an endoscopic catheter in standing sedated horse:
  - ○ ensure no CNS communication – contrast radiography/CT:
    - ♦ death reported when haematoma invaded cribiform plate.
    - ♦ damage to infraorbital nerve and chemical sinusitis.
  - ○ endoscopy and/or sinusoscopy.
  - ○ repeated every 3–4 weeks until ablated – usually 2–5 times.
- ablation in lesions <5 cm diameter in standing sedated horse:
  - ○ transendoscopic laser.
  - ○ cryogenic ablation.
  - ○ may need repeated weekly treatments.
  - ○ electrocautery snare excision.
- surgical resection via a large frontonasal flap in standing sedated horse:
  - ○ profuse haemorrhage (Fig. 1.35).

Prognosis

- guarded – recurrence is common (15- 50% of cases within 1–2 years):
  - ○ better post-CT assessment as previously undetected lesions can now be treated.
- follow-up endoscopy every 6 months to detect early recurrence.

Sinus and nasal neoplasia

Definition/overview

- uncommon.
- clinical signs vary considerably depending on the site and extent of the mass.
- radiographic and endoscopic examination of the head, plus biopsy for histopathology.
- surgical removal may be possible via facial flap approaches, but recurrence is common.

Aetiology/pathophysiology

- many tumours are malignant and/or locally invasive.
- more common in older animals.
- benign tumours damage areas by local expansion.

- nasal passages and paranasal sinuses:
  - primary tumours of these structures.
  - invasion from adjacent structures such as mouth and palate.
- most commonly reported tumours are:
  - SCC ○ adenocarcinoma ○ fibroma.
  - chondroma ○ lymphoma.
  - osteoma ○ osteosarcoma.
  - haemangiosarcoma.
- odontogenic tumours derived from tooth-forming elements are rare:
  - usually occur in young animals.

Clinical presentation

- varies with location and extent of mass:
  - early localised cases may be incidental or present as localised infections.
- secondary sinusitis due to drainage problems.
- nasal discharge:
  - often foul-smelling, bloody, purulent and usually unilateral.
- expansion of mass may lead to facial swelling, airway obstruction, and exophthalmos.
- mouth tumours may present with halitosis and occasionally dysphagia.

Differential diagnosis

- other causes of secondary sinusitis, including:
  - maxillary cysts, chronic primary sinus empyema, PEH and nasal polyps.

Diagnosis

- full clinical examination plus oral examination and lymph node palpation (Fig. 1.36):

- endoscopy and/or sinoscopy plus biopsy for histopathology.
- head radiography may identify:
  - poorly defined solid soft tissue masses in the sinuses (Fig. 1.37).
  - mineralised tumours of dental origin.
- transocular ultrasonography for orbital masses.
- CT/MRI may allow a more detailed evaluation.

Management

- surgical excision may be possible via bone flap surgery if limited in extent and benign.
- small nasal tumours have been treated by endoscopic laser ablation or intralesional formalin.

Prognosis

- determined by the chronicity, extent, and severity of the lesion:
  - late diagnosis often limits success with high recurrence rates and poor prognosis.

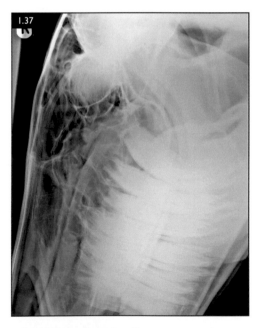

FIG. 1.37 Laterolateral radiograph of the head of case in Fig. 1.36. Note the soft tissue radiodensity in the ventral part of the rostral and caudal maxillary sinus surrounding the cheek teeth roots and with an irregular outline dorsally.

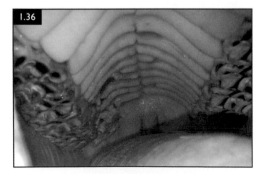

FIG. 1.36 Intraoral view of a palatine SCC adjacent to the right upper arcade of cheek teeth.

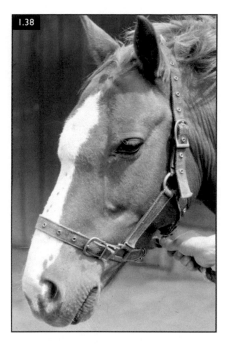

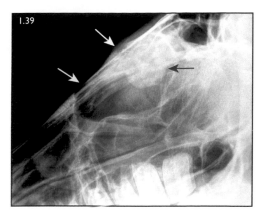

FIG. 1.39 Laterolateral radiograph of the paranasal sinuses of a horse with a sinus cyst. Note dorsally the thinning of the frontal bone by pressure from the underlying cyst (yellow arrow) plus more caudally a reactive suture periostitis (white arrow). Within the conchofrontal sinus there is sinus empyema and a circular area of increased density (red arrow) that at surgery was found to be calcified pus and cyst lining.

FIG. 1.38 Marked facial swelling over the frontal sinuses as a result of a sinus cyst.

- well circumscribed benign lesions may be more successfully treated.

Paranasal sinus cysts

Definition/overview
- swelling caudal to the rostral edge of the facial crest:
  - invariably caused by an expansile mass within the paranasal sinuses.
  - paranasal sinus cysts are a frequent cause.

Aetiology/pathophysiology
- aetiology and pathophysiology are unknown.
- fluid-filled structures that are either single- or multiloculated:
  - epithelial lining that produces a yellow, mucoid-like fluid.
- usually develop in the maxillary sinus, including ventral conchal sinus:
  - can expand into the frontal sinus.
- facial remodelling is partly due to widespread osteoclasts present within the cyst.

Clinical presentation
- can occur in the first year of life or, more commonly, in adult horses.
- facial swelling over the maxillary and conchofrontal sinuses is common (Fig. 1.38).
- unilateral nasal discharge due to obstruction of drainage ostia and secondary sinusitis.
- nasal obstruction due to conchal swelling is frequent.
- incidental finding during exploratory sinus surgery.
- expansile pressure of lesion distorts the outline of the sinus and nasal turbinates.
- exophthalmia occurs occasionally due to pressure from the cyst behind the orbit.

Differential diagnosis
- other expansile lesions of the paranasal sinuses:
  - fibrous dysplasia in the young horse, PEH, SCC, and primary sinusitis.

Diagnosis
- radiography of the head reveals:
  - soft tissue or fluid density within the sinus (Fig. 1.39).

- typical rounded appearance indicative of an encapsulated lesion:
  - ◆ associated fluid accumulation may obscure this outline.
- distortion of the normal sinus outline and structures.
- soft tissue mineralisation.
- ventrodorsal projections, nasal septum or vomer bone deviation.
- CT scans allow much more accurate definition of the extent of the lesion.
- trephination of the sinus usually results in a flow of typical clear yellow fluid.
- nasal endoscopy may reveal:
  - rounded masses in the middle meatus.
  - confined to the sinuses:
    - ◆ diffuse narrowing or obstruction of the meatus due to turbinate expansion.

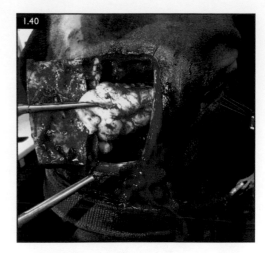

FIG. 1.40 Resection of a sinus cyst in a standing sedated horse.

Management
- surgical removal via a large facial bone flap (Fig. 1.40):
  - either in the standing sedated horse or under GA.
  - any small cyst remnants left do not appear to cause any significant complications.

Prognosis
- excellent with surgical removal, with a very low incidence of recurrence.

Intranasal foreign bodies

Definition/overview
- uncommon condition usually caused by the aspiration of pieces of wood, seeds, and other vegetative material.
- clinical signs in acute cases include nasal discomfort with intense and persistent sneezing, facial rubbing, and epistaxis.
- chronic cases have increasingly purulent and malodorous unilateral nasal discharge.
- diagnosis:
  - rostral nasal passage sites by direct visual examination.
  - endoscopic examination of entire nasal passages will identify the foreign body.
  - radiopaque foreign bodies may be visible on head radiographs.

- treatment by endoscopically guided retrieval in the standing sedated horse followed by a short course of systemic antibiotics and NSAIDs is usually effective.

Iatrogenic trauma of the nasal passages

Definition/overview
- common complication of nasogastric intubation or nasal endoscopy.
- epistaxis due to iatrogenic trauma to the nasal turbinates (particularly ethmoturbinates):
  - mild or profuse during passage or withdrawal of endoscope or tube.
- history of the passage of an endoscope or nasogastric tube.
- further investigation only if epistaxis does not stop or recurs without further nasal intubation:
  - endoscopy seldom successful in the face of acute haemorrhage.
- no treatment is necessary as haemorrhage is invariably self-limiting:
  - tie the horse up so that blood contamination is limited to one area.
  - light sedation and head elevation.
  - bleeding often stops spontaneously within 10–15 mins.

- excellent prognosis.
- prevention is important:
  - avoid using an inappropriate stomach tube:
    - polyurethane tube that does not vary in rigidity with temperature.

- side openings encourage kinking of the end of the tube:
  - form a sharp edge across the turbinates.
  - press tube or endoscope ventrally when it is passed into the ventral meatus.

PHARYNX AND LARYNX

Nasopharyngeal cicatrix

Definition/overview

- rare condition where web of fibrous tissue transverses the nasopharynx causing constriction and obstruction.
- outbreaks have been recorded and there is an association with grazing.
- more frequent in hot climates and reported mainly in Texas in the USA.

Aetiology/pathophysiology

- unknown cause:
  - recently implicated *Pythium* – a fungal infection.
  - caused by inflammation rather than pythiosis.
- post-inflammation, secondary healing can result in a web of scar tissue forming over the floor of the nasopharynx.
- most cases associated with deformity of other laryngeal or pharyngeal cartilages:

Clinical presentation

- poor performance, abnormal respiratory noise and dyspnoea.
- can be asymptomatic.
- more common in horses >5 years old and possibly females.

Differential diagnosis

- other causes of respiratory noise and poor performance.

Diagnosis

- endoscopy (Fig. 1.41):
  - web of fibrous tissue within the nasopharynx:
    - involving the soft palate alone or entire circumference of pharynx.
    - may cause constriction.

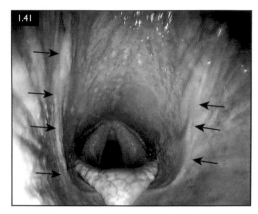

FIG. 1.41 A mild case of nasopharyngeal cicatrix (outlined by arrows).

- other abnormalities often present:
  - arytenoid chondropathy.
  - epiglottic deformity.
  - guttural pouch ostia deformity.

Management

- treatment may not be necessary if no loss of performance.
- mild cases frequently respond to laser ablation of the scar tissue.
- cutting of the cicatrixes and bougie dilation have been used in a few cases.
- treatment of other associated lesions may be required.
- medical treatment generally ineffective.
- severe webbing or marked swelling of the arytenoid cartilages:
  - permanent tracheostomy or insertion of a permanent tracheotomy tube.
- prevention in Texas has included removal of access to pasture.

Prognosis

- recurrence following treatment is very common.

- horse moved to a different climate:
  - outlook is fair.

Pharyngeal cysts

Definition/overview

- developmental cysts are rare:
  - most common in subepiglottic position (see page 32).
  - occasionally on dorsal pharynx or soft palate:
    - former may be remnants of the craniopharyngeal duct or Rathke pouch.
    - latter may have a salivary origin.
- usually incidental endoscopic findings.

Aetiology/pathophysiology

- speculated to be of embryological origin.
- more commonly reported in Thoroughbreds and Standardbreds.

Clinical presentation

- incidental finding on endoscopy.
- can be associated with respiratory noise and obstruction in some horses.

Differential diagnosis

- pharyngeal lymphoid hyperplasia and other pharyngeal masses.

Diagnosis

- endoscopy (Fig. 1.42).

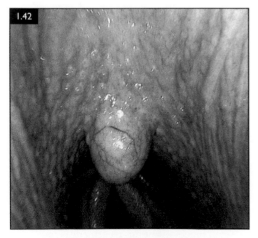

FIG. 1.42 A dorsal pharyngeal cyst on endoscopy.

Management

- surgical resection or transendoscopic laser ablation of the cyst.
- intralesional injections of formalin using a procedure similar to that described for PEH.

Prognosis

- good with no recurrence recorded.

Subepiglottic cyst

Definition/overview

- congenital condition of variable severity:
  - life-threatening respiratory obstruction of the newborn foal.
  - clinical signs of dorsal displacement of the soft palate.
  - incidental finding in an adult horse.

Aetiology/pathophysiology

- failure of glossoepiglottic duct to fully atrophy due to unknown cause.
- recognised in all breeds – most reported in Thoroughbreds and Standardbreds.
- smooth-walled cyst (1–5 cm diameter) filled with straw-coloured sticky fluid:
  - occasionally multilobular.
  - forms between base of the tongue and epiglottis (within loose mucosa).

Clinical presentation

- severity varies enormously:
  - severe respiratory obstruction at birth or shortly afterwards:
    - emergency management may be necessary including nasotracheal intubation or tracheotomy.
  - respiratory noise in a foal often when turned out:
    - intermittent and sudden onset as the cyst precipitates an epiglottic entrapment or dorsal displacement of the soft palate.
  - dysphagia in foal or young horse:
    - coughing, especially during eating.
    - bilateral nasal discharge of mucoid material containing food.
    - suckling foal, reflux of milk from the nares.
    - onset may be sudden.

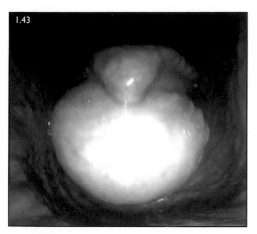

FIG. 1.43 Large subepiglottic cyst.

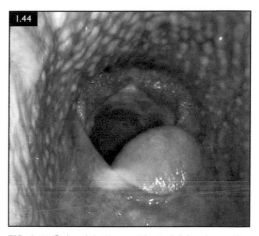

FIG. 1.44 Subepiglottic cyst just visible above the (dorsally displaced) soft palate.

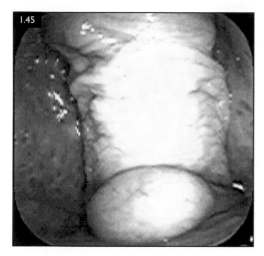

FIG. 1.45 Oral endoscopic examination showing a subepiglottic cyst.

- o poor performance, often with respiratory noise and/or choking up at exercise:
  - ◆ young or adult horse.

Differential diagnosis

- varies depending on the clinical presentation:
  - o other causes of permanent dorsal displacement of the soft palate.
  - o other causes of dysphagia in the young horse including:
    - ◆ fourth branchial arch defects, soft palate hypoplasia, and cleft palate.

Diagnosis

- endoscopy:
  - o often, cyst is clearly visible (Fig. 1.43).
  - o several deglutition sequences should be observed:
    - ◆ frequently cyst will 'pop' into view above the soft palate and then disappear back underneath it (Fig. 1.44).
  - o manipulation of the subepiglottic mucosa with forceps under local anaesthetic solution may help reveal the cyst.
  - o endoscopy via the mouth is rarely required (Fig. 1.45):
    - ◆ often under GA.
- lateral radiography of the oropharynx (especially if taken with the mouth open):
  - o rounded soft tissue density (Fig. 1.46).

Management

- surgical excision.

Prognosis

- excellent following complete removal, as recurrence is rare.

Pharyngeal lymphoid hyperplasia

Definition/overview

- extremely common condition of the young horse (<2 years old):

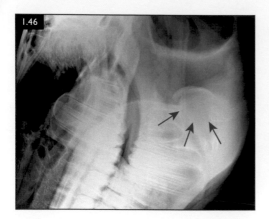

FIG. 1.46 Laterolateral radiograph of the pharynx of a horse. The rounded subepiglottic cyst (arrows) is visible ventral to the soft palate.

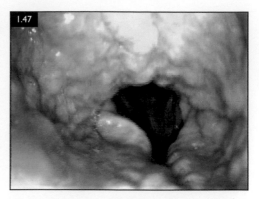

FIG. 1.47 Marked pharyngeal follicular lymphoid hyperplasia over the entire pharynx.

- ○ normal developmental process rather than a genuine disease.
- unusual to result in airway obstruction except in severe cases.
- respiratory noise is a frequent finding.

Aetiology/pathophysiology

- normal response of the pharyngeal lymphoid tissue to hypertrophy in response to:
  - ○ exposure to antigenic stimuli, including viruses and bacteria.
  - ○ other respiratory irritants, such as dust and spores.
  - ○ young horses travelling, entering training and mixing with peers.
- pharyngeal tissues respond by secreting mucus and local immunoglobulins.
- hypertrophy resolves as horse and its immune system mature:
  - ○ condition is rare after 5 years of age.

Clinical presentation

- incidental finding detected on routine endoscopy:
  - ○ usually, no interference with health or performance.
- abnormal respiratory noise in extensive/ severe cases with reduced performance.

Differential diagnosis

- includes all the other causes of respiratory noise.

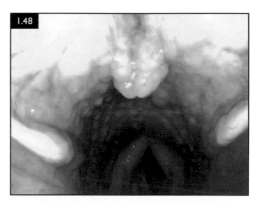

FIG. 1.48 Pharyngeal follicular lymphoid hyperplasia coalescing into a polyp.

Diagnosis

- endoscopic examination is diagnostic (Figs. 1.47, 1.48):
  - ○ grading system (1–4) has been established:
    - ♦ grades 3 and 4 may be associated with clinical signs.

Management

- not usually necessary as improves with maturity.

Prognosis

- very good as the condition spontaneously resolves with maturity.

Foreign bodies of the pharynx

Definition/overview

- rare with two distinct types recognised:
  - oropharyngeal foreign bodies
    – ingested.
  - nasopharyngeal foreign bodies
    – inhaled.

Aetiology/pathophysiology

- thorns and twigs can be inhaled or even implanted directly.
- oral foreign bodies are usually sharp, metal objects.
- penetration by the object can lead to infection in surrounding tissues, including the retropharyngeal region.

Clinical presentation

- nasal/nasopharyngeal foreign bodies can present with:
  - marked epistaxis, particularly at exercise, due to damage to the nasal turbinates.
  - coughing.
  - distressed horse with palpable throat pain and resistance to flexion of throat region.
  - longer-standing cases may have a purulent and foul-smelling nasal discharge.
  - swelling in the retropharyngeal region with secondary deeper infection.
- oropharyngeal foreign bodies usually present with:
  - sudden-onset oral phase dysphagia.
  - coughing and nasal return of food and saliva.
  - marked dropping of food and visible difficulty or reluctance to swallow.

Differential diagnosis

- Guttural pouch mycosis and strangles are the most important differential diagnoses.
- Oropharyngeal foreign bodies can be a diagnostic challenge:
  - signs of dysphagia in multiple conditions including dental disease.

Diagnosis

- endoscopy often diagnostic for pharyngeal foreign bodies:

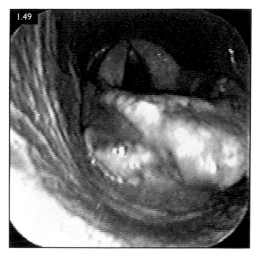

FIG. 1.49 Marked subepiglottic swelling and ulceration caused by an oropharyngeal foreign body. A twig with numerous thorns was removed digitally through the mouth, under GA.

  - assessment of the nasal turbinates for laceration and source of the haemorrhage.
- retropharyngeal FBs, especially of wooden consistency:
  - may require ultrasonography, radiography or even CT/MRI to locate them.
- oropharyngeal FBs similarly difficult to diagnose:
  - endoscopy may reveal:
    - swelling of the epiglottis/ subepiglottic tissues (Fig. 1.49).
    - permanent dorsal displacement of the soft palate.
  - radiography may reveal:
    - subepiglottic swelling and a radiodense foreign body.
  - oral palpation using a suitable gag in the sedated horse may reveal:
    - foreign body if not too far caudal.
  - mouth endoscopy and palpation of the oropharynx under GA may be necessary in some cases.

Management

- removed, often without complication, usually under GA:
  - oropharyngeal by digital manipulation.
  - nasopharyngeal by using grasping forceps under endoscopic visualisation.

- o significant haemorrhage can result from the removal of either:
  - ◆ packing the defect to control haemorrhage is unwise.
  - ◆ pharyngeal packing can result in respiratory obstruction in recovery from anaesthesia.
  - ◆ haemorrhage is seldom life-threatening.
- antibiotics and anti-inflammatory drugs to control postoperative swelling.

Prognosis

- good as long as the foreign body is completely removed.

Dorsal displacement of the soft palate (DDSP) – intermittent

Definition/overview

- Dorsal displacement of the soft palate (DDSP) can be intermittent or persistent:
  - o intermittent usually occurs during exercise and is a common cause of:
    - ◆ dynamic respiratory obstruction.
    - ◆ exercise intolerance.
    - ◆ abnormal respiratory noise.
- principally a racehorse disease, but eventers and hunters are occasionally affected.
- soft palate becomes dislocated from the normal subepiglottic position and obstructs the airway (Fig. 1.50).

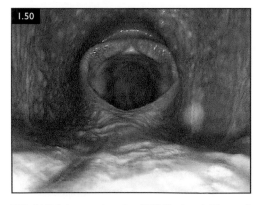

FIG. 1.50 A horse showing DDSP at rest. The soft palate is dorsal to the epiglottis, obscuring its normal outline, and the free border of the soft palate is clearly visible.

- requires dynamic 'overground' endoscopy for diagnosis.
- variety of conservative and surgical treatments for this condition.

Aetiology/pathophysiology

- cause of DDSP at exercise is not entirely clear but probably a neuromuscular weakness.
- during galloping exercise, generation of significant pressure changes in the upper airway during inspiration and expiration.
- nasopharynx can only stabilise itself in the face of these intraluminal pressure changes by skeletal muscle contraction (no bony or cartilaginous support):
  - o some of these muscles act on the hyoid apparatus and larynx affecting:
    - ◆ their position, shape and tension in the nasopharynx (extrinsic factors).
  - o skeletal muscles in the palate and nasopharynx can affect the dynamic stability of the nasopharynx (intrinsic factors).
- neuromuscular weakness of the extrinsic and/or intrinsic muscles:
  - o may lead to loss of palatal support in the face of pressure changes.
  - o cause of neuromuscular weakness is still unknown:
    - ◆ lack of individual ability or fitness.
    - ◆ other acquired factors.
- DDSP may occur secondarily to other primary conditions affecting the horse:
  - o general unfitness.
  - o cardiovascular disorders.
  - o lower airway disease
  - o recurrent laryngeal neuropathy.
  - o palatal problems, including clefts, injuries, ulceration, and cysts.
  - o pharyngeal paralysis.
  - o severe abnormalities of the epiglottis:
    - ◆ deformities, entrapment, inflammation or subepiglottic cysts
  - o pharyngeal discomfort caused by:
    - ◆ lymphoid hyperplasia, inflammation, infections, swellings or excess discharges.
  - o more controversially, conditions that lead to mouth pain and/or mouth breathing:
    - ◆ such as dental disease and biting problems:

- o neck position, especially in dressage or show animals.
- o resolution of primary problem may lead to spontaneous improvement in DDSP.

Clinical presentation

- horse performing well but suddenly dramatically slows down and makes:
  - o vibrant 'gurgling' respiratory noise ('choking up'):
    - ♦ may not produce this at home but will suddenly 'go backwards' in the last furlong or so of a race when under maximal pressure.
    - ♦ upon relocation of the palate by the horse, noise disappears and horse resumes galloping without problem.
  - o billowing of the cheeks also noted in some cases due to mouth breathing.
- wide variation on this classical presentation:
  - o up to 30% of cases may not make an audible respiratory noise.
  - o noise may be harsher, leading to confusion with other respiratory obstructions.
  - o many horses will develop DDSP at the start of exercise and perform moderately throughout, leading to a suspicion of limited ability.

Differential diagnosis

- all other causes of dynamic respiratory obstruction should be considered especially:
  - o recurrent laryngeal neuropathy.
- other primary problems that affect the horse's performance, including limited athletic ability.

Diagnosis

- history, clinical signs, and endoscopic examination, initially at rest, to rule out some of the primary problems:
  - o intermittent DDSP during resting endoscopy is common in normal horses:
    - ♦ DDSP or palatal/pharyngeal flaccidity at rest not predictive for DDSP at exercise.

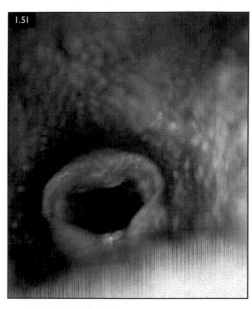

FIG. 1.51 DDSP and collapse of the ventral wall of the nasopharynx, or billowing of the soft palate at exercise, observed by overground endoscopy during fast gallop exercise.

- o persistent displacement, either with or without attempts at swallowing, are suspicious and should be investigated further.
- o occlude nostrils of the horse and observe whether pharyngeal collapse or DDSP occurs in response to the lower airway pressure.
- palpation of the larynx.
- definitive diagnosis requires endoscopic examination at exercise either on a treadmill or using 'overground' videoendoscopy (Fig. 1.51):
  - o requires an exercise test that produces the obstruction, which can be difficult if it only occurs during racing.

Management

- any primary or predisposing conditions need to be treated.
- conservative measures include:
  - o period of rest followed by increasing the fitness of the horse.
  - o approach may be as effective as surgical treatment.
- other traditional techniques include:
  - o tongue tie to stop the horse retracting its tongue:

- ◆ recent research has failed to show any benefit.
- ○ Australian or 'figure-of-eight' nosebands have been used to stop the horse opening its mouth during exercise.
- ○ spoon bit and Cornell collar.
- ○ many of these devices are subject to regulations under the rules of racing or competition of the relevant organisations.
- most common surgical procedure used for DDSP is the laryngeal advancement or 'tie-forward' procedure:
  - ○ permanent suture placed either side between thyroid cartilage and basihyoid bone.
  - ○ replaces function of thyrohyoid muscle.
  - ○ success rate in excess of 80%.
- other surgical techniques that have been used but with significant complications and limited success rates include:
  - ○ myotomy of the sternothyrohyoid muscles or tenotomy of the insertion of the muscle onto the thyroid cartilage of the larynx – the Llewellyn procedure.
  - ○ staphylectomy:
    - ◆ resection of tissue from free border of soft palate via a laryngotomy.
  - ○ ventriculectomy and cordectomy and subepiglottic resection.
- following treadmill observation that billowing of the palate preceded DDSP (Fig. 1.51), surgical techniques to stiffen the palate were developed:
  - ○ thermal palatoplasty:
    - ◆ photocautery using a laser.
    - ◆ actual cautery using red hot irons (Fig. 1.52).
  - ○ published results do not appear to be better than any other surgery.

Prognosis

- almost all procedures used to treat DDSP have the same success rate – 60%.

Dorsal displacement of the soft palate – permanent

Definition/overview

- less common than the intermittent form.
- caused by either physical or neurological abnormalities.

Aetiology/pathophysiology

- multiple causes of permanent DDSP:
- physical obstruction of the subepiglottic space including:
  - ○ subepiglottic cysts   ○ palatal cysts.
  - ○ foreign bodies.
  - ○ severe pharyngeal lymphoid hyperplasia.
- neurological abnormalities, in particular pharyngeal paralysis:
  - ○ most commonly caused by guttural pouch mycosis.

Clinical presentation

- marked respiratory stertor at exercise, including at trot or even walk.
- markedly diminished performance.
- pharyngeal phase dysphagia leading to:
  - ○ coughing.
  - ○ nasal return of food material and saliva.

Differential diagnosis

- no specific list of differential diagnoses.
- other relevant conditions include cleft palate and palatal hypoplasia in the foal, and oesophageal obstruction (choke) in the adult horse.

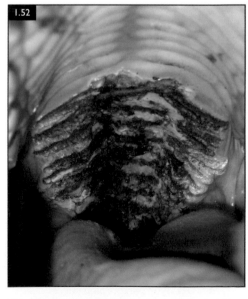

FIG. 1.52 The soft palate of a horse following thermal palatoplasty by actual cautery.

Diagnosis

- endoscopy:
  - DDSP not resolved despite repeated swallowing (Fig. 1.53).
  - always include a guttural pouch examination.
  - oral endoscopy, possibly under GA (Fig. 1.54).
- radiography:
  - confirms diagnosis by identifying soft palate dorsal to the epiglottis.
  - identification of soft tissue masses ventral to epiglottis, causing physical DDSP.

Management

- treat any underlying disease that is identified:
  - guttural pouch mycosis or subepiglottic cysts.
- unidentified causes:
  - prolonged use of anti-inflammatory and antibiotic treatment.
  - if unsuccessful, staphylectomy surgery has been suggested.
  - laryngeal tie-forward surgery alone or in combination with staphylectomy:
    - ♦ success rates of over 80% are reported.

Prognosis

- physical cause that can be treated, usually an excellent prognosis.
- neurological causes are associated with a guarded prognosis:
  - some pharyngeal function may return after guttural pouch mycosis treatment.
- other causes of pharyngeal paralysis carry a poor prognosis.

Nasopharyngeal collapse (NPC)

Definition/overview

- dynamic pharyngeal collapse has become apparent since treadmill endoscopy:
  - dorsal, ventral, lateral, dorsal and lateral, or complete pharyngeal collapse have been observed.
- ventral nasopharyngeal collapse (palatal instability) implicated as precursor to DDSP.

Aetiology/pathophysiology

- nasopharynx is an unsupported muscular tube and can contract completely.
- without appropriate muscular tone the pharynx is unable to resist the changes in airway pressure at exercise.
- neuromuscular weakness will result in collapse of the nasopharynx, similar to pathogenesis of DDSP.

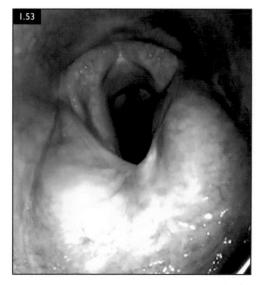

FIG. 1.53 Permanent DDSP. The apparent swelling is the outline of the epiglottis underneath the palate.

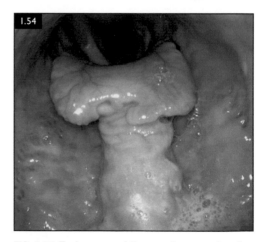

FIG. 1.54 Endoscopy of the oropharynx, showing a deformed apex of the epiglottis in a horse under GA.

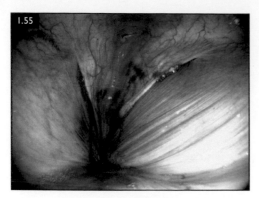

FIG. 1.55 Pharyngeal collapse resulting in dyspnoea, secondary to haemorrhage and swelling into the guttural pouch.

- possible causes for dynamic collapse have focused on pharyngeal inflammation:
  - previous evidence of pharyngeal lymphoid hyperplasia.
  - inflammation in the region of the pharyngeal nerves in the guttural pouch.
  - no causal relationship has been established.
- ventral pharyngeal collapse is associated with tensor veli palatine muscle dysfunction.
- other causes of dynamic pharyngeal collapse include:
  - rostral respiratory tract obstructions leading to increased negative pressure in the pharynx.
  - myopathies causing weakness.
  - neuropathies.
- physical compression from peripharyngeal pathology can cause persistent collapse:
  - guttural pouch empyema can result in dorsal pharyngeal collapse.
  - retropharyngeal lymph node swelling can lead to caudal and lateral collapse.
- physical positioning of the head in some disciplines:
  - competition horses required to perform 'in an outline' (ventral flexion of the poll).

Clinical presentation

- persistent pharyngeal collapse associated with surrounding swelling will present with significant dyspnoea (Fig. 1.55):
  - horse may have marked stertor at rest and stand with the head extended.
- dynamic pharyngeal collapse presents as a dynamic airway obstruction of the performance horse:
  - associated signs of exercise intolerance and abnormal respiratory noise.
- collapse of the ventral nasopharynx, or billowing of the soft palate:
  - specific obstruction noted on dynamic endoscopy.

Differential diagnosis

- presenting signs of dynamic pharyngeal collapse may lead to a tentative diagnosis of DDSP but cannot reliably rule out other airway obstructions of the performance horse.
- principal differential diagnosis of persistent pharyngeal collapse is nasal occlusion or severe recurrent obstructive lower airway disease.

Diagnosis

- persistent pharyngeal collapse readily diagnosed by resting endoscopy:
  - area of the swelling provides information as to the location of the swollen tissue.
  - examine guttural pouches to assess swelling in this area.
  - oral examination:
    - fracture of sixth cheek tooth can result in severe swelling and respiratory obstruction.
- radiography may be helpful in the diagnosis of persistent pharyngeal collapse.
- dynamic pharyngeal collapse requires overground endoscopy for diagnosis (Fig. 1.56):
  - ensure horse exercised with head in regular position.
  - define whether ventral, dorsal and/or lateral, or circumferential.
  - identification of concomitant conditions.

Management

- persistent pharyngeal collapse requires treatment of the underlying condition:
  - drainage of guttural pouch empyema or retropharyngeal abscesses.

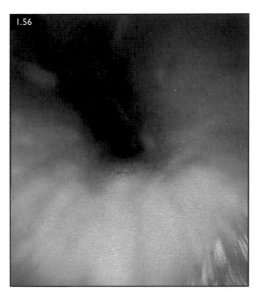

FIG. 1.56 Overground endoscopy of dynamic pharyngeal collapse at exercise, in a 9-year-old Warmblood stallion used for dressage.

- o relief of guttural pouch tympany.
- dynamic dorsal or lateral pharyngeal collapse does not have a specific treatment:
  - o treatment with rest and anti-inflammatory medications.
  - o time to mature in young horses.
- collapse of the ventral nasopharynx can be treated in the same way as DDSP.

Prognosis

- persistent pharyngeal collapse caused by a treatable condition has excellent prognosis:
  - o no long-term 'stretching' or other distortion of the pharynx.
- dynamic dorsal and lateral pharyngeal collapse is stated to have a good prognosis:
  - o most horses improve with maturity and resolution of inflammation.
  - o no detailed case studies are available, and this may be overly optimistic.
- ventral pharyngeal collapse has a prognosis similar to DDSP:
  - o little evidence that surgical stiffening of the palate is of any benefit.

Recurrent laryngeal neuropathy (RLN)

Definition/overview

- probably the most important cause of upper airway obstruction in the horse.
- equine idiopathic RLN is associated with the length of the recurrent laryngeal nerve, and hence is more frequent in large horses:
  - o left side of the larynx is almost invariably affected, as the left nerve is longer.
- RLN causes neurogenic atrophy in several laryngeal muscles, including the main adductor, the cricoarytenoideus dorsalis (CAD).
- loss of muscles' function causes loss of abduction of the ipsilateral arytenoid cartilage and airway obstruction:
  - o spectrum of the disease varies enormously.

Aetiology/pathophysiology

- RLN is a pathological diagnosis.
- idiopathic equine RLN is a distal axonopathy:
  - o precise cause of axonopathy is not known.
  - o genetic predisposition seems highly likely.
  - o 'die back' of the recurrent nerve from the distal (laryngeal) end:
    - ◆ large-diameter myelinated nerve fibres are preferentially affected.
    - ◆ results in neurogenic atrophy of the intrinsic musculature of the larynx:
      - – only laryngeal muscle not innervated/affected is cricothyroid muscle.
      - – first observed in adductors such as cricoarytenoideus lateralis (CAL):
        - ◇ seldom significant.
      - – atrophy next in CAD – main abductor of larynx:
        - ◇ clinically significant.
- other, less frequent, causes of damage to the RLN include:
  - o infections:
    - ◆ guttural pouch mycosis or equine protozoal myelopathy.
  - o trauma.

- o perivascular injection of irritant substances.
- o toxicoses (including lead and organophosphates).

Clinical presentation

- spectrum of the disease varies enormously.
- invariably an athletic horse performing poorly:
  - o usually associated with inspiratory respiratory stertor.
- abnormal sounds range from soft musical whistle to harsher roaring sound:
  - o inspiratory.
  - o usually gets louder and longer with increased work.
  - o disappears very quickly after the animal stops.
  - o expiratory noise is usually normal and often vibrant – 'high blowing'.
- more severe cases can present with dyspnoea and even collapse.
- RLN following perivascular injection often in association with Horner syndrome.
- RLN caused by guttural pouch mycosis often detected incidentally during endoscopic examination for another presenting sign, notably dysphagia or epistaxis.

Differential diagnosis

- other upper airway obstructions of the exercising horse, including:
  - o axial deviation of the aryepiglottic folds.
  - o pharyngeal collapse, epiglottic retroflexion or arytenoid chondritis.
  - o DDSP has some features that are similar, but others that are distinctly different:
    - ♦ usually presents with low-frequency expiratory noise only at extreme exercise.

Diagnosis

- examination at exercise:
  - o ridden or lunge at the canter on both reins.
  - o ensure horse is taking one breath per stride to determine phase of respiration:
    - ♦ head moving down – expiring.

- ♦ head moving up – inspiring.
  - o inspiratory 'whistle' or 'roar'.
- adductor function fails initially and affected horses are unable to close their glottis:
  - o detected as an audible expiration at a time when no respiration expected:
    - ♦ horse threatened suddenly, or forcibly stimulated to contract the abdominal musculature:
      - – may let air through glottis resulting in a grunt
      - – 'grunt to a stick test'.
- palpation of the larynx:
  - o scars, especially ventrally from previous laryngotomy or trauma.
  - o assess lateral and dorsal larynx for symmetry or anatomical defects.
  - o assess the muscular processes on either side concurrently:
    - ♦ prominent on one side may indicate atrophy of the CAD.
- endoscopy at rest:
  - o unsedated horse.
  - o ideally, pass endoscope up both nostrils and assess separately:
    - ♦ negate eccentric positioning within nasopharynx.
  - o allow horse to relax and observe larynx for a few minutes:
    - ♦ bilaterally symmetrical abduction of the arytenoids during inspiration.
  - o asymmetry of the rima glottides is obvious in severe cases:
    - ♦ more difficult to assess:
      - – subtle milder cases.
      - – asynchronous arytenoid movement at rest.
  - o assess abduction of arytenoids after:
    - ♦ repeated swallowing:
      - – induced by water through biopsy channel/transendoscopic catheter.
    - ♦ nasal occlusion for 10–20 seconds.
  - o grade positional and functional symmetry of arytenoid cartilages:
    - ♦ Havermeyer scale (Table 1.1).
  - o position on the resting scope not reliable indicator of function at exercise:
    - ♦ diagnosis of clinically significant RLN at exercise only possible at rest if full loss of abduction.
- exercising endoscopy:

TABLE 1.1 Havemeyer system for classification of laryngeal neuropathy

ENDOSCOPIC FINDING	HAVERMEYER SCALE	LANE SCALE	US SCALE
Symmetrical at rest, full synchronous movement	Grade I	1	1
Some asynchronous movement, full abduction easily attained	Grade II.1	2	2a
Some asymmetry at rest, full abduction attained and maintained	Grade II.2	3– to 3	2b
Asymmetry at rest, full abduction attained but not maintained	Grade III.1	3 to 3+	3
Asymmetry at rest, full abduction not attained	Grade III.2	4– to 4	3
Asymmetry with little arytenoid movement	Grade III.3	4+	3
Total paralysis of the arytenoid	Grade IV	5	4

- o essential for complete and accurate assessment of laryngeal function at exercise.
- o high-speed treadmill endoscopy or overground endoscopy.
- o grading scale of function as per Rossignol:
  - ♦ Grade A: symmetrical full abduction of arytenoid cartilages (Fig. 1.57).
  - ♦ Grade B: asymmetrical abduction – one cartilage slightly less abducted (Fig. 1.58).
  - ♦ Grade C: asymmetrical abduction – one cartilage collapsing ipsilaterally.
  - ♦ Grade D: asymmetrical abduction – one cartilage collapsing to contralateral side (Fig. 1.59).
- o identify other concomitant problems.

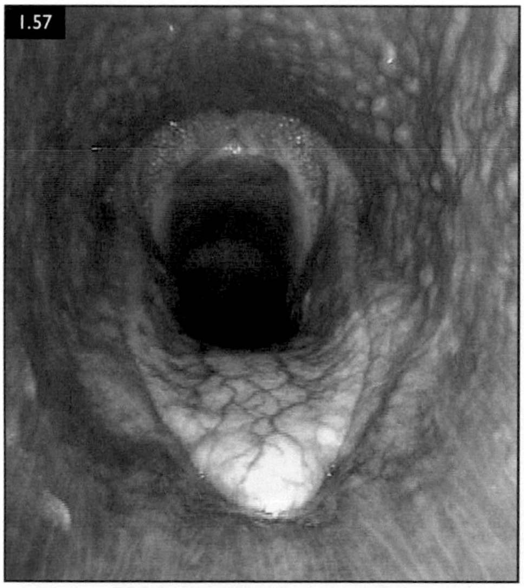

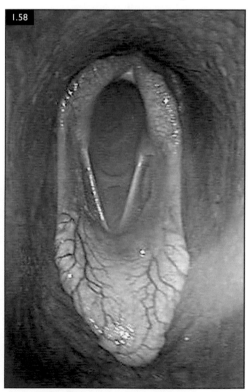

FIG. 1.57 Dynamic overground endoscopy showing symmetrical full abduction of the arytenoid cartilages.

FIG. 1.58 Grade III.2 RLN, showing asymmetry of the arytenoid cartilages, in a horse shortly before undergoing overground endoscopy.

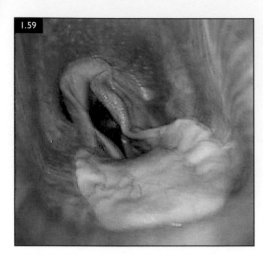

FIG. 1.59 Collapse of the left arytenoid cartilage over to the right side of the larynx during exercise.

- ultrasonography can be useful:
  - transcutaneous using a high-frequency probe from lateral aspect:
    - laryngeal cartilage symmetry and identification of any defects.
    - assess CAL and CAD muscles for atrophy and fibrosis (Fig. 1.60).
  - transoesophageal using a specific probe:
    - more accurate assessment of CAD through the oesophagus.

Management

- depends on the degree of the neuropathy and the athletic potential of the horse:

  - maximum demand for air in racehorses, followed by eventers.
- grade of II.1 or lower is *usually* considered within normal limits.
- grade II.2 and III.1 RLN *usually* have normal exercise tolerance:
  - treatment for vocal cord collapse may be indicated.
- grades III.2 and higher are *usually* significant:
  - result in collapse of the arytenoid cartilage during strenuous exercise.
- **poor correlation between the degree of RLN observed at rest, and the ability of the horse to maintain abduction of the arytenoid cartilage at exercise:**
  - treatment guided by careful assessment of all clinical signs and diagnostic tests.
- grades III.3 and IV RLN are *usually* associated with severe respiratory obstruction at exercise and surgery is necessary for all but the most sedentary horses.
- surgical techniques include:
  - vocal fold and ventricle resection (Hobday/Williams procedure).
  - Laryngoplasty (tie-back):
    - may be combined with above.
    - under GA or in standing sedated horse.
    - wide range of complications.
  - CAD reinnervation:
    - nerve-pedicle grafting.
    - under GA or in the standing sedated horse.

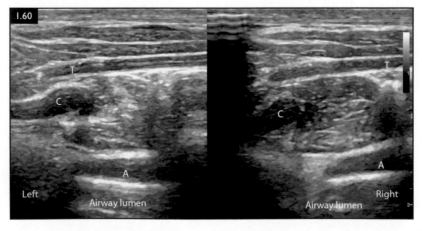

FIG. 1.60 Ultrasonographic image showing fibrosis of the left cricoarytenoideus lateralis muscle (arrow). T = thyroid cartilage; C = cricoid cartilage; A = arytenoid cartilage.

- ◆ needs early diagnosis of RLN – prior to development of muscle fibrosis.
    - ◆ 3–12 months for reconditioning of the muscle.
  - ○ arytenoidectomy:
    - ◆ useful where the tie-back has failed.
  - ○ permanent tracheotomy:
    - ◆ severe and bilateral cases.
    - ◆ non-competition horses.

Prognosis

- guarded, as an incurable, progressive disease.
- all surgical procedures can have significant complications.

Vocal fold collapse

Definition/overview

- part of the RLN complex recognised using exercising endoscopy.
- may be a precursor of arytenoid collapse.
- common in cases of laryngeal dysplasia.

Aetiology/pathophysiology

- recurrent laryngeal nerve also innervates the vocalis muscle of the vocal cord.
- function of this muscle is for vocalisation:
  - ○ adjacent laryngeal ventricle increases resonance.
- reduced tension and collapse in the vocal fold is caused by:
  - ○ loss of tone in the vocalis muscle.
  - ○ loss of abduction of arytenoids will further slacken the fold.
  - ○ loss of function of cricothyroid muscle also results in vocal fold collapse.
- vocal cord collapse is a common presenting sign of laryngeal dysplasia:
  - ○ reduced tension in the vocal fold caused by absence or hypoplasia of the cricothyroideus muscle.

Clinical presentation

- poor performance associated with respiratory noise.

Differential diagnosis

- other dynamic respiratory obstructions of the performance horse should be considered.

- most important differential is whether it is associated with collapse of the arytenoid cartilage.

Diagnosis

- requires dynamic endoscopy (Fig. 1.61).
- majority of cases are diagnosed based on a musical inspiratory noise associated with a moderate (grade II.1 to III.1) RLN at rest.

Management

- vocal cord collapse is very successfully treated surgically:
  - ○ ventriculocordectomy via a ventral laryngotomy:
    - ◆ 'Hobday' procedure, either under GA or standing sedation/local anaesthesia.
  - ○ vocal cordectomy in the standing sedated horse by transendoscopic laser ablation.

Prognosis

- resolution of the respiratory noise following cordectomy for a horse with vocal fold collapse is very good (Fig. 1.62).

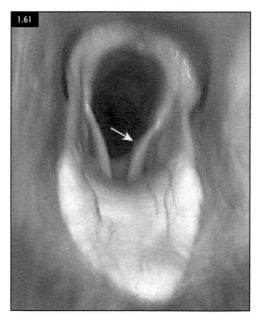

FIG. 1.61 Dynamic overground endoscopy of a horse with bilateral collapse of the vocal cords (arrow illustrating the left cord).

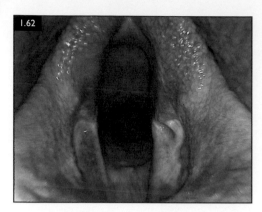

FIG. 1.62 A horse that is racing successfully having undergone a left ventriculocordectomy.

- improvement in performance is more guarded:
  - vocal cord can contribute a large amount of respiratory noise.
  - collapse of the arytenoid results in the major respiratory obstruction.
  - RLN is a progressive condition:
    - ♦ further respiratory noise and obstruction may develop.

Arytenoid chondritis

Definition/overview

- important cause of airway obstruction due to:
  - inflammation, thickening, and distortion of the arytenoid cartilage.
  - leads to exercise intolerance and an abnormal respiratory noise.
- diagnosed on endoscopy.
- medical treatment is sometimes effective in mild cases.
- partial arytenoidectomy in surgical treatment of more severe cases.

Aetiology/pathophysiology

- progressive inflammatory process develops within the corniculate process of the arytenoid cartilage:
  - due to its limited blood supply, difficult to resolve once established.
  - leads to distortion of the cartilage, dystrophic mineralisation, protruberances of damaged cartilage and/or infected granulation tissue, and fistula formation.

  - tracts may drain mucopurulent material.
  - decreased abduction of the affected arytenoid (Fig. 1.63).
- cause is unknown:
  - may include trauma to cartilage and/or infection following mucosal damage.
- usually unilateral.

Clinical presentation

- presentation similar to other respiratory obstructions of the racehorse:
  - poor performance associated with a stridor-like inspiratory noise.
  - acute onset or chronic and insidiously progressive.
- severity of signs varies with the degree of damage and subsequent obstruction:
  - severe and bilateral cases, clinical signs may be evident at rest or walk.
- coughing is common.

Differential diagnosis

- other respiratory obstructions of the racehorse, particularly RLN.

Diagnosis

- endoscopic examination is diagnostic but requires care:
  - **easily confused with RLN, particularly in left-sided case of chondritis.**
  - limited movement of affected arytenoid cartilage.

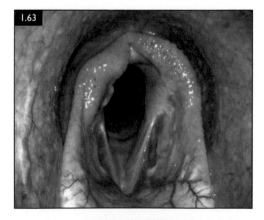

FIG. 1.63 Chondritis of the right arytenoid cartilage. There is limited abduction, distortion of the corniculate process and a discharging sinus on the axial margin.

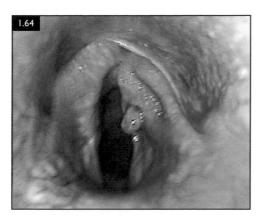

FIG. 1.64 Granuloma on the left arytenoid cartilage, associated with minimal abduction and mild displacement of the rostral palatopharyngeal arch. Horse had undergone tie-back surgery 6 months previously.

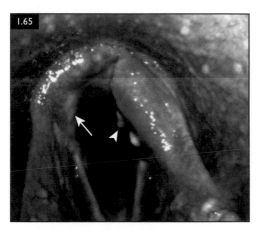

FIG. 1.65 'Kissing lesion' (arrow) on the right arytenoid cartilage with a discharging granuloma on the left arytenoid cartilage (arrowhead).

- o swelling of the corniculate process:
  - ♦ may be associated with mild rostral displacement of palatopharyngeal arch.
- o most reliable finding is a small discharging sinus, usually on the axial border of the cartilage, often associated with a granuloma (Fig. 1.64).
- o 'kissing' lesion', a small reddened or ulcerated area, is commonly identified on the contralateral corniculate process (Fig. 1.65).
- o bilateral cases may have a very narrowed rima glottidis.

- palpation over the affected arytenoid may increase clinical signs of airway obstruction and noise.
- lateral radiographs of the larynx may reveal focal mineralisation.

Management

- prolonged course of antibiotics and NSAIDs (6 weeks):
  - o may control the condition and reduce swelling/discharge from the arytenoid cartilage for a reasonable period in some established cases.
  - o usually associated with improvement in arytenoid motility.
  - o significant axial granulomas and kissing lesions do not usually resolve.
- granulomas and kissing lesions can be removed surgically:
  - o transendoscopic laser surgery.
  - o conventional surgery via a laryngotomy.
- surgical management of arytenoid chondritis is by arytenoidectomy:
  - o partial when all arytenoid removed apart from the muscular process.
  - o subtotal where a rim of corniculate cartilage is left *in situ*.
  - o performed through a laryngotomy and associated with a number of complications.

Prognosis

- partial arytenoidectomy has a guarded to fair prognosis for return to athletic activity.
- conservative approach warrants a guarded prognosis:
  - o majority of mildly affected cases will be able to perform, probably at a lower level.

Laryngeal dysplasia (fourth branchial arch defect syndrome 4-BAD)

Definition/overview

- embryologically the larynx is derived from the fourth and sixth branchial arches.
- variety of laryngeal abnormalities caused by hypo- or aplasia of structures that derive from the fourth branchial arch are recognised:

- ○ fourth branchial arch defects (4-BAD).
- ○ one of the common presentations, rostral displacement of the pharyngeal arch, is sporadically described as a distinct condition.
- condition is unusual but more common than is generally recognised and frequently missed.

Aetiology/pathophysiology

- incidence of approximately 2 Thoroughbred horses per 1000.
- no genetic link has been identified.
- likely aetiology is embryological damage.
- congenital condition and not progressive.
- predeliction for 4-BAD to affect the right side of the larynx.
- many left-sided cases may be misdiagnosed as RLN.

Clinical presentation

- structures involved alter the clinical condition:
  - ○ wing of the thyroid cartilage and associated cricothyroid muscle are missing:
    - ◆ presentation may be similar to RLN.
    - ◆ collapse of vocal fold during high-speed exercise.

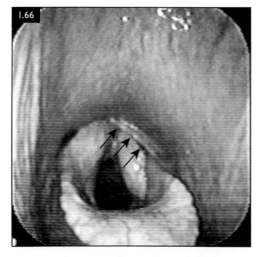

FIG. 1.66 A horse with a fourth branchial arch deformity. There is asymmetrical abduction of the arytenoid cartilages and unilateral rostral displacement of the palatopharyngeal arch (arrows).

- ◆ endoscopy at rest may reveal asymmetry of the rima glottidis, raising suspicion of RLN.
- ◆ right-sided RLN is diagnosed consider:
  - – guttural pouch mycosis, perivascular injection, other trauma or 4-BAD.
  - ○ crico- and thyropharyngeus muscles are absent:
    - ◆ rostral displacement of palatopharyngeal arch (RDPPA) will develop.
    - ◆ visible endoscopically (Fig. 1.66):
      - – upper oesophageal sphincter is incompetent.
      - – results in aspiration of air into the proximal oesophagus.
      - – cases may present with eructation, recurrent tympanitic colic or dysphagia.

Differential diagnosis

- most important differential is RLN:
  - ○ particularly important if surgical correction is considered.
  - ○ laryngoplasty is frequently impossible in horses with 4-BAD.
- eructation may be misdiagnosed by owners as 'wind sucking' or 'crib biting'.

Diagnosis

- can be challenging.
- most reliable technique is palpation of the larynx:
  - ○ reveals abnormalities in almost all cases.
  - ○ most consistent finding is absence of the wing of the thyroid cartilage:
    - ◆ complete ring of the cricoid can be palpated.
    - ◆ feels like a large tracheal ring.
    - ◆ always compare sides of the larynx.
- ultrasonography can confirm hypoplasia of the wing of the thyroid cartilage (Fig. 1.67).
- CT and MRI have been used to confirm abnormalities of the cartilage skeleton.
- endoscopy may reveal:
  - ○ asymmetry of the arytenoid cartilages or it can be normal.
  - ○ rostral displacement of the palatopharyngeal arch may be visible:

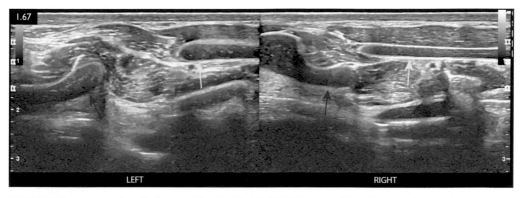

FIG. 1.67 Ultrasonography of a horse with left-sided 4-BAD. The cricoid cartilage (red arrows) are normal, but the left thyroid cartilage (yellow arrows) is shorter and does not overlap the cricoid, compared with the normal right side.

- ♦ rim of tissue partly obscuring or overlying the dorsal aspect of the arytenoid cartilages, either unilateral or bilateral.
  - ○ occasionally horses show no abnormalities at rest:
    - ♦ dynamic endoscopy is necessary to reveal dynamic rostral displacement of the palatopharyngeal arch (RDPPA) or dynamic vocal fold collapse (Fig. 1.68).
- • radiography of the larynx and proximal trachea may reveal:
  - ○ air in the proximal oesophagus, if RDPPA is visible endoscopically:
    - ♦ 'teardrop' appearance.

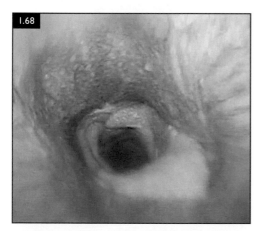

FIG. 1.68 Dynamic overground endoscopy of a horse with right-sided rostral displacement of the palatopharyngeal arch.

Management

- • no effective treatment for RDPPA and the abnormality is permanent.
- • many horses with laryngeal dysplasia maintain arytenoid abduction at exercise but have bilateral collapse of the vocal cords:
  - ○ bilateral ventriculectomy and cordectomy may be effective in such cases.
  - ○ arytenoidectomy of the affected side has been reported in a small number of cases.

Prognosis

- • poor.
- • permanent congenital abnormalities and almost all horses are ineffective athletes.
- • some horses will respond to bilateral ventriculocordectomy.

Epiglottitis

Definition/overview

- • result of infection becoming established within cartilage.
- • primarily associated with racehorses:
  - ○ anecdotal association with all-weather surfaces.

Aetiology/pathophysiology

- • inflammatory process within the elastic cartilage of the epiglottis:

   o less likely to become permanently established in the epiglottic cartilage than in the arytenoid.

Clinical presentation

- respiratory noise and poor performance are usual presenting signs.
- occasional cases present with dysphagia.

Differential diagnosis

- pharyngeal foreign bodies, which can be associated with significant epiglottic swelling, epiglottic entrapment, and general pharyngitis.

Diagnosis

- endoscopic examination is diagnostic:
  - epiglottis is swollen and normal crenated outline is lost (Fig. 1.69).
  - often reddened and presented in a more vertical orientation than normal.
  - occasionally, abscess on the dorsal surface of the epiglottis, identified as a rounded swelling.
  - purulent discharge can be noted from the cartilage occasionally if there is ulceration of the mucosal surface (Fig. 1.70).

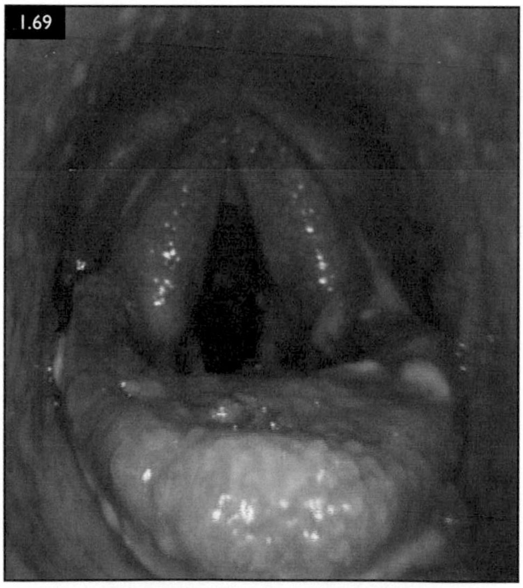

Management

- prolonged course of antibiotics, possibly in association with NSAIDs, is indicated.
- corticosteroids may be indicated if swelling is severe enough to result in respiratory obstruction at rest.

Prognosis

- fair.
- recurrence of the swelling and discharge is less usual than in arytenoid chondritis.
- permanent distortion of the epiglottis is a frequent outcome, which may predispose to DDSP (Fig. 1.71).

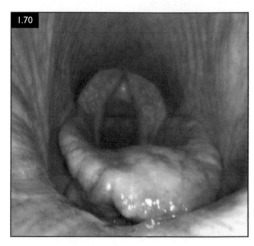

FIG. 1.70 Purulent discharge from the apex of the epiglottis in a horse with chronic epiglottitis.

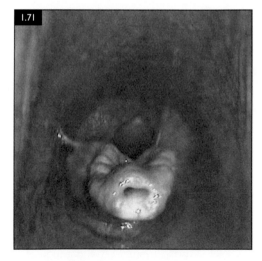

FIG. 1.69 Swollen and inflamed epiglottis in a race-horse with epiglottitis.

FIG. 1.71 Chronic distorted epiglottis following treatment for epiglottitis.

Epiglottic entrapment

Definition/overview

- frequent condition where the cartilage of the epiglottis becomes enveloped by the underlying glossoepiglottic mucosa and aryepiglottic folds.
- cause of the entrapment is often unclear but careful examination is vital to differentiate any secondary causes.
- entrapments vary in stability:
  - some horses have permanent entrapments.
  - others are more intermittent and can be missed on a single examination.
- diagnosis is by endoscopy usually at rest:
  - incidence at rest is suggested as 0.75–3.3%.
- variety of surgical techniques are available for treatment.

Aetiology/pathophysiology

- often unknown aetiology:
  - inflammation of aryepiglottic folds and loose subepiglottic tissue may be a factor in some cases.
  - congenital epiglottic hypoplasia and subepiglottic cyst cases are predisposed.
  - recorded in association with cleft or hypoplastic palate in foals.
- how the glossoepiglottic and aryepiglottic folds become caught over the end of the epiglottis is not known.

Clinical presentation

- vibrant respiratory noise:
  - inspiratory, expiratory, or both.
- obstruction to the airflow varies with:
  - degree of entrapment and associated swelling and inflammation.
  - any secondary DDSP.
- associated poor performance and other signs of DDSP.
- occasional cases present with:
  - dysphagia, including coughing after eating.
  - headshaking.
  - asymptomatic.

Differential diagnosis

- DDSP is the primary differential.

Diagnosis

- endoscopic examination is diagnostic:
  - assess the epiglottis carefully:
    - stable entrapments are easily diagnosed (Fig. 1.72).
    - normal epiglottis has a crenated edge, with pronounced vasculature.
    - entraped epiglottis has a smooth edge and no vasculature (covering mucosa).
    - coverage of the epiglottis is variable.
    - long-standing cases:
      - caudal edge of entrapment may ulcerate.
      - apex of the epiglottis may erode through the entrapment (Fig. 1.73).
  - intermittent entrapments are more of a diagnostic challenge:
    - most entrapments are precipitated by deglutition, not by exercise:
      - careful assessment of several deglutition sequences is indicated.
      - dynamic endoscopy rarely necessary for diagnosis:
        - ◇ most cases diagnosed at rest.
- radiography of the pharynx can reveal the blunted outline of an entrapped epiglottis, epiglottic hypoplasia and subepiglottic cysts.

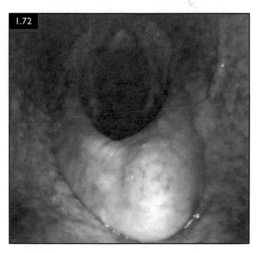

FIG. 1.72 Stable non-ulcerated epiglottic entrapment.

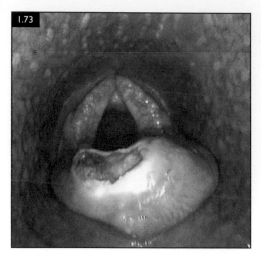

FIG. 1.73 Epiglottic entrapment with significant ulceration of the entrapping glossoepiglottic mucosa.

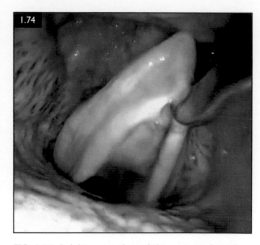

FIG. 1.74 Axial transection of the entrapping glossoepiglottic mucosa using a hook knife passed through the mouth under GA (hence upside down).

Management

- intermittent cases can be managed successfully by anti-inflammatory medication:
  - usually administered as a nasal spray using a canine urinary catheter.
  - combination of DMSO, hydrocortisone, and propylene glycol are often used.
- most cases are managed surgically:
  - stable entrapments in the standing sedated horse:
    - custom-built hook knife passed via contralateral nasal passage.
    - hooks entrapping membrane.
    - knife is withdrawn, and membrane transected in the midline.
    - guarded or closed hook knives limit the risks of iatrogenic damage.
  - incised via a transendoscopic laser following topical local anaesthesia.
- some surgeons prefer to perform the procedure under GA (Fig. 1.74):
  - same hook knife passed via the mouth, under oral endoscopic examination.
- transection does not release the entrapment:
  - resection via a laryngotomy is necessary.

Prognosis

- good with most cases making a rapid and uneventful recovery.

- recurrence in small percentage of cases managed by simple transection.
- excision of the glossoepiglottic mucosa can result in chronic coughing due to low-grade dysphagia in some horses.
- iatrogenic trauma to the epiglottis or pharyngeal structures, especially in standing procedures, is a serious complication.

Axial or medial deviation of the aryepiglottic folds (ADAF)

Definition/overview

- aryepiglottic mucosal folds extend between the lateral epiglottis and the corniculate process of the arytenoid cartilages.
- important cause of dynamic airway obstruction in the racehorse.
- recognised since the advent of dynamic endoscopy.

Aetiology/pathophysiology

- unknown.
- frequently associated with other airway obstructions, commonly/not invariably DDSP:
  - associated with loss of palatal seal:
    - air leaks from oropharynx to nasopharynx.

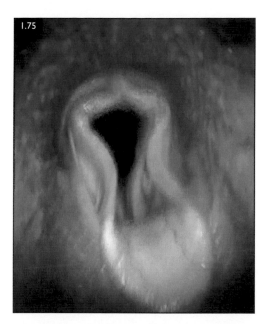

FIG. 1.75 Dynamic overground endoscopy of a horse with ADAF.

- axial deviation of the right aryepiglottic fold is commonly identified with arytenoid collapse (RLN).

Clinical presentation

- presents as a typical airway obstruction of the performance horse or racehorse.
- history of poor exercise performance associated with a harsh inspiratory noise:
  - no characteristic feature of the inspiratory noise.
- no known breed or gender bias but may be a higher incidence in young horses (2–3 years old).

Differential diagnosis

- all the causes of inspiratory noise and poor performance in the racehorse should be considered.
- **care should be taken with a diagnosis of ADAF alone, as many cases are associated with other respiratory obstructions.**

Diagnosis

- dynamic endoscopy is required to establish a diagnosis of ADAF:
  - deviation towards the midline, of one (usually right side) or both of the aryepiglottic mucosal folds (Fig. 1.75).
  - degree of deviation varies between cases:
    - determines the degree of clinical signs and possible treatment options.
  - other concurrent URT endoscopic findings include:
    - axial collapse of the vocal cords.
    - left laryngeal hemiplegia.
    - intermittent DDSP.
    - right laryngeal dysfunction.
    - dorsal pharyngeal collapse.

Management

- surgical resection of the aryepiglottic folds is the treatment of choice for moderate to severe cases or where there are no concurrent abnormalities:
  - ideally performed by transendoscopic laser ablation of the folds.
  - resection can be performed via a laryngotomy incision under GA.
- postoperatively, topical antibiotic, and anti-inflammatory pharyngeal sprays may be used.

Prognosis

- fair.
- aryepiglottic folds appear to re-form quite rapidly, although their subsequent function and stiffness is unknown.

Epiglottic retroflexion

Definition/overview

- not recognised prior to the advent of dynamic endoscopy.
- during retroflexion, the epiglottis is aspirated into the trachea:
  - soft palate is observed tightly clasped around the larynx.

Aetiology/pathophysiology

- presumed cause is a neuromuscular weakness of the geniohyoid muscle.
- not known if this is the limiting factor in a horse's athletic ability or the result of acquired disease.
- described as a complication of 'tie-forward' surgery.

Clinical presentation

- poor performance associated with a vibrant respiratory noise.

Differential diagnosis

- most other dynamic respiratory obstructions of the performance horse, especially DDSP.

Diagnosis

- dynamic endoscopy (Fig. 1.76).
- no distinctive features of the condition at rest.

Management

- epiglottic resection results in severe dysphagia.
- permanent tracheotomy can be considered to bypass the larynx.
- tie-down – suture from epiglottis to thyroid cartilage has been described but limited results are available.

Prognosis

- poor.
- some success has been reported with surgical augmentation.
- some return of function may develop with rest.

Iatrogenic ventral glottic stenosis

Definition/overview

- complication of ventriculocordectomy:
  - adhesion formation in the ventral larynx.

Aetiology/pathophysiology

- mucosa-covered, fibrous band of tissue forms, stretching across the laryngeal lumen.
- usually iatrogenic after bilateral ventriculocordectomy:
  - particularly common following laser surgery:
    - extended 'die back' following the thermal injury of laser.
    - reported after unilateral laser cordectomy.
  - following conventional surgery, usually bilateral cordectomy is the cause.

- rarely after severe external laryngeal trauma.

Clinical presentation

- usually presents as a deterioration in respiratory noise following laryngeal surgery.

Differential diagnosis

- natural progression of RLN or incorrect initial diagnosis of respiratory obstruction.

Diagnosis

- endoscopic examination is diagnostic (Fig. 1.77):

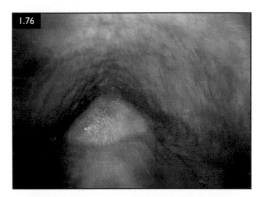

FIG. 1.76 High-speed treadmill endoscopy view of epiglottic retroflexion. The soft palate is in a normal position, implying that the epiglottis is not pivotal in preventing DDSP. (Photo courtesy Saf Barakzai)

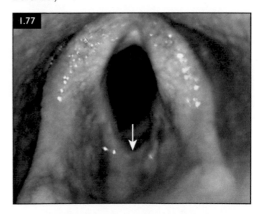

FIG. 1.77 Web larynx, or iatrogenic ventral glottic stenosis. The horse had undergone a laser Hobday under sedation, and subsequently developed an adhesion (arrow) from the right vocal cord to the previous scar.

○ fibrous adhesion joining the site of the two vocal cords is present.
○ degree of glottic stenosis is variable.

Management

- difficult condition to treat:
  ○ exacerbated by difficulty of client management with any iatrogenic condition.
  ○ most successful procedure is the creation of a mucosal flap on one side of the larynx, folded back and sutured to itself, leaving the other side to granulate.

Prognosis

- good if the second surgery is successful.
- recurrence of the cicatrix is a frequent complication.

Ventroaxial/medial luxation of the apex of the corniculate process (VALACP)

Definition/overview

- respiratory obstruction at exercise, not appreciated prior to dynamic endoscopy.
- apex of the corniculate processes appears to separate, allowing one side to luxate ventrally, giving the larynx a 'heart-shaped' appearance (Fig. 1.78).

Aetiology/pathophysiology

- association with RLN is proposed, but not proven.
- elongated transverse arytenoid ligament has been proposed as the cause.

Clinical presentation

- clinical signs are typical of respiratory obstruction at exercise.
- cannot be distinguished from the other causes by history.
- incidental finding in some cases.

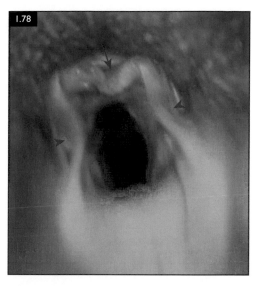

FIG. 1.78 Dynamic overground endoscopy of a racehorse showing ventroaxial luxation of the corniculate process of the arytenoid cartilage (VALACP, red arrow) combined with some axial deviation of the aryepiglottic folds (ADAF, arrowheads).

Differential diagnosis

- primary differential diagnoses are RLN and laryngeal dysplasia.

Diagnosis

- dynamic endoscopy is essential for diagnosis.
- VALACP has been identified in horses at rest after swallowing, but this is unusual.

Management

- no effective treatment has been developed.

Prognosis

- poor, and respiratory obstruction is usually persistent.
- if incidental, excellent prognosis.

TRACHEA

Tracheal trauma

Definition/overview

- lacerations of the neck occasionally involve the trachea or the oesophagus:
  - control of haemorrhage from a major vessel within the neck is the priority with such cases.
- assessment of any neurological compromise such as recurrent laryngeal function and damage to the vagosympathetic trunk is important.
- may be open or closed wounds in the trachea.

Aetiology/pathophysiology

- external trauma as the result of a kick, wire injuries, fence posts, metal objects or falls.

Clinical presentation

- accompanying wound in the neck with open lacerations to the trachea:
  - initially may be severe haemorrhage.
  - subcutaneous emphysema and/or frothing of the blood in the area if the trachea is perforated.
  - later may be pyrexia, disseminating cellulitis, increased swelling, tracheal compression, and respiratory obstruction.
- closed injuries to the trachea due to blunt trauma present with:
  - no skin wound.
  - may be rapidly developing severe subcutaneous emphysema with a leaking trachea:
    - 'parchment'-type crepitus, typical of emphysema on palpation.
  - secondary inflammatory oedema.
  - possible tracheal obstruction from external compression by swellings and/ or wall injury.

Differential diagnosis

- no specific differential diagnosis:
  - more relevant is the potential involvement of other structures:

- common carotid artery lies dorsolateral to the trachea.
- vagosympathetic trunk deep to it.
- oesophagus is usually left of, and dorsal to, the trachea.
- recurrent laryngeal nerve dorsal to the trachea, in the deep tissues of the neck.

Diagnosis

- direct examination and sterile palpation of the wound.
- endoscopic examination of the trachea (Fig. 1.79).
- radiography and ultrasonography will often reveal:
  - gas in the soft tissues of the neck.
  - possible deformity of the tracheal outline or rings (Fig. 1.80).
  - subcutaneous emphysema is common following lacerations to the chest and pectoral area and does not necessarily indicate tracheal laceration.

Management

- debride any laceration and establish ventral drainage.
- **closure of the wound is usually contraindicated and can result in severe abscessation with further compression and damage.**

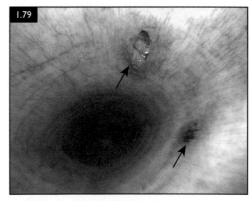

FIG. 1.79 Endoscopic view of a laceration of the dorsal trachea (arrows). The horse presented with subcutaneous emphysema, and it was postulated that blunt trauma had resulted in laceration of the dorsal trachea from crushing the trachea against the cervical vertebrae.

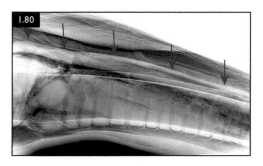

FIG. 1.80 Laterolateral radiograph of the upper neck from the same horse as Fig. 1.79. The emphysema is visually exciting, outlining the oesophagus (arrows), but does not help isolate the source of the gas.

- healing by secondary intention should be encouraged by regular careful wound management and antibiotic/anti-inflammatory medications.
- trachea usually heals well with second-intention healing.
- closed wounds:
  ○ pressure bandages.
  ○ systemic/topical anti-inflammatories.
  ○ systemic antibiotic.
  ○ severe respiratory obstruction:
    ♦ temporary tracheotomy distal to the injury may be required.
- primary surgical repair of tracheal injuries is possible in some cases.
- suction decompression of subcutaneous emphysema, using wide-bore needles, is surprisingly effective.

Prognosis

- fair.
- lacerations to trachea will heal with no long-term problems if treated appropriately and early.
- extensive subcutaneous emphysema can tract caudally into the thorax or mediastinum leading to life-threatening complications.
- tracheal lacerations can result in disturbance of the airflow and respiratory noise, due to tracheal stenosis, particularly if there is extensive damage to the tracheal rings:
  ○ airway stenosis is usually not significant.

Tracheal foreign bodies

Definition/overview

- equine trachea has an amazing ability to clear itself of debris:
  ○ foreign bodies are quite common but seldom significant.
- foreign bodies of significance are those that may get stuck in the trachea, notably twigs and thorns (rare occurrence) (Fig. 1.81).

Aetiology/pathophysiology

- most commonly inhaled but ingested material can sometimes enter the trachea.
- foreign materials with barbs or thorns tend to work their way distally and are prevented from being coughed up.
- wedged in the airway, will cause pain and a foreign body reaction:
  ○ significance of the reaction depends on the location of the fragment.
  ○ lodged in distal trachea or bronchial tree may lead to severe necrotising pneumonia.

Clinical presentation

- sudden onset of coughing with subsequently bilateral mucopurulent nasal discharge.
- possible LRT disease.
- long-term cases may have chronic coughing with malodorous breath.

Differential diagnosis

- other causes of bilateral nasal discharge and coughing should be considered.

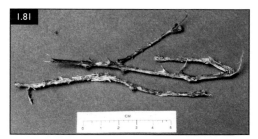

FIG. 1.81 Several twigs with thorns removed from the trachea of a horse under GA, using an endoscopic snare. (Photo courtesy Geoff Lane)

Diagnosis

- endoscopic examination is almost invariably diagnostic:
  - beyond the carina of the trachea can usually be examined by anaesthetising the carina with 20–30 ml of local anaesthetic.
  - followed by passing a long (>2 m scope) further along the bronchi, following the purulent discharge.

Management

- surgical removal is difficult, so most foreign bodies are removed by using an endoscopic technique.
- most proprietary endoscopic tools, such as biopsy forceps and instrument cages, are too flimsy for use in the horse and therefore a snare often has to be manufactured:
  - heavy duty fishing line passed via the endoscope biopsy channel.
  - snaring the foreign body can be extremely challenging:
    - may take hours with the horse under sedation.
  - beneficial to pass the endoscope via a distal tracheotomy:
    - increases the reach of the endoscope and removes the need to withdraw the object through the nostrils.
  - foreign body may break up upon removal and require additional procedures to remove the remaining fragments.
- broad-spectrum antibiotics are administered perioperatively, and other medications determined by the degree of involvement of the LRT.

Prognosis

- object located and removed completely; prognosis is excellent.
- any bronchitis or pneumonia can usually be resolved with appropriate treatment once the foreign body is removed.
- inability to retrieve the object is a frequent complication, in which case the prognosis is grave.

Tracheal collapse

Definition/overview

- uncommon condition seen in a variety of situations.
- idiopathic dorsoventral collapse, frequently intrathoracic, almost always in small ponies and donkeys, especially Shetlands and miniature ponies.
- lateral collapse (scabbard trachea) of the cervical trachea is reported in the Thoroughbred and crosses.
- typically presents with dyspnoea and stridor.
- diagnosis achieved by external tracheal palpation, endoscopy, and lateral neck and thoracic radiographs.
- both conservative and surgical treatments have been successfully used.

Aetiology/pathophysiology

- tracheal collapse can develop secondary to conditions such as:
  - external compression from enlarged lymph nodes, abscesses and tumours (mediastinal).
  - trauma to, or around, the trachea.
  - temporarily due to severe expiratory dyspnoea as a result of pulmonary disease.
  - during standing sedation if animals rest their necks on bars at the front of stocks.
- lateral tracheal flattening (scabbard trachea) in the first few tracheal rings is common in the Thoroughbred and crosses but is often incidental.
- dorsoventral tracheal collapse in ponies:
  - most common form and due to a tracheal cartilage ring deformity.
  - precise aetiology is not known:
    - some cases in young animals may be developmental.
    - cases in older animals could be degenerative in origin.
  - usually associated with flattening of the tracheal cartilage rings (reducing dorsoventral distance), with resultant stretching of the dorsal tracheal ligament.
  - other sorts of deformity may occur concurrently at different sites.

Clinical presentation

- may be asymptomatic in many small ponies and donkeys:
  - limited workload or mild changes.
- affected ponies usually present with a history of respiratory distress, including significant respiratory stertor and coughing.
- pony or horse may be normal at rest and only show clinical signs during exertion or during hot or humid weather.
- EIPH may occur in severe cases because of increased thoracic pressures.
- scabbard trachea of the Thoroughbred may often be asymptomatic but can present as poor performance with respiratory noise.

Differential diagnosis

- primary differential diagnosis for dorsoventral tracheal collapse of the pony is recurrent airway obstruction or summer pasture-associated airway obstruction.

Diagnosis

- palpation of the trachea:
  - dorsoventral deformity:
    - sharpened edge to the lateral aspects, especially in the cranial part of the neck.
    - more difficult to palpate:
      - distally where the defects are most common.
      - thick skinned, fat small ponies.
  - scabbard trachea deformity:
    - distinctive ridges on the ventral midline of the deformed trachea in the upper cervical region.
- diagnosis is usually confirmed by endoscopy (Fig. 1.82):
  - dorsoventral deformity:
    - markedly wider, flatter, and restricted trachea.
    - particularly associated with coughing or deep breathing:
      - inspiratory narrowing cervical lumen.
      - expiratory narrowing intrathoracic lumen.
    - mucosal lining may be red and inflamed.
  - scabbard deformity:
    - slight lateral flattening of the upper tracheal lumen.
    - often an adequate airway space.
- lateral radiographs of the distal cervical and thoracic trachea may be helpful:
  - must be timed to coincide with the part of the respiratory cycle for the tracheal collapse to occur.

Management

- initially conservative treatment is recommended including:
  - restricting exercise.
  - keeping the animal cool in hot weather.
  - treating concurrent respiratory tract disease.
- acute severe cases may benefit from intranasal oxygen and cooling regimes.
- systemic corticosteroids will reduce any mucosal swelling in the trachea as well as control any concurrent lung inflammation.
- medical therapy may result in only short-term improvement.
- surgery to stent the collapsing trachea has been reported but is seldom practical due to the extent of the tracheal collapse and possible intrathoracic location.
- scabbard trachea in the Thoroughbred is often incidental and usually not treated.

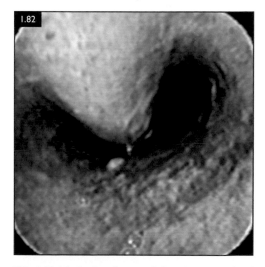

FIG. 1.82 Marked collapse of the dorsal tracheal ligament in a pony, concurrent with coughing. The pony was managed with corticosteroids and was found dead in the field a few months later.

o it can be managed by permanent tracheotomy if permitted by the relevant regulatory authorities and if the horse is destined for an athletic career.

o resection and anastomosis of the cervical trachea has been reported.

Prognosis

- guarded to poor as the dorsoventral tracheal collapse is generally a progressive condition with no reliable surgical solution.
- medical management results in short-term improvement only in some cases.
- small ponies that do very little work can cope with the problem in the short term.
- collapse secondary to other diseases may only partially or temporarily improve even if the underlying condition is resolved.
- scabbard trachea is incurable but is seldom progressive.

Tracheal stenosis

Definition/overview

- rare condition either:
  o secondary to tracheal surgery or trauma.
  o primary congenital deformity.
- occasional cases associated with external compression by mediastinal tumours or streptococcal mediastinal abscesses.

Aetiology/pathophysiology

- congenital stenotic defects are very rare.
- most common cause is tracheotomy surgery.

Clinical presentation

- mild stenosis may be asymptomatic.
- poor performance with harsh respiratory noise is the typical presentation.
- history of prior tracheotomy surgery is not always available.

Differential diagnosis

- most upper airway obstructions can be included in the differential diagnosis.

Diagnosis

- palpation and auscultation of the trachea.
- endoscopic examination is definitive (Fig. 1.83).

Management

- surgical techniques to ablate the stenotic area are available:
  o laser surgery.
  o tracheal resection and anastomosis, and external tracheal prosthesis.
  o resection of the mass is effective in the short term (Fig. 1.84):
    ♦ recurrence of the stenosis is quite common.
- second permanent tracheotomy tube, slightly further caudally in the neck, may be an alternative solution.

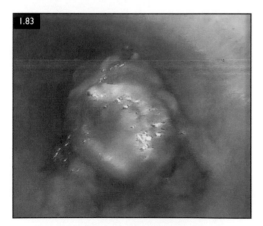

FIG. 1.83 Granulating lesion, subsequent to a previous tracheotomy incision, obstructing much of the trachea.

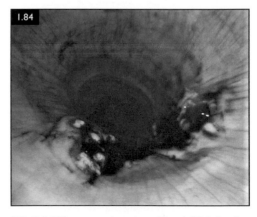

FIG. 1.84 The same horse as Fig. 1.83 following resection of the mass by a tracheotomy incision.

Prognosis

- guarded for tracheal surgery.
- good for permanent tracheotomy (complications of managing the tube).

- resolution of the stenosis without surgery is hopeless.

GUTTURAL POUCH

Guttural pouch empyema

Definition/overview

- accumulation of purulent material within the guttural pouch.
- uncommon condition but a differential diagnosis for unilateral purulent nasal discharge.
- commonly recognised site for *Streptococcus equi equi* (strangles) colonisation:
  - **any purulent material in this region should be viewed as contagious and probably strangles related, unless proven otherwise.**

Aetiology/pathophysiology

- usually, *Streptococcus* species upper airway infection, which localises in the pouch:
  - primary infection.
  - secondary to an URT viral infection or other guttural pouch disease.
- pouch appears unable to clear these organisms as effectively as elsewhere in the upper airway.
- horses can become chronic carriers or prolonged shedders of strangles:
  - infection remains subclinical.
  - or associated with frank empyema of the pouch:
    - ♦ remains as liquid pus accumulation.
    - ♦ or the pus can inspissate:
    - ♦ tends to form multiple rounded accumulations (chondroids) (Fig. 1.85).
    - ♦ streptococcal infection becomes less significant.
    - ♦ anaerobic infection may become more relevant.

Clinical presentation

- unilateral, or predominantly unilateral, purulent nasal discharge:

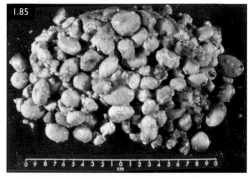

FIG. 1.85 Accumulation of chondroids removed surgically from a pony with guttural pouch empyema. Culture of the chondroids revealed no significant growth.

- chronic history for up to a year despite treatment.
- distension of the pouch is frequent:
  - swelling in the parotid region is seldom noted clinically.
  - distension into the airway, especially the nasopharynx:
    - ♦ may cause dyspnoea and an abnormal respiratory noise.

Differential diagnosis

- primary differential diagnosis is sinusitis:
  - many cases have been treated with a presumptive diagnosis of sinusitis.
- discharge from the lower airway can occasionally appear down one nostril.

Diagnosis

- endoscopy usually provides a definitive diagnosis:
  - unilateral dorsal pharyngeal swelling (nasopharynx) in some cases (Fig. 1.86).
  - purulent discharge from the guttural pouch ostia may be present (Fig. 1.87):

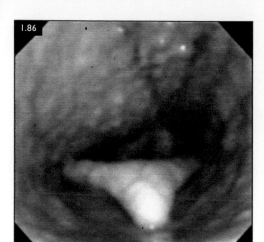

FIG. 1.86 Unilateral pharyngeal collapse associated with empyema of the right guttural pouch.

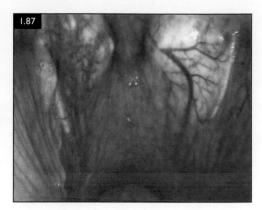

FIG. 1.87 Purulent material discharging from the right guttural pouch ostium.

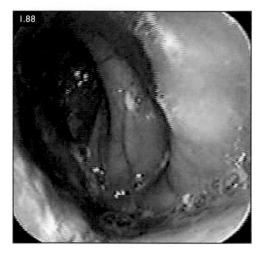

FIG. 1.88 Endoscopic view of guttural pouch empyema with liquid purulent material, showing thickening of the lining of the pouch. Culture of the fluid yielded pure *Streptococcus equi equi*.

> ♦ not diagnostic as normal for horses to aspirate some material from the nasopharynx into the openings of the guttural pouch during swallowing.
> ○ opening to pouch is in the dorsal pharynx under a cartilage flap:
> > ♦ essential endoscope is passed up the ventral nasal meatus to enter the pouch.
> ○ pouch visibility is often quite obscured by purulent material:
> > ♦ pouch lining is markedly thickened (limits identification of normal structures) (Fig. 1.88).
> ○ contralateral pouch may be normal or involved.
> • lateral radiographs of the guttural pouch are diagnostic for:
> ○ fluid or soft tissue infiltration of the pouch.
> ○ chondroids visualised occasionally but associated fluid accumulation can obscure their outline.

Management

- catheterisation of the guttural pouch and lavage is indicated:
  - care must be taken in selecting the agent to lavage the pouch.
  - irritant materials such as iodine or peroxide may cause serious neurological damage due to the cranial nerves passing through the pouch.
  - lavage with antibiotic solutions is also dangerous:
    - ♦ material lavaged from the pouch may be ingested:
      - – may result in antibiotic-induced severe diarrhoea.
      - – gel-based repositol penicillin preparations are available for instillation into the pouch as an alternative.
  - warm water is relatively non-irritant, cheap and surprisingly effective.

- systemic antibiotic treatment is recommended (based on culture and sensitivity):
  - antibiotic of choice is usually penicillin.
- following a period of lavage, further examination is indicated:
  - pouch is clear but thickened and inflamed:
    - ♦ withdraw catheter and continue systemic antibiotic treatment.
  - still purulent material in the pouch:
    - ♦ inspissation of pus and chondroid formation likely.
    - ♦ further lavage attempted.
    - ♦ antibiotic treatment altered to include anti-anaerobe therapy (metronidazole).
- chondroids can seldom be broken down by lavage:
  - removed endoscopically with a 'basket' (time consuming).
  - surgical removal often necessary.

Prognosis

- good for simple empyema:
  - most cases resolve satisfactorily with lavage.
  - how many remain chronic intermittent shedders of *Streptococcus equi equi* is not known.
- guarded following chondroid formation:
  - complete removal is difficult to achieve.
  - recurrence has been noted even when surgery was initially successful.

Guttural pouch tympany

Definition/overview

- uncommon condition of the foal.
- congenital dysfunction of the pharyngeal opening of the pouch:
  - build-up of excessive amounts of air in the guttural pouch.
- unilateral or bilateral.

Aetiology/pathophysiology

- unclear but probably a congenital defect.
- ostia are usually patent but do not function correctly:
  - act as a one-way valve leading to accumulation of air in the pouch.

Clinical presentation

- foals usually present with marked swelling of the parotid region.
- palpation reveals a tympanic swelling that is quite painless (Fig. 1.89).
- dysphagia or dyspnoea may be present if the swelling has become extreme.

Differential diagnosis

- clinical presentation is quite characteristic.
- most likely differential diagnosis is a retropharyngeal abscess:
  - palpation will reveal a firm painful mass.

Diagnosis

- radiography is the most valuable technique to confirm the diagnosis (Fig. 1.90):

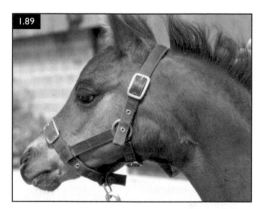

FIG. 1.89 A foal with guttural pouch tympany, showing swelling in the pharyngeal region.

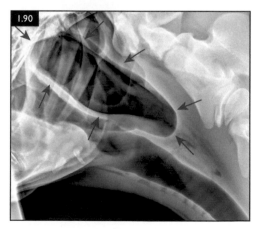

FIG. 1.90 Radiograph showing a gas-distended guttural pouch (arrows).

- lateral radiograph will reveal extreme distension of the guttural pouch.
- endoscopy will initially reveal marked dorsal pharyngeal swelling (Fig. 1.91):
  - entry into the guttural pouch causes collapse of the pouch.
  - no abnormalities of the internal structures are noted.

Management

- majority of cases managed very successfully by chronic catheterisation of the guttural pouch:
  - large-bore (28Ch) Foley catheter is placed within the affected guttural pouch(es) and left *in situ* for 2–6 weeks.
  - usually results in sufficient alteration of the ostium to prevent it forming a one-way seal in the future.
- salpingopharyngeal fistula can be created, using a transendocopic laser:
  - establish communication into the guttural pouch (Fig. 1.92).
  - simple and effective with minimal complications.
  - unilateral cases can be managed by creation of a fistula in the septum between the two pouches, but this is a more demanding procedure.

Prognosis

- excellent with almost all cases resolving with chronic catheterisation.
- recurrence is rare.

Guttural pouch mycosis

Definition/overview

- important but rare condition.
- clinical signs vary depending on the structures involved in the guttural pouch:
  - most common and important is severe epistaxis.

Aetiology/pathophysiology

- fungal infection of the guttural pouch.
- mycotic plaque forms on the pouch wall and is highly erosive.
- where the plaque occurs leads to damage to different structures (Fig. 1.93):
  - internal carotid artery is frequently involved:

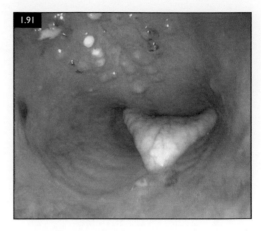

FIG. 1.91 Endoscopy of a foal with guttural pouch tympany showing marked dorsal pharyngeal swelling.

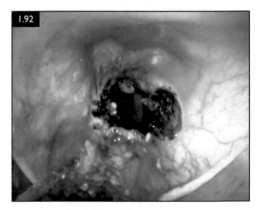

FIG. 1.92 Transendoscopic laser creation of a salpingopharyngeal fistula, from the pharyngeal recess into the guttural pouch.

- plaque forms on roof of medial compartment caudal and medial to the temporohyoid articulation (Fig. 1.94).
  - pharyngeal branch of vagus nerve and recurrent laryngeal nerve are involved in some cases.
  - less commonly the plaque is more lateral:
    - damage to branch of external carotid artery (external maxillary artery) (Fig. 1.95).

Clinical presentation

- most common presentation is severe epistaxis:

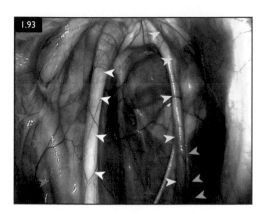

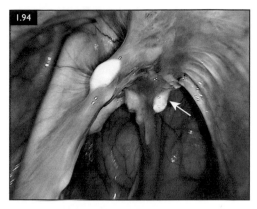

FIG. 1.93 Normal guttural pouch, showing the stylohyoid bone (white arrowheads) that divides the pouch into medial (right) and lateral compartments. The internal carotid artery (yellow arrowheads) is in the medial pouch, along with the neural fold containing the glossopharyngeal and hypoglossal nerves, and the cervical sympathetic trunk (red arrowheads). The vagus nerve branches off medially from this fold (green arrowheads). The external maxillary artery and its numerous branches are in the lateral pouch (orange arrowheads).

FIG. 1.94 Resolving guttural pouch mycosis, after 6 weeks of treatment with antifungal agents, showing the location of the plaques in the dorsal pouch over the sigmoid flexure of the internal carotid artery (arrow).

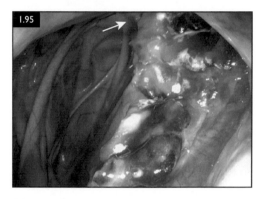

FIG. 1.95 Guttural pouch mycosis of the lateral compartment, showing the normal unaffected sigmoid flexure of the internal carotid artery (arrow), and the mycotic plaque lateral to the stylohyoid bone (obscured).

- horses are usually discovered after a haemorrhage:
  - ◆ stable heavily contaminated with blood.
- following the initial bleed, horses will usually continue to discharge dark blood from principally one nostril.
- if untreated, a second severe bleed usually occurs a few hours or days later.
- first bout of epistaxis is seldom fatal:
  - ◆ horses will often bleed three times before dying.
  - ◆ highly variable and should not be relied upon.
- next common presentation is acute-onset, often severe, pharyngeal phase dysphagia:
  - coughing when eating and discharge of food, mucus, and saliva from both nostrils.
  - discharge is often stained with dark blood.
- other cranial neuropathies can include:
  - laryngeal hemiplegia, facial paralysis and Horner syndrome:
  - right-sided RLN should always raise suspicion of guttural pouch mycosis.

- pain in the caudal head/cranial neck region can occur, leading to head carriage and position changes.

Differential diagnosis

- principal other cause of severe epistaxis is nasal trauma:
  - external – a severe blow to the head.
  - internal – trauma:
    - ◆ iatrogenic such as a stomach tube.
    - ◆ accidental (twig or fence splinter up the nasal passage).
- EIPH can be severe but has a history of strenuous exercise immediately beforehand.

- dysphagia has multiple causes:
  - pharyngeal phase dysphagia is generally neurogenic in origin.
  - various poisonings, such as lead, can cause neurogenic damage.
  - masses below the epiglottis can cause permanent DDSP and dysphagia.

Diagnosis

- endoscopy is the principal diagnostic aid:
  - **care must be exercised during examination.**
  - examination of the nasopharynx usually reveals a large blood clot distending the ostium of the pouch (Fig. 1.96):
    - ♦ blood in the pharynx from other causes often aspirate some into the ostia during swallowing.
    - ♦ small trickle of blood from the ostium is not necessarily significant.
  - decision has to be made as to whether to examine the pouch itself:
    - ♦ endoscopy may dislodge a blood clot and precipitate a fatal haemorrhage.
    - ♦ information gained by examining the pouch can be limited.
    - ♦ visibility is frequently obscured by blood.
    - ♦ principal aim of the examination is to localise the fungal plaque:
      - – dorsomedial mycosis usually internal carotid haemorrhage.
      - – lateral mycosis usually external maxillary haemorrhage.
- important to assess laryngeal motility in all patients:
  - frequently affected in horses with mycosis.
  - often results in total paralysis of the larynx (Grade IV).
  - lesser grades of hemiparesis are more likely to be idiopathic RLN.
- dysphagic patients usually exhibit permanent DDSP:
  - repeated attempts at swallowing should be observed by flushing water into the nasopharynx.
  - should result in active contraction of the pharynx and bilateral opening of the guttural pouch ostia, followed by replacement of the soft palate in a subepiglottic position.

- radiography can be used:
  - lateral radiograph of the parotid region may reveal fluid lines in the guttural pouch, or more irregular blood clots forming soft tissue densities.

Management

- medical management can be pursued in all patients.
- medical management is more appropriate in dysphagic patients and consists of:
  - topical administration of antifungal agents such as enilconazole:
    - ♦ via Foley catheter implanted in the guttural pouch under endoscopic control.
  - pouch is irrigated daily with an antifungal solution.
  - some clinicians use antifungal powders (nystatin) to insufflate into the pouch to improve contact of the medication with the fungal lesion.
- urgent surgery is recommended for all haemorrhaging patients:
  - fatal haemorrhage usually results before antifungal medication has worked.
  - several techniques are available:
    - ♦ simple ligation of the internal carotid and occipital arteries.
    - ♦ proximal and distal vascular occlusion:
      - – embolisation coils under fluoroscopic control.
      - – catheterisation of selected vessels using embolectomy or Foley catheters.

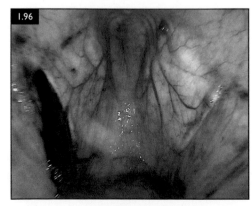

FIG. 1.96 Large blood clot from the right guttural pouch ostium, typical of haemorrhage due to guttural pouch mycosis.

Prognosis

- excellent if appropriate arterial occlusion is achieved in the absence of neurological disease.
- intraoperative complications are common and warrant a guarded prognosis initially.
- prognosis for return of neurological function is guarded:
  - many horses improve following resolution of the mycosis, but deficits can remain.
  - particular importance in performance horses that present with RLN.

Temporohyoid osteoarthropathy

Definition/overview

- rare but increasingly recognised condition.
- involves bony proliferation and pain associated with the temporohyoid articulation.
- disease is very variable in presentation.

Aetiology/pathophysiology

- precise cause is not known.
- postulated the condition is a septic arthritis of the temporohyoid joint following an extension of middle ear disease:

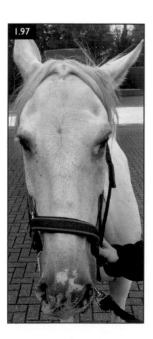

FIG. 1.97 A horse with temporohyoid osteoarthropathy, showing drooping ear, drooping eyelid and left deviation of the muzzle, typical of facial neuropathy. The horse also has a corneal ulcer.

- no evidence of middle ear infection in most cases.
- some horses do have a history of prior 'strangles' infection.
- course of the disease is unpredictable:
  - usually presented with an acute history.
  - ankylosis of the temporohyoid joint is prevented by the constant movement of the stylohyoid bone via the tongue.
  - results in continuing inflammation around the joint.
  - swelling presses on nerves adjacent to the joint, particularly the facial and vestibulocochlear.
  - movement can also result in pathological fracture of the basisphenoid bone.

Clinical presentation

- often acute despite the apparently chronic nature of the disease.
- variable clinical signs can include:
  - oral phase dysphagia.
  - head shyness.
  - non-descript pain in the parotid area.
  - difficulty in ridden exercise.
  - altered head carriage and reluctance to flex the neck.
- relatively consistent feature is quite marked pain on squeezing the mandibles together, leading to severe reaction from the horse.
- facial neuropathy is often quite marked (Fig. 1.97).
- corneal ulceration due to neurological compromise of blinking.

Diagnosis

- endoscopy of the guttural pouch is the most reliable way of establishing a diagnosis:
  - usually, swelling, and inflammation associated with the temporohyoid articulation (Fig. 1.98):
    - signs can be difficult to interpret (somewhat subjective).
    - compare with the contralateral side.
  - fracture of the stylohyoid bone can be observed as marked thickening of the bone.
  - purulent or serous discharge can be noted from the articulation (Fig. 1.99).

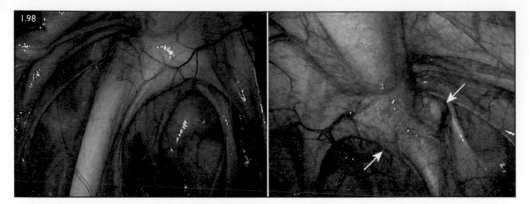

FIG. 1.98 Endoscopy of both guttural pouches, showing marked swelling of the temporohyoid articulation, associated with marked reddening and mucosal inflammation on the right (affected) side (arrows).

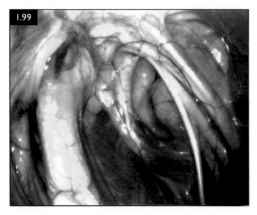

FIG. 1.99 Serous discharge from the temporohyoid joint of a horse with dysphagia. This horse responded to a prolonged course of antibiotics and anti-inflammatory agents.

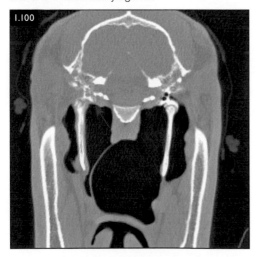

FIG. 1.100 CT scan showing thickening and destruction of the right temporohyoid articulation (arrow), compared with the normal left joint.

- other diagnostic aids often used due to the confusing nature of the clinical signs.
- diagnosis is possible using CT:
  - marked thickening around the temporohyoid joint usually observed (Fig. 1.100).
- radiography may be of benefit:
  - fractures of the stylohyoid bone.
  - dorsoventral views can reveal sclerosis of the petrous temporal bone relative to the contralateral side.
  - many cases show no radiographic abnormalities.
- scintigraphy may reveal an increased uptake of radioisotope in the region of the temporohyoid articulation on dorsal views of the head.

Management

- antibiotic treatment can be sufficient in some cases (clinical signs frequently recur).
- surgery is recommended in most cases and is designed to reduce the movement, and hence pain, emanating from the temporohyoid articulation:
  - resection of the ceratohyoid is recommended.
  - can be conducted in the standing sedated horse.

Prognosis

- following ceratohyoidectomy is good:
  - majority of horses make a rapid and full recovery.

Medical conditions of the upper respiratory tract

VIRAL DISEASES

Equine influenza (EIV)

Definition/overview

* highly contagious respiratory disease with high morbidity and low mortality.
* usually, a self-limiting URT disease but complications include:
  * secondary bacterial respiratory infections.
  * lower respiratory tract disease.
  * myocarditis.
  * post-viral fatigue syndromes.
* severe or fatal disease is very unusual except in debilitated horses or neonatal foals.
* affects naïve horses of any age:
  * typically seen in young horses when first introduced into training yards.
* large, economically devastating outbreaks can occur:
  * susceptible groups of horses.
  * when new viruses with sufficient antigenic differences from vaccine strains enter groups of vaccinated horses.
* causes pyrexia, depression, nasal discharge, and a persistent harsh, dry cough.
* horses usually recover with rest and symptomatic treatment.
* EIV is an 'Office International des Epizooties' (OIE)-listed disease:
  * vaccination against EIV is compulsory under the rules of most racing authorities and the Fédération Equestre Internationale (FEI).

Aetiology/pathophysiology

* type A orthomyxoviruses with two major surface proteins:
  * neuraminidase (N) and haemagglutinin (H).
  * equine influenza viruses possess either:
    * H7N7 (formerly known as A/ Equine 1 viruses):
      - not circulated in Europe for many years and may be extinct.

* H3N8 (formerly known as A/ Equine 2) is now predominant cause of disease:
  - American lineage evolved into three further lineages:
    ◇ Florida, Kentucky, and South American.
  - dominance of Florida lineage that evolved into two clades:
    ◇ Florida Clade 1 and 2.
    ◇ Clade 2 now dominate.
* influenza viruses undergo gradual 'antigenic drift':
  * create sufficient antigenic differences.
  * vaccine- (or disease-) induced antibodies fail to neutralise the new virus:
    * result in vaccine breakdown.
  * OIE periodically recommends which strains should be included in vaccines:
    * regular fine-tuning of vaccine strains of questionable importance.
    * effective protection by 'out-of-date strains', especially when used as whole killed virus antigen with suitable adjuvants.
* virus transmitted from infected horses by aerosol (across distances up to 50 m) or by respiratory droplets:
  * directly from horse to horse.
  * indirectly via fomites, including hands.
  * virus survival in the environment is short-lived and not important in transmission.
* virus infects respiratory epithelial cells, causing:
  * destruction of ciliated columnar cells and loss of epithelial integrity.
  * exposure of cough receptors.
  * increased mucus production and decreased mucociliary clearance.
* infection is usually restricted to the URT:
  * small minority of horses (mainly foals or immunocompromised animals):
    * clinically apparent pulmonary disease occurs.
* virus-induced impairment of mucociliary clearance can allow:

- secondary bacterial infection to develop.
- mostly resident airway microbes:
  - *Streptococcus equi* subsp. *zooepidemicus*.
  - members of the genera *Pasteurella*, *Actinobacillus*, and *Haemophilus*.
- persistent infections do not occur, and latency is not established:
  - EIV replication is restricted to respiratory epithelial cells.
  - virus does not appear capable of invasion and causing viraemia.

Clinical presentation

- incubation period of 1–3 days and duration of less than 3 weeks.
- sudden onset of acute URT infectious disease signs:
  - pyrexia (up to 41.1°C [106°F]) with depression and anorexia.
  - serous nasal discharge that becomes mucopurulent.
  - lymphadenopathy:
    - mainly submandibular and occasionally retropharyngeal lymph nodes.
  - persistent, dry, harsh, hacking cough.
- complications more likely to occur in horses that are exercised and/or kept in unhygienic stable air environments:
  - secondary bacterial LRT infections (pneumonia and pleuropneumonia).
  - vasculitis, myocarditis, and chronic post-viral fatigue syndromes.
- clinical disease in horses with incomplete immunity:
  - partially completed or lapsed vaccination programmes.
  - usually mild and difficult to differentiate clinically from other causes of infectious URT disease.
- disease generally more severe in foals, yearlings, young adult horses, and in immune naïve populations.

Differential diagnosis

- all other viral and bacterial causes of infectious URT disease, especially:
  - equine herpesviruses and equine viral arteritis (EVA) virus.
  - *S. equi* subsp. *equi*.

Diagnosis

- clinical signs are suggestive, but not diagnostic.
- leucopenia with lymphopenia and/or neutropenia and increase in serum amyloid A (SAA) are suggestive of viral disease.
- laboratory methods to confirm a diagnosis:
  - detection of **virus RNA** on nasal or nasopharyngeal swabs:
    - quantitative ('real-time') polymerase chain reaction (qPCR).
    - current diagnostic method of choice:
      - rapid results and very high sensitivity and specificity.
  - **virus isolation** is an important part of surveillance:
    - allows collection of representative strains for H antigen (HA) sequencing:
      - enables monitoring of genetic drift of HA.
      - not used for diagnosis of clinical cases:
        - ◊ slow and yields false-negative results.
  - **virus antigen detection** has been superseded by qPCR testing:
    - still offered by some laboratories.
    - patient-side ELISA tests for detection of human influenza A viruses:
      - cross-react with equine influenza A viruses.
      - used at some competitions for rapid initial diagnosis.
  - **serology** carried out using:
    - haemagglutination inhibition (HAI) test was the standard diagnostic test.
    - single radial haemolysis (SRH) is more useful for monitoring response to vaccination and in epidemiological studies:
      - SRH titres provide a measure of protective immunity:
        - ◊ horses with titres >150 mm^2 generally gives clinical and virological protection against homologous viral challenge.

◇ horses with titres >85mm^2 and <150 mm^2 give clinical protection.

Management

- usually, a self-limiting disease provided clinical cases are properly managed.
- affected horses should be rested for 3 weeks:
  - ○ if stabled, kept in a dust-free environment with good air hygiene.
- continued training and poor air hygiene:
  - ○ delay recovery.
  - ○ predispose to secondary infection.
  - ○ may cause chronic post-viral fatigue syndromes.
- **broad-spectrum antimicrobials are often administered but should be avoided unless bacterial super-infection has been diagnosed.**
- NSAIDs may be used to control pyrexia if required.
- other treatments may be employed but are usually unnecessary:
  - ○ clenbuterol to improve ciliary clearance.
  - ○ nebulised bronchodilators or mucolytics.
- strict infection control should be employed to prevent spread of infection to adjacent yards:
  - ○ suspension of movement on and off infected premises.
  - ○ within the affected yard, barrier precautions should be established to try and prevent spread:
    - ◆ virus is easily inactivated by many disinfectants, including:
      - – 1% bleach   70% ethanol iodine-based disinfectants.
      - – quaternary ammonium disinfectants.
      - – peroxygen disinfectants and phenolics.
- infected horses typically shed the virus for 6–7 days:
  - ○ maintain isolation until no more clinical signs and body temperature is normal for at least 5 days.
  - ○ qPCR testing can be used to confirm the end of virus shedding if required.

Prevention

- controlled principally by **vaccination**:
  - ○ variety of vaccines are available including:
    - ◆ inactivated (whole killed virus) and subunit canary pox recombinant vaccines:
      - – all delivered by intramuscular injection.
    - ◆ North America, an intranasal modified live virus vaccine is available.
  - ○ current OIE recommendations are that vaccines should contain:
    - ◆ strains of American Florida Clade 1 and Clade 2.
    - ◆ vaccines containing genetically 'out of date' strains can provide effective protection against currently circulating strains.
- vaccination is required by many organisations:
  - ○ mandatory in racing and equestrian sports since the 1980s.
  - ○ primary vaccination course consists of:
    - ◆ two injections 21–92 days apart.
    - ◆ third dose given 150–215 days later.
- annual boosters are given thereafter.
- horses may not race until 8 days after any vaccination.
- depending on the specific regulator, boosters may be required every 6 months.
- immunity gap may occur in young Thoroughbreds between the second and third vaccinations of the primary course:
  - ○ decrease of SRH antibody titres below those required for clinical protection.
- faced with an epizootic:
  - ○ immunity maximised by third vaccination of primary course 2–3 months after second vaccination.
  - ○ subsequent boosters at 6-monthly intervals (off-label use of vaccines).
- mares may be vaccinated 8–4 weeks before foaling:
  - ○ provides optimum levels of colostral antibody.
  - ○ foals born to vaccinated mares should not be vaccinated before 4 months of age.

Prognosis

- good for full recovery.

Equine herpesvirus infections (EHV)

Definition/overview

- viruses ubiquitous in horse populations worldwide:
  - major economic and welfare impacts on all sectors of the horse industry.
- morbidity is high but mortality is generally low:
  - may be high in some outbreaks of neurological disease.
- EHV-1 causes respiratory disease, abortion, neurological, and ocular disease.
- EHV-4 is generally (but not exclusively) associated with respiratory disease.
- EHV-2 and EHV-5 have uncertain clinical significance.
- prevalence of EHVs in Thoroughbred populations approaches 100%:
  - prevalence of EHV respiratory disease varies from 10–60%.
  - mainly associated with EHV-4.
- natural immunity is short-lived:
  - EHV-1 and EHV-4 establish lifelong latent infections.
  - reactivate periodically and spread virus to new, susceptible horses.
- control is by management precautions and vaccination.
- EHV-1 is an OIE listed disease:
  - equine herpesvirus myeloencephalopathy (EHM) is considered an emerging disease in the USA.

Aetiology/pathophysiology

- nine equine herpesviruses (EHV-1 to EHV-9):
  - EHVs 1 to 5 are associated principally with horses:
    - alpha herpesviruses, EHV-1 and EHV-4, are respiratory viruses:
      - regarded as the two most important EHVs that infect horses.
    - EHV-3 causes venereal disease (see page 42, Book 2).

- EHV-2 and EHV-5 are gamma herpesviruses:
  - high prevalence but uncertain clinical significance.
  - EHVs 6 to 8 (asinine herpesviruses 1 to 3) associated mainly with donkeys.
- source of EHV infection either through:
  - direct or indirect contact.
  - aerosolised virus in respiratory secretions from infected or reactivating horses.
  - uterine fluids from aborted mares are highly contagious.
  - EHM cases shed virus via the respiratory route and are contagious to other horses.
- EHV-1 has a tropism for epithelial, endothelial, lymphoid, and neuronal cells.
- infection of URT epithelium followed by endothelial and lymphoid cells in the lamina propria:
  - leads to a cell-associated (CD+ T lymphocyte) viraemia.
  - viraemia leads to a leucopenia, principally a lymphopenia.
  - leucocytosis, mainly a lymphocytosis, on recovery.
  - virus disseminated throughout the body:
    - uterine endothelium.
    - CNS and eye.
- infection of vascular endothelium results in thrombosis and ischaemia, causing:
  - abortion, paresis/paralysis, and chorioretinal disease.
  - virus may cross the chorioallantois to reach the fetus or:
    - placental ischaemia may lead to sudden abortion of a virus-negative fetus.
  - EHV-4 usually establishes productive infection in epithelial cells only.
  - EHV-2, 4 and 5 generally do not cause a viraemia.
- lifelong latency is established following primary infection in:
  - circulating T-lymphocytes and trigeminal ganglion neurons.
  - reservoir of virus that, through periodic reactivation from latent infected horses:
    - maintains EHV in the horse population.

♦ reactivation in response to stress (e.g. transport) or induced by high doses of corticosteroids.

♦ reactivation results in shedding of infectious virus in nasal secretions:

– usually, asymptomatic.

– occasionally, clinical disease, including abortion and/or neurological disease.

Clinical presentation

- incubation period with EHV-1 and EHV-4:
  ○ following experimental infection is short (<48 hours).
  ○ longer incubation periods of up to 10 days suspected in the field.
- severity of URT disease varies:
  ○ mild or subclinical in horses previously exposed to the virus.
  ○ more obvious in naïve horses and usually more clinically apparent with EHV-4:
    ♦ depression and biphasic pyrexia of 10 days' duration.
  ○ nasal discharge is initially serous becoming mucopurulent.
  ○ some coughing and lymphadenopathy.
  ○ ill-defined poor performance syndrome in some horses.
  ○ chronic post-viral fatigue syndrome is suspected in some recovered horses:
    ♦ poorly defined and difficult to diagnose.
  ○ EHV-1 viraemia persists for up to 20 days.
  ○ animals usually recover within 21 days of infection.
- EHV-1 or EHV-4 infected neonatal foals can show severe disease:
  ○ due to a viral pneumonitis and liver disease.
  ○ respiratory distress, jaundice, and high mortality in neonates.
- EHV-2 and EHV-5 have been detected in nasal swabs and tracheal aspirates from many clinically normal horses, especially young horses:
  ○ both linked to poor performance in some studies.
  ○ subclinical infections may predispose the horse to other infections.

○ detected in gastric mucosa and uterine flushings:
  ♦ unknown role in gastric and in uterine disease.
- EHV-2 has been linked to outbreaks of respiratory disease in young horses and also to keratoconjunctivitis.
- EHV-5 has been linked to equine multinodular pulmonary fibrosis (EMPF).

Differential diagnosis

- EHV respiratory tract disease, includes all other causes of infectious URT disease with or without abortion, especially influenza virus and EVA.

Diagnosis

- definitive diagnosis requires laboratory investigations:
  ○ serology.
  ○ virus isolation.
  ○ detection of virus antigen, or DNA.
  ○ EHV respiratory disease closely resembles other causes of infectious URT disease.
- increased SAA, leucopenia and lymphopenia followed by a leucocytosis and lymphocytosis on recovery suggestive of viral infection:
  ○ concurrent abortions or neurological disease raises the index of suspicion.
- single high (>1:80) or rising complement fixation titre (CFT) against EHV-1 or EHV-4 on paired serum samples 10–14 days apart, is diagnostic:
  ○ elevated virus neutralising antibody titres are also diagnostic.
  ○ remain elevated for months after infection:
    ♦ may not necessarily indicate recent infection.
- detection of virus DNA on nasal or nasopharyngeal swabs using qPCR:
  ○ **preferred diagnostic test because it is rapid, sensitive, and specific.**
- confirming the diagnosis in horses that do not exhibit detectable shedding of infectious virus is challenging:
  ○ seroconversion on the CFT provides good evidence of infection.
  ○ considered diagnostic even if qPCR tests are negative.
- latently infected horses and viraemic horses can be identified by:

- qPCR detection of virus DNA in leucocytes.
- estimates of virus load help to differentiate:
  - lytic (high virus load) from latent infection cycles (low virus load).
- EHV-1-associated neurological disease:
  - xanthochromia in a CSF sample is suggestive.
- infected tissues, such as placental or central nervous system tissue, can be tested by:
  - PCR, virus isolation, and histopathology.
- virus antigens can be detected in infected tissues by immunocytochemistry:
  - useful test for placental and fetal tissues to confirm EHV abortion.
- virus isolation:
  - demonstration of cytopathic effect on susceptible cell lines.
  - slow and has yielded frequent high false-negative results.

Management

- affected horses should be separated from the herd:
  - maintained in strict barrier housing conditions.
  - until 14–21 days after resolution of respiratory or neurological clinical signs.
  - strict hygiene maintained around aborted mares for 28 days because uterine fluids are highly infectious.
- confirmed to no longer be shedding virus by qPCR testing if required:
  - helps with decision making at the end of outbreaks.
- easily inactivated by many disinfectants, including:
  - 1% bleach   o 70% ethanol.
  - iodine-based disinfectants.
  - quaternary ammonium disinfectants.
  - peroxygen disinfectants and phenolics.
- uncomplicated URT disease:
  - rest and stabling in a clean, dust-free environment.
  - NSAIDs can be used to control pyrexia.
  - broad-spectrum antimicrobials are often administered:
    - **unnecessary unless bacterial super-infection has been diagnosed.**

- other respiratory medicines (e.g. mucolytics and beta-2 agonists) are not required.
- immunostimulants:
  - inactivated *Propionibacterium acnes*, mycobacterial cell wall abstracts, or interferon-alpha.
  - used by some practitioners in horses with suspected chronic post-viral disease.
  - products may not be licensed in all countries and not indicated for acute disease.
- neurological disease cases:
  - supportive care should be provided.
  - nucleoside analogue antiviral drugs can be used in these cases:
    - p/o or i/v acyclovir and p/o valacyclovir.
    - poor bioavailability in horses.
    - currently lacking convincing clinical benefits in horses.
- **Vaccination:**
  - against EHV-1 and EHV-4 assists in disease control:
    - decreases nasal virus shedding.
    - reduces spread of the virus, and frequency of abortion.
  - current vaccines are licensed for control of respiratory disease and abortion.
  - **no vaccines have marketing authorisation for control of neurological disease:**
    - all have demonstrated the ability to reduce virus replication in vaccinated horses and so may be helpful in preventing neurological disease.
  - use of vaccines to aid control of neurological disease constitutes off-label use:
    - requires informed consent from the owner or keeper in Europe.

Prognosis

- respiratory disease:
  - good.
  - some horses may develop chronic fatigue/poor performance syndromes.
- abortion:
  - mares that have aborted usually successfully breed in the next season.
- neurological disease:

- varies significantly.
- severely affected horses (recumbent) sometimes require euthanasia.
- less severely affected horses can make a full recovery.

Equine viral arteritis (EVA)

Definition/overview

- causes respiratory disease and abortion.
- shares many clinical features in common with EHV-1 infection.
- stallions become carriers:
  - shedding infectious virus in semen.
  - main reservoir of infection and transmission of virus to susceptible horses.
- disease is OIE listed and is notifiable in many countries.
- can be controlled by vaccination.

Aetiology/pathophysiology

- caused by a togavirus and has worldwide distribution.
- virus mainly transmitted directly from horse to horse by:
  - aerosolised respiratory secretions.
  - venereally from carrier stallions to mares.
- indirect transmission via fomites is possible.
- initial virus replication in the respiratory tract followed by cell-associated viraemia:
  - disseminates virus to the reproductive tract.
  - virus replicates in the walls of small arteries and veins causing a vasculitis.
  - in stallions, persistent infection of the accessory sex glands, mainly the ampulla:
    - infectious virus is shed in semen for several years.
    - semen quality and fertility are not affected.
  - mares are infected via venereal or respiratory routes at the time of covering:
    - leads to early embryonic death.
  - infection of pregnant mares at any time of gestation via the respiratory route:
    - leads to fetal death.

- serological surveys have revealed marked breed differences in the incidence of seropositive horses and carrier stallions:
  - Standardbreds have a significantly higher incidence than other breeds.
  - reflecting differences in stud management and practice.

Clinical presentation

- incubation period on average of 7 days but highly variable (up to 21 days).
- initial clinical signs of pyrexia, depression, and anorexia.
- respiratory disease may develop, but in many mares and stallions, may be mild or subclinical:
  - respiratory signs, if present, are typical of infectious URT disease and include:
    - nasal discharge, lymphadenopathy, and coughing.
- marked conjunctivitis and lacrimation may occur.
- clinical signs relating to vasculitis include:
  - conjunctival and periorbital oedema.
  - scrotal and preputial oedema.
  - oedema of the limbs in some horses.
- usually, no clinical signs relating to early embryonic death.
- abortion leads to an autolysed expelled fetus.
- carrier stallions are clinically normal and show normal libido and fertility.

Differential diagnosis

- all other causes of infectious respiratory disease and abortion, especially EHV-1 infections.

Diagnosis

- clinical features of EVA disease are not pathognomonic:
  - outbreak of respiratory disease associated with marked conjunctivitis, oedema, and infertility or abortion is highly suggestive.
- leucopenia with lymphopenia followed by leucocytosis with lymphocytosis on recovery is suggestive of a viral infection.
- confirmation of diagnosis requires:
  - demonstration of virus, virus antigens, or virus nucleic acids in nasal swab or semen samples.

- o rising virus neutralising antibody titre on paired serum samples taken 10–14 days apart is diagnostic.
- many laboratories perform an EVA PCR on nasal swabs as part of an equine URT disease PCR panel.

Management

- disease is notifiable in many countries and suspected or confirmed cases must be reported.
- clinical cases should be isolated and maintained with strict barrier conditions until no new clinical EVA cases are observed for 3–4 weeks.
- virus is easily inactivated by many disinfectants, including:
  - o 1% bleach   o 70% ethanol.
  - o iodine-based disinfectants.
  - o quaternary ammonium disinfectants.
  - o peroxygen disinfectants and phenolics.
- affected horses require little veterinary attention:
  - o clinical disease is often mild and self-limiting or subclinical.
  - o NSAIDs can be used to control pyrexia and improve welfare.
  - o antibiotics and other respiratory medicines are not indicated.
- prevention and control of EVA in many countries is based on testing and exclusion, restriction of movement of affected horses or quarantine:
  - o for example, in the UK, horses imported from a country where EVA is known or suspected to occur are:
    - ♦ isolated on arrival for 21 days.
    - ♦ blood samples taken on arrival and 14 days later are tested for antibodies.
  - o mares and stallions are tested for antibodies before breeding.
  - o disease can be controlled by vaccination but, because of the notifiable status, the vaccine can only be used under the supervision of regulatory agencies in many countries:
    - ♦ veterinary certification of vaccination is usually required.
    - ♦ distinguish vaccinated horses from infected and convalescent horses:
      - – important that the horse is confirmed seronegative before vaccination.

- – EVA-positive stallions and mares can still be used for breeding, albeit following strict rules.

Prognosis

- good for recovery from clinical disease.
- EVA causes major economic loss because of breeding failure.

Adenovirus

- infections are common, based on serology:
  - o believed to cause subclinical disease only.
- clinical disease only been seen in immunocompromised animals:
  - o specifically Arabian foals with severe combined immunodeficiency (SCID):
    - ♦ bronchopneumonia.
- clinical significance of adenovirus infections in young horses in training is uncertain:
  - o currently no data to suggest that infection impacts on training, causes poor performance, or predisposes to other, more serious, respiratory disease.

Rhinovirus

- equine rhinoviruses are divided into equine rhinitis A virus (ERAV), equine rhinitis B virus type 1 (ERBV1) and equine rhinitis B virus type 2 (ERBV2).
- globally widespread and are serologically very common in horses.
- horses typically become infected when younger, while being trained and raced.
- viruses are believed to be able to cause URT disease and fever:
  - o clinically indistinguishable from the other respiratory viruses.
  - o many cases the disease will be subclinical.
- role in the development of inflammatory airway disease is currently unknown.
- shed through nasal secretions:
  - o ERAV also sheds in faeces and urine.
  - o ERAV develops a viraemia whereas ERBV does not.
- infection confirmed with serology and PCR.

Other viral infections

African horse sickness (AHS)

- endemic in southern Africa and causes high morbidity/mortality in susceptible horses.
- notifiable disease in many countries and OIE listed.
- caused by an orbivirus related to blue-tongue virus of sheep:
  - virus requires an insect vector, *Culicoides imicola*, for transmission.
  - geographical distribution of the vector extends into Europe.
  - it is possible that climate change may eventually extend its range.
- severity of clinical signs varies considerably:
  - peracute disease is sudden death due to pulmonary oedema.
  - acute disease is death from pulmonary oedema and myocardial failure.
  - subacute disease there is myocarditis, signs of heart failure and death in around 50% of cases.
  - least severe form of the disease ('horse sickness fever'):
    - ♦ horses with some immunity to the virus.
    - ♦ resistant species (zebras and donkeys).
    - ♦ transient URT disease and low mortality.

- vaccination can be used to control the disease.

Hendra virus (formally known as equine morbillivirus)

- zoonotic henipavirus of the family Paramyxoviridae.
- Hendra virus infections in horses and humans recognised since 1994 in Australia:
  - Queensland and the north of New South Wales.
- Fruit bat reservoir and transmission requires very close contact with bat uterine secretions or body fluid exposure from infected horses.
- infections can cause fatal pneumonia and encephalitis:
  - no pathognomonic clinical signs (wide range of signs).
  - significant diagnostic challenge for attending veterinarians.
- high morbidity and mortality but not all horses die from the infection.
- fatal infections of Australian equine veterinarians have occurred.
- Hendra virus infection is a notifiable disease in Australia and is OIE listed.
- vaccination can be used to prevent the disease:
  - many equine referral hospitals in Queensland refuse to take unvaccinated horses.

BACTERIAL DISEASE

Strangles

Definition/overview

- highly contagious bacterial infection of the URT:
  - most severe form ('classical strangles') has abscessation of the lymph nodes draining the URT.
  - variety of other, potentially fatal, sequelae including disseminated abscessation and purpura haemorrhagica.
- alternative manifestation is a mild, transient URT disease without abscesses:
  - referred to as 'atypical strangles'.

- more mild 'atypical' cases than severe 'classical' cases in most outbreaks.
- strangles affects naïve horses and ponies of all ages and types:
  - younger animals kept in large open populations most likely to become affected.
- some horses develop chronic infections of the guttural pouch and become carriers:
  - reservoirs of infection, and source of contagion to other horses.
- reportable disease in the USA and many other countries.
- the Horserace Betting Levy Board in the UK has established guidelines on strangles

(http://www.hblb.org.uk and follow the links).

Aetiology/pathophysiology

- caused by Lancefield Group C *Streptococcus equi* subsp. *equi*:
  - closely related to the other common equine Group C streptococcus:
    - *Streptococcus equi* subsp. *zooepidemicus*.
    - differentiated by:
      - sugar fermentation tests, PCR, and multilocus sequence typing (MLST).
  - *S. equi* possesses a variety of virulence determinants including:
    - surface M protein (major immunogenic and antiopsonic protein).
    - antiphagocytic hyaluronic acid capsule.
    - most pathogenic isolates are capsulated and possess full-length M proteins.
- infection is acquired by:
  - direct horse-to-horse transmission of infected respiratory tract secretions.
  - indirectly via infected droplets on water troughs and buckets, feeding utensils, hands, veterinary equipment, and tack.
- aerosol transmission does not appear to be important.
- bacterial survival in the environment is short-lived:
  - <1 week if cultures are dessicated or exposed to UV light.
  - can survive for a few weeks (possibly up to 2 months) in water troughs or in droplets of water or pus on wood and tack.
- bacteria colonise:
  - nasopharynx.
  - other regions of the URT including the paranasal sinuses and guttural pouches.
  - produce typical clinical signs of URT infectious disease.
- bacteria may cross the respiratory epithelium and reach drainage lymph nodes:
  - mainly submandibular and retropharyngeal lymph nodes.

- persist, despite efficient neutrophil recruitment to the site, and cause abscesses.
  - retropharyngeal lymph node abscesses may become very large:
    - compress the airway, causing dyspnoea (hence the term 'strangles').
    - may rupture either externally or internally into the guttural pouch:
      - causing guttural pouch infection and empyema.
      - chondroids (balls of inspissated pus containing viable bacteria) may develop in chronic cases of empyema.
  - occasional parotid lymph node abscesses develop.
- persistent (months to years) guttural pouch infection may develop in a small proportion (<10%) of recovered horses:
  - carrier animals, which are often asymptomatically infected.
  - may shed bacteria intermittently in respiratory tract secretions.
- bacteria do not disseminate beyond the head in most cases:
  - disseminates widely via the blood/lymph circulations in small number of horses:
    - metastatic abscessation ('bastard strangles').
    - abdomen (abdominal viscera and peritoneum).
    - thorax (lungs, pleura, and mediastinum).
    - central nervous system and the eye.
    - skeletal and cardiac muscle, and tendon and joint sheaths.
- *S. equi* antigens in the circulation can trigger purpura hemorrhagica:
  - immune-mediated vasculitis causing:
    - petechial haemorrhages.
    - subcutaneous and visceral oedema.
    - sometimes skin sloughs of the extremities.
- atypical strangles:
  - transient URT disease with lymphadenopathy.
  - no abscessation or other complications:
  - not clear why there are two forms of the disease, but probable factors include:
    - infectious dose and frequency.

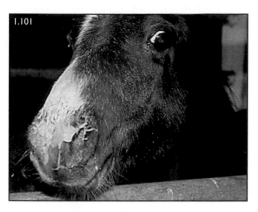

FIG. 1.101 *S. equi* infection ('strangles') causes a moderate to profuse bilateral mucopurulent nasal discharge.

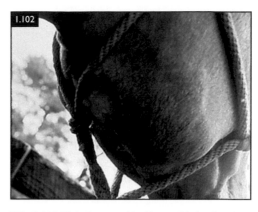

FIG. 1.102 This horse with *S. equi* infection has a draining submandibular lymph node abscess. (Photo courtesy Paul Lunn)

- bacterial strain differences.
- horse genetic differences.
- previous immune exposure of the horse.
  - bacteria isolated from atypical cases retain their virulence and can cause more severe disease in other horses.

Clinical presentation

Severe 'classical' disease

- incubation period:
  - variable (1–14 days), even following experimental challenge.
- clinical signs:
  - pyrexia (up to 42°C [107.6°F]) earliest clinical sign and persists for up to 2 weeks.
  - affected horses are depressed and anorexic for 1–2 weeks.
  - nasal discharge (Fig. 1.101) increasingly purulent and persists for 2–3 weeks.
  - lymph node enlargement is palpable from 2–3 days after infection:
    - abscesses usually develop 2–3 weeks later (Fig. 1.102).
    - large, unruptured retropharyngeal abscesses (Fig. 1.103) can cause:
      - moderate to marked airway compression.
      - ventral deviation of the trachea and occlusion of the nasopharynx.

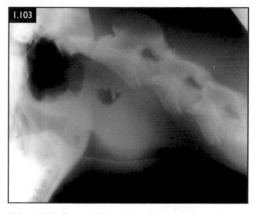

FIG. 1.103 *S. equi* infection. Non-ruptured retropharyngeal lymph nodes can be become large enough to compress the nasopharynx and trachea, causing dyspnoea. This radiograph shows ventral deviation of the trachea caused by a large non-ruptured retropharyngeal lymph node abscess. (Photo courtesy Paul Lunn)

      - difficulties with swallowing ('choke' like).
      - inspiratory dyspnoea and possibly stertorous inspiratory noise.
  - guttural pouch empyema causes intermittent, mostly unilateral purulent nasal discharge:
    - usually no guttural pouch swelling externally.

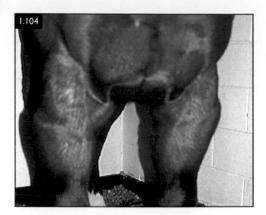

FIG. 1.104 Purpura haemorrhagica can be characterised by large plaques of proximal limb and ventral trunk oedema. (Photo courtesy Paul Lunn)

♦ pouch may be painful on percussion or palpation.
o metastatic abscessation presents with signs relating to where abscesses develop:
♦ plus, more generalised signs including weight loss, intermittent pyrexia, and anorexia.
o purpura haemorrhagica cases show:
♦ widespread subcutaneous oedema (Fig. 1.104).
♦ petechial haemorrhages.
♦ possible skin sloughs.
♦ clinical signs relating to visceral injury.

Mild 'atypical' disease

• transient and self-limiting.
• clinical signs:
o resembles URT viral infectious disease with:
♦ pyrexia, depression, lymph node enlargement, and nasal discharge.
♦ frequently only recognised as S. equi infection if samples are collected for microbiology.
o more serious sequelae associated with 'classical' disease do not develop.
o these horses are epidemiologically important in an outbreak:
♦ shed bacteria, are a source of contagion to others and may become carriers.

Carriers

• clinical signs for carriers are variable:

o guttural pouch carriage is subclinical in most cases:
♦ sometimes there is intermittent uni- or bilateral nasal discharge.
o usually some guttural pouch pathology, but often subtle:
♦ obvious empyema is less common.
♦ pouches may appear normal on endoscopy and be infected.
♦ carriers only identified by sampling and testing the pouches.
o paranasal sinuses can act as carrier sites, with/without signs of sinus disease.

Differential diagnosis

• other causes of upper respiratory infectious disease including:
o equine influenza virus.
o EHV-1 and -4.
o equine rhinovirus, and EVA virus.
• abscesses may be caused by other bacteria, particularly S. equi subsp. zooepidemicus.
• enlarged lymph nodes occur in other types of inflammatory, infectious or neoplastic processes.

Diagnosis

• classical disease:
o history and clinical findings of an outbreak of URT infectious disease with abscesses are characteristic of S. equi infections.
• milder ('atypical') disease:
o history and clinical examination findings are not diagnostic.
o resembles other types of URT infectious disease.
• confirmation of strangles by demonstrating the presence of S. equi:
o microbiological culture is no longer considered the gold standard:
♦ low recovery of S. equi and resultant high rate of false-negative results.
o superseded by qPCR:
♦ qPCR at least 3 times more sensitive than culture.
♦ sensitivities and specificities greater than 95%.
♦ no advantage in combining qPCR testing with culture.

- performed on:
  - nasal swabs:
    ◇ usually adequate in acute clinical cases.
  - nasopharyngeal swabs or lavages.
  - preferred sample for initial diagnosis of clinical cases
  ○ needle aspirates from lymph node abscesses or lymphadenopathy are useful.
  ○ samples can be negative for *S. equi* in typical cases:
    - shedding of bacteria can be intermittent resulting in single samples from infected horses yielding negative test results.
- serology using the dual antigen (SEQ2190/'Antigen A' and SeM/'Antigen C') duplex iELISA:
  ○ very sensitive and specific means of demonstrating exposure to *S. equi*.
  ○ horse must not have been vaccinated.
  ○ titres remain elevated for several months.
  ○ test very useful at the end of an outbreak to identify horses exposed to infection and which may be carriers.
  ○ used for screening horses before entry into stables to identify recent infection or carrier animals and can be used in combination with quarantine.

  ○ up to 2 weeks for seroconversion to occur:
    - horses with intermediate, or 'grey zone', titres should have a second sample collected 10–14 days later to confirm their serological status.
- Singlex ELISA serological tests measuring antibody to SeM as a single antigen:
  ○ not sufficiently reliable to be used for clinical diagnosis.
  ○ cross reactivity between M proteins from *S. equi* and *S. zooepidemicus*.
  ○ SeM antibody titres are raised in cases of:
    - purpura haemorrhagica or metastatic abscessation.
    - may identify horses at risk for purpura haemorrhagica.
- endoscopy can be used to:
  ○ confirm guttural pouch abnormalities.
  ○ identify retropharyngeal lymph node abscesses bulging under the floor of the medial compartment of the pouch.
  ○ sampling of the pouch using lavages (Fig. 1.105).
- ultrasonography can be used to investigate retropharyngeal abscesses and to perform guided aspiration and drainage (Figs. 1.106, 1.107).
- radiography is an alternative means of assessing the retropharyngeal region and the guttural pouches:

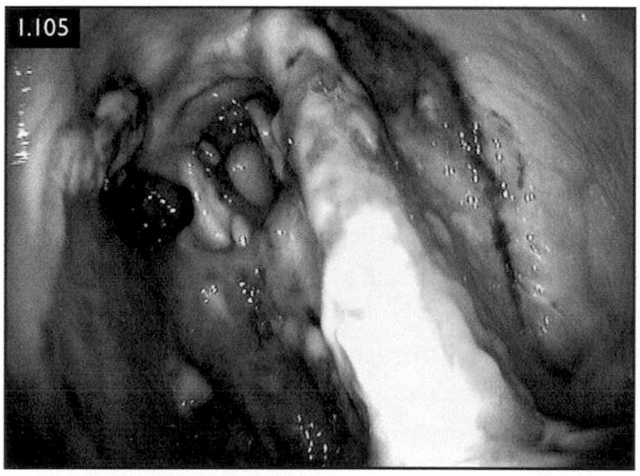

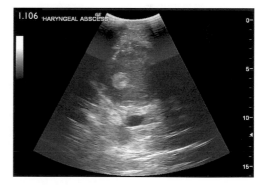

FIG. 1.105 Strangles infection in a guttural pouch showing the medial compartment on the left side of the picture and the lateral compartment on the right side. In between is the stylohyoid. The mucosal lining of the guttural pouch is thickened and inflamed. The pouch contains a small amount of mucopurulent secretions and multiple stone-shaped inspissated pus (chondroids).

FIG. 1.106 An ultrasonographic image of a retropharyngeal abscess following an infection with strangles (left is dorsal and right ventral). The abscess measures approximately 9 cm deep from the skin into the throat area. It has a heterogenous echogenicity and a capsule can be identified around it. Medially (ventral on image) you can identify a hypoechoic circular structure – the carotid artery.

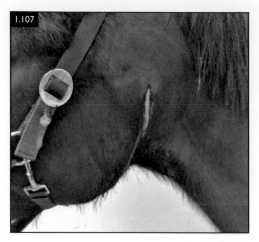

FIG. 1.107 Purulent secretion draining from the retropharyngeal abscess after a stab incision through the skin. The optimal point of incision was determined using ultrasonography.

- can be used for identifying pus or chondroids in the guttural pouches and paranasal sinuses.
- identifying carriers is not cheap or easy:
  - requires detection of bacteria in either nasopharyngeal or guttural pouch samples.
  - serology using the duplex iELISA is cost effective and highly sensitive/specific method of separating groups of horses:
    - those which have been exposed to infection:
      - need follow-up sampling to determine their carrier status.
    - those which have not and do not need follow-up sampling.
  - preferred, and most cost effective, method of identifying carriers is:
    - collection of guttural pouch lavages endoscopically from both pouches plus a nasopharyngeal swab.
    - test these by qPCR (samples combined to reduce costs).
  - if guttural pouch endoscopy is not feasible, carriers can be identified using:
    - series (at least three) of nasopharyngeal swabs or nasopharyngeal washes.
    - collected at weekly intervals and submitted for qPCR testing.
    - nasal swabs are not suitable.

Management

- three aims of managing an outbreak of strangles are:
  - prevent spread of infection to new premises.
  - limit the spread of infection within the infected premises.
  - ensure that carriers are identified and treated at the end of the outbreak.
- movement of horses on and off the infected premises should be suspended:
  - reduces the risk of infection spreading elsewhere.
- personnel should be briefed about the risk of indirect transmission and precautions taken with hand washing, clothing, footwear, and tack.
- management of clinical cases requires strict isolation and barrier nursing:
  - suspicion of *S. equi* infection:
    - premises segregated into different risk groups in separate areas, which can be in buildings or outside.
    - separation zone of at least 5 m (ideally 10 m) maintained between groups.
  - designate a red (infected) group, a yellow (in-contact) group and a green (not exposed) group:
    - colour code each area, including feed utensils, forks, brushes and barrows etc, using electrical tape.
  - in many livery/shared yards, it is not possible to safely designate a green group because of co-handling and mixing of horses.
  - rectal temperatures should be monitored, and recorded, from all horses twice daily:
    - once a diagnosis is confirmed by laboratory tests, any horses developing fever (even a single fever spike) should be considered infected.
  - horses may be moved from green to amber groups and from amber to red based on fever or other clinical signs.
  - movement of personnel **always** from green to amber to red.
  - horses must never move from red to amber or amber to green while the outbreak is in progress.

Treatment

- **antimicrobial treatment of clinical cases is controversial:**
  - some clinicians advocate never using antibiotics because they:
    - prolong the clinical disease.
    - reduce immunity.
    - increase risk of metastatic abscessation.
  - no evidence to support these concerns in the literature.
- antimicrobials and NSAIDs may be used to:
  - promote welfare in early cases with pyrexia and depression, especially foals.
  - cases with respiratory distress, metastatic abscessation, purpura haemorrhagica and guttural pouch carriers.
  - antimicrobial of choice is penicillin (22.000–44.000 IU/kg i/m q12h or i/v q6h).
  - other antimicrobials e.g. cephalosporins are effective:
    - not an appropriate choice under antimicrobial stewardship.
  - trimethoprim–sulphonamide combinations are an inappropriate choice.
  - in-contact horses can also be treated with antimicrobials provided:
    - they can be moved to a clean area and are not subsequently exposed.
    - this approach is fraught with problems and should be avoided in most outbreaks.
  - antimicrobials should not be used in horses with developing abscesses:
    - managed by hot fomentation and encouraged to burst.
    - extended courses of NSAIDs should be avoided.
    - large retropharyngeal abscesses may require drainage:
      - needle or surgical technique under ultrasound guidance (Fig. 1.107).
- nasal shedding may not begin until 1–2 days after onset of fever:
  - transmission can be limited by isolation of early cases.
  - nasal shedding persists for 2–3 weeks in most cases.
- screening for carriers should begin 4–6 weeks after the end of the outbreak.
- carriers can be successfully treated by guttural pouch lavage and antimicrobial treatment using penicillin instilled locally into the guttural pouch:
  - any chondroids that are present should be removed endoscopically.
  - liquid, or semi-liquid, pus in the affected pouch, should be lavaged daily:
    - approximately 2 litres of saline via an indwelling Foley catheter.
    - until there is no visible pus.
    - thereafter antimicrobial treatment is started.
  - benzyl penicillin is instilled into the pouch after lavage at weekly intervals until the pouch is negative on qPCR:
    - formulated as a gel with gelatin (Table 1.2).
    - or a proprietary penicillin poloxamer gel with reverse thermodynamic properties (liquid when cold and semi-solid when warm).
    - **note that some clinicians have reservations about using instilled gels.**
  - some carriers can be challenging to control the inflammation and infection in the guttural pouch.

Prevention

- relies on management measures.
- new arrivals should be kept quarantined and tested for exposure to *S. equi* using the duplex iELISA if available:

TABLE 1.2 Recipe to make 50 ml penicillin gel for guttural pouch infusion

- Add 2 g of gelatin to 40 ml sterile water
- Heat or microwave to dissolve the gelatin
- Cool gelatin to 45–50°C
- Add 10 ml sterile water to 10,000,000 IU sodium penicillin G
- Combine penicillin solution and cooled gelatin
- Dispense into syringes and leave overnight at 4°C to set

Note: The mixture must be warmed to body temperature before infusion.
Source: Verheyen K, Newton JR, Talbot NC *et al.* (2000) Elimination of guttural pouch infection and inflammation in asymptomatic carriers of *Streptococcus equi*. *Equine Vet J* 32:527–532.

- seropositive horses tested for *S. equi* carriage before admission to the stables:
  - ◆ qPCR testing of guttural pouch lavages plus nasopharyngeal swabs.
  - horses should have two serology samples performed:
    - ◆ first on entry to quarantine.
    - ◆ second 10–14 days later.
    - ◆ ensures that horses exposed just before entry to quarantine are identified.
- new cases should be isolated, investigated, and treated promptly.
- premises with endemic infection should screen all horses for carriage using the duplex iELISA test if available:
  - identify horses that have been exposed and require screening to identify carriers.
- quaternary ammonium disinfectants, 1% bleach, 70% ethanol, iodine-based disinfectants and phenolics are effective disinfectants:
  - disinfectants become easily inactivated by organic debris.

- cleaning of grossly contaminated environments or surfaces with water and detergent should precede disinfection.
- live attenuated intramucosal vaccine has been available in Europe since January 2005.
- bacterin, M protein, and live attenuated intranasal vaccines are available in the USA and Australia.

Prognosis

- variable:
  - mild disease ('atypical strangles') is good.
  - more severe disease ('classical strangles') depends on whether complications develop.
  - majority of horses recover once abscesses have resolved.
  - up to 10% of cases develop complications, which delays recovery or may be fatal.

Medical conditions of the lower respiratory tract

INFECTIOUS CONDITIONS

Rhodococcus equi pneumonia

Definition/overview

- *Rhodococcus equi* is a primary respiratory pathogen that causes:
  - suppurative bronchopneumonia and lung abscesses in foals between 1 and 6 months old (Fig. 1.108).
  - pneumonia in older foals and adults is rare.
- may also cause extrapulmonary abscesses:
  - mainly in the abdomen and in bones of affected foals.
- bacteria replicate in soil and the gastrointestinal tract of foals.
- high bacterial numbers are exhaled in the breath from infected foals.

- most foals with milder pulmonary disease recover and progress to useful athletic careers.
- prognosis for abdominal and bone abscesses is guarded.
- currently no effective *R. equi* vaccine.

Aetiology/pathophysiology

- Gram-positive pleomorphic coccobacillus:
  - may appear cytologically as a rod or coccus.
- soil-living, environmental organism:
  - replicates efficiently in hot, dry, dusty conditions.
  - prefers light or sandy soils.
- after ingestion, the organism replicates in the intestinal tract:
  - large numbers of bacteria are shed in faeces, especially in foals.

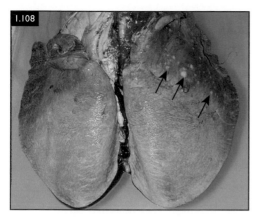

FIG. 1.108 Dorsoventral view of the lungs of a foal with *R. equi* infection as seen at necropsy. Multifocal abscesses (arrows) are visible in the lung parenchyma.

- densely stocked mare/foal paddocks can harbour large quantities of the bacteria.
- pulmonary infection occurs from inhalation of bacteria-laden dust.
- intestinal tract and abdominal infection can occur following ingestion of:
  - sufficient infectious dose from soil.
  - bacteria-laden pus secondary to pulmonary disease.
- abscesses develop at other sites by haematogenous dissemination from the lung or gut.
- abscess formation when *R. equi* establishes an intracellular infection and persists within macrophages:
  - ability to survive within macrophages conferred by a plasmid encoding a group of 'virulence-associated proteins' (Vap proteins A–G).
  - act to prevent phagosome–lysosome fusion and hence prevent respiratory-burst killing of infected cells.
  - virulent strains in foals are Vap A positive.
- causes suppurative bronchopneumonia, lung abscesses, and mediastinal and tracheobronchial lymph node abscessation:
  - lung abscesses are most commonly discrete or diffuse.

- 'miliary' abscesses can occur.
- abscesses in the gut develop mainly in:
  - wall of the jejunum, caecum, and colon.
  - mesenteric lymph nodes.
  - more rarely occur in any other abdominal viscera.
- causes osteomyelitis in long bones and vertebrae.

Clinical presentation

- occur in foals between 1 and 6 months old:
  - disease in younger and older foals, or adults, is rare.
  - exposure probably occurs within the first 2 weeks of life.
  - clinical signs appear several weeks later.
- usually insidious in onset and slowly progressive:
  - some foals present with acute-onset severe pulmonary disease.
- signs include pyrexia, depression, anorexia, coughing, and variable nasal discharge:
  - depending on extent of pulmonary disease, may be wheezing and crackling on auscultation.
  - pulmonary consolidation, if extensive, may be detectable by auscultation/percussion.
- extrapulmonary signs are present in up to two-thirds of necropsied animals:
  - abdominal abscesses cause pyrexia, depression, diarrhoea, colic, and weight loss.
  - synovitis, commonly in the tarsocrural and stifle joints:
    - ♦ marked joint effusion, with minimal lameness other than a stiff gait.
  - osteomyelitis is extremely painful and causes severe lameness:
    - ♦ affected bones may fracture.
    - ♦ vertebral abscesses may progress to cause neurological signs.

Differential diagnosis

- other causes of juvenile pneumonia should be considered including:
  - acute interstitial pneumonia
  - bacterial bronchopneumonia:

- ♦ *Streptococcus zooepidemicus*, *S. pneumoniae*, *Actinobacillus* spp., *Pasteurella* spp., *Klebsiella* spp., and *Bordetella bronchiseptica*.
- ○ parasitic bronchopneumonia.
- ○ *Pneumocystis jiroveci* infection in immunosuppressed individuals.

Diagnosis

- foals develop leucocytosis with neutrophilia and an increase in plasma fibrinogen.
- increased SAA levels are not a reliable finding.
- ultrasonography and radiography for detection of pulmonary abscesses (Fig. 1.109):
  - ○ diagnosis cannot be made based on imaging alone:
    - ♦ *Streptococcus zooepidemicus* can cause similar clinical signs/lung abscesses.
- definitive diagnosis by tracheal aspirate samples:
  - ○ demonstration of septic airway inflammation on cytology (Fig. 1.110).
  - ○ *R. equi* on bacterial culture.
- PCR assays for detecting the *VapA* gene provide increased sensitivity over culture:
  - ○ interpreted along with clinical signs and imaging.
  - ○ may yield positive results in foals without clinical disease.
- serology and faecal culture are unreliable:

- ○ seroconversion and GI tract colonisation in the absence of disease are common.

Management

- intracellular persistence of *R. equi* makes antimicrobial treatment difficult.
- **macrolide antimicrobials combined with rifampin are recommended:**
  - ○ concentrated in macrophages and target site of bacterial persistence.
  - ○ combination therapy is recommended to reduce development of resistance.
  - ○ long-term (1–2 months) oral combination therapy with:
    - ♦ erythromycin (estolate 25 mg/kg p/o q6h, phosphate 37.5 mg/kg p/o q12h):
      - – plus rifampin (5–10 mg/kg p/o q12–24h).
    - ♦ newer alternative to erythromycin is azithromycin:
      - – allows reduced-frequency dosing.
      - – 10 mg/kg p/o q24h for 5 days, then q48h.
      - – possibly reduced side effects.
    - ♦ clarithromycin (7.5 mg/kg p/o q12h), in combination with rifampin:
      - – widely used with superior clinical efficacy compared to erythromycin.
  - ○ treatment can be expensive and adverse reactions may occur:

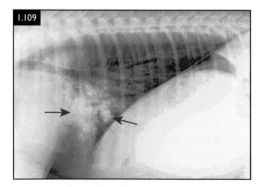

FIG. 1.109 Thoracic radiograph of a foal with *R. equi* infection. Multifocal abscesses (arrows) are visible as opacities within the lung field. (Photo courtesy John Prescott)

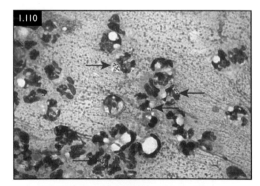

FIG. 1.110 Cytology of tracheal aspirate fluid from a foal with *R. equi* infection. Variably preserved neutrophils are the predominant cell type. Intracellular rod-shaped bacteria are visible (arrows). (Photo courtesy Dorothee Bienzle)

- fatal clostridial diarrhoea or hyperthermia:
  - hyperthermia most common with erythromycin.
- foals lose the ability to sweat properly.
- provide adequate shade, fans, etc. during periods of increased environmental temperature and humidity.
- foals with severe pulmonary signs may require:
  - hospitalisation.
  - oxygen therapy.
  - inhalation and systemic therapy with bronchodilators.
  - fluid therapy.

Monitoring and prevention

- close surveillance of foals for signs of respiratory disease, including:
  - regular haematology screens to identify foals with:
    - raised total WBCs, neutrophilia, and raised fibrinogen.
  - allows early identification of affected foals.
- enzootically infected farms:
  - serial monitoring of thoracic ultrasonograms:
    - help to detect foals in the early stages of the disease.
    - many foals with ultrasonographic changes will clear the infection without developing clinical signs of disease.
    - recommended that foals with minor changes be monitored more frequently:
      - only treated if disease becomes clinical.
    - **not all foals require treatment.**
    - increasing numbers of resistant isolates have been identified with increased antimicrobial use.
- measures to reduce exposure to *R. equi* include:
  - maintaining young foals (<4 weeks old) on clean grass paddocks.
  - avoid dusty, overcrowded dirt paddocks with little grass:
    - reduces environmental burden and risk of infection in the first weeks of life.

- affected foals should be removed from pasture (high numbers of bacteria in faeces).
- high-risk facilities:
  - hyperimmune equine plasma can be administered to newborn foals at birth and again at 3–4 weeks of age to reduce the risk of respiratory infection early in life.

Prognosis

- poor for foals with severe pulmonary disease or resistant isolates, even if treated aggressively.
- foals with less severe disease, the prognosis is moderate to good.
- foals that recover do progress into training and have an effective athletic life:
  - racing performance in Thoroughbreds does not seem to be affected.
- generally poor for foals with extrapulmonary abscesses.

Bacterial pneumonia

Definition/overview

- inflammation of the lungs due to bacterial colonisation of the pulmonary parenchyma.
- most cases are secondary to viral respiratory infection, although primary bacterial infections can occur.

Aetiology

- common pathogens isolated from bacterial pneumonia in adult horses include:
  - *Streptococcus zooepidemicus.*
  - beta-haemolytic *Streptococcus* spp.:
    - *Streptococcus equi* and *Streptococcus pneumoniae* are less common causes.
  - Gram-negative organisms such as *Pasteurella* spp., *Escherichia coli*, *Klebsiella* spp., *Enterobacter* spp., and *Pseudomonas* spp:
    - sole cause of pneumonia.
    - more commonly isolated in combination with streptococcal pneumonias.
  - anaerobic bacteria such as *Bacteroides* spp. and *Clostridium* spp. Mainly

found in complicated cases with pleuropneumonia.
- bacterial pneumonia of neonatal foals with bacterial sepsis is usually caused by:
  - *Streptococcus* spp., *E. coli*, or *Actinobacillus* spp.
  - aspiration of milk is a common cause of pneumonia for young foals that are weak or have congenital abnormalities:
    - bacterial populations are mixed in these cases.
- *Rhodococcus equi* is more common, in older foals, especially from endemic farms or areas.

Pathophysiology

- immune defence mechanisms of the upper airways prevent most bacteria from reaching the lungs under normal conditions.
- any bacteria penetrating the respiratory system to the level of the lungs are rapidly destroyed and removed by cellular and humoral defences of the LRT.
- commensal bacteria of the URT may invade the lungs if:
  - respiratory immune defences are damaged or otherwise impaired:
    - viral respiratory infection.
    - stressors such as prolonged transport of an animal.
- aspiration pneumonia is a relatively common sequela to episodes of choke (oesophageal obstruction) in adult horses.
- response to infection of the lungs causes:
  - inflammatory cells, especially neutrophils, to be recruited to combat infection:
    - may contribute to tissue destruction and loss of organ function.
  - accumulation of cellular debris, serum exudate, and fibrin within the airways, further impairs gas exchange.

Clinical presentation

- common clinical signs include:
  - fever (sometimes intermittent).
  - depression.
  - nasal discharge   o coughing.
  - tachypnoea   o exercise intolerance.

Differential diagnosis

- viral, fungal, and parasitic pneumonias should be considered.
- equine asthma (e.g. inflammatory airway disease [IAD], heaves).
- primary or secondary pulmonary neoplasia, such as lymphosarcoma.

Diagnosis

- based on history, physical examination, and laboratory and radiographic findings.
- auscultation:
  - lung sounds may include:
    - increased bronchovesicular sounds, crackles and/or wheezes.
  - friction rubs in complicated cases involving the pleura.
- thoracic percussion may reveal:
  - areas of lung consolidation or abscessation.
  - fluid accumulation within the pleural cavity (pleuropneumonia).
- haematology:
  - WBC count is usually elevated (mature neutrophilia with/without band cells).
  - hyperfibrinogenaemia is common.
  - increased total plasma proteins in chronic cases (hyperglobulinaemia).
- thoracic radiographs (Fig. 1.111) are usually confirmatory:
  - helpful for assessing treatment response.
  - prognostic indicator.

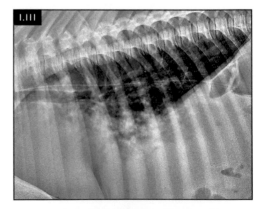

FIG. 1.111 Aspiration pneumonia in a foal. The ventral (dependent) accessory and middle lung lobes are consolidated. An alveolar pattern obscures the caudal vena cava, heart and diaphragm. Note the presence of a radiopaque feeding tube in the oesophagus.

- thoracic ultrasonography (Fig. 1.112) may show:
  - areas of consolidated or atelectatic lung.
  - and/or parenchymal abscess(es):
    - depends on their location in the affected lung.
- tracheobronchial aspirates should be obtained:
  - collected using a bronchoscope and a protected aspiration catheter:
    - **only with no signs of respiratory distress.**
  - or via transtracheal aspiration.
  - samples submitted for bacterial culture, Gram-staining, and cytology.

Management

- therapy based on culture/sensitivity results of samples collected from the lower airways:
  - streptococcal pneumonias respond well to therapy with penicillin.
  - mixed bacterial infections are common:
    - broad-spectrum antimicrobials are more desirable.
    - penicillin/aminoglycoside combinations often used before culture results.
  - azotaemia or severe dehydration is present:

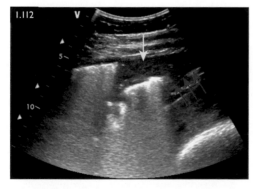

FIG. 1.112 Thoracic ultrasonography reveals loss of normal pleural surface in the caudoventral lung field. The uniformly hypoechoic lung at the tip of the yellow arrow is suggestive of consolidated lung parenchyma. Hyperechoic 'B-line' comet tails are present at the border of aerated and non-aerated lung. Red arrows indicate the border of the diaphragm.

- fluoroquinolone can be considered.
  - provides Gram-negative coverage while avoiding nephrotoxic side effects.
  - enrofloxacin should be restricted to adults because of known musculoskeletal side effects in foals.
  - other antibiotics that offer a moderately broad spectrum of activity against Gram-negative and Gram-positive organisms include:
    - second- and third-generation cephalosporins.
    - ampicillin, and/or trimethoprim–sulphonamide.
    - metronidazole is additionally used if anaerobic infection is suspected.
- NSAIDs are indicated to control inflammation and pain if kidney function is normal.
- other treatments may include:
  - moderate intravenous fluid administration to hydrate respiratory secretions to facilitate clearance from the respiratory tract.
  - prolonged rest from strenuous exercise is critical.
  - treatment failure or relapse may occur if the duration of medical treatment and adequate rest are not enforced.

Prognosis

- good if uncomplicated cases are managed promptly with adequate antimicrobial therapy and rest.
- may dramatically change with complications such as:
  - pulmonary abscessation and/or extension of the infection into the pleural space.

Bacterial pleuritis/ pleuropneumonia

Definition/overview

- bacterial colonisation of the pulmonary parenchyma can result in pneumonia and/or pulmonary abscess formation.
- extension of the infection and inflammatory process to the pleural space results in pleuritis or pleuropneumonia.

Aetiology/pathophysiology

- most common organisms associated with pneumonia include:
  - *Streptococcus zooepidemicus* or other beta-haemolytic *Streptococcus* spp.
  - can be complicated with infection by Gram-negative bacteria such as:
    - *Pasteurella* spp., *Escherichia coli*, *Enterobacter* spp., *Klebsiella* spp., and *Pseudomonas* spp.
    - anaerobes such as *Bacteroides* spp. and *Clostridium* spp. may be involved but are less common.
    - *Mycoplasma felis* has been identified as a cause of pleuritis in horses.
- pleuropneumonia may occur spontaneously, but common risk factors include:
  - recent transportation.
  - viral infection.
  - oesophageal obstruction (choke).
  - GA.
- inflammation and infection in bacterial pleuropneumonia leads to:
  - large amounts of fluid containing bacteria, neutrophils, fibrin, and cellular debris accumulating in the pleural cavity.
  - layers of fibrin develop over the visceral and parietal pleura:
    - adherence of pleura by fibrin.
    - loculation of fluid.
    - inelastic fibrin membrane over the pleural surfaces:
      - may limit lung expansion within the thoracic cavity during respiration.

Clinical presentation

- acute stage of disease may include:
  - fever, depression, and increased respiratory rate (shallow pattern).
  - exercise intolerance, nasal discharge, and intermittent coughing.
  - other signs:
    - rapid weight loss, sternal and/or limb oedema, and gait stiffness.
    - horses may stand with abducted elbows due to pleural pain:
      - elicited by palpation of the thoracic wall.
      - signs may be mistaken for colic or laminitis.

- chronic pleuropneumonia:
  - signs may be limited to intermittent fever, weight loss, and exercise intolerance.

Differential diagnoses

- other infectious pneumonias, including viral, fungal, and parasitic.
- heaves.
- primary lung neoplasia is uncommon:
  - thoracic lymphoma or metastatic tumours as differential for pleural fluid.

Diagnosis

- history, clinical signs, and physical examination usually suggestive:
  - careful auscultation of the thorax may detect abnormalities even in early disease:
    - crackles or wheezes.
    - decreased lung sounds in the ventral lung field.
    - mucus movement within the trachea.
    - pleural friction rubs.
  - bilateral chest percussion is essential and helps determine the presence and amount of pleural fluid within each hemithorax:
    - pain response may be elicited during percussion in acute cases.
- inflammatory leucogram (neutrophilia +/– band neutrophils) and hyperfibrinogenaemia are common.
- thoracic ultrasonography is the preferred diagnostic tool for characterisation of pleural fluid (Fig. 1.113):
  - consolidated or atelectatic lung may also be visible depending on its location.
  - assess the entire field of both lungs to detect:
    - abscesses, loculation of fibrinous fluid, or adhesions.
  - provides information regarding prognosis and response to treatment.
- thoracocentesis indicated:
  - characterise the pleuropneumonia.
  - isolate organism(s) involved.
  - therapeutic measure.
  - pleural fluid:

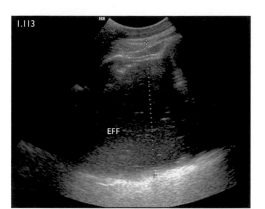

FIG. 1.113 Transthoracic ultrasonography of a horse with pleuropneumonia reveals the presence of pleural effusion (labelled EFF) between the parietal and visceral pleura in the left hemithorax. A similar effusion was detected in the right hemithorax.

♦ cytology with Gram staining for bacterial organisms:
– extra- and intracellular bacteria may be visible.
♦ increased cellularity (>10–20 × 10^9 cells/l):
– mainly of neutrophils is consistent with pleuropneumonia.
♦ fluids cultured both aerobically/ anaerobically for identification/ sensitivity:
– *Mycoplasma* culture may be useful.
• thoracic radiography (Fig. 1.114) may be used to:
○ roughly estimate extent of pulmonary involvement with pleuropneumonia.

○ optimise lung parenchyma visualisation when performed after thoracic drainage.
• tracheobronchial aspirate should be performed as described for bacterial pneumonia.
• alternatively, bronchoscopy may be performed in horses that are not showing signs of significant respiratory distress:
○ obtain samples of airway exudates from the distal trachea and mainstem bronchi for cytology and culture (Fig. 1.115).
○ specialised protected aspiration catheters are required to obtain sterile samples.

Management

• broad-spectrum antimicrobial therapy is required.
• antimicrobials commonly used initially are:
○ penicillin combined with an aminoglycoside, ceftiofur or trimethoprim-sulfamethoxazole.
○ metronidazole is commonly used to provide added efficacy against anaerobes.
○ culture and sensitivity testing should be carried out to verify drug selection.
○ prolonged antimicrobial treatment is required in most cases:
♦ transition to an oral antimicrobial after the initial period of treatment.
• pleural drainage is indicated if pleural fluid is present:

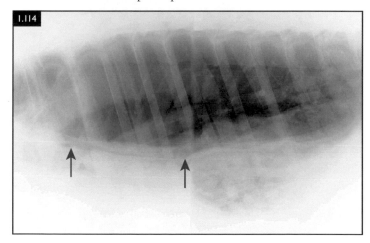

FIG. 1.114 Lateral chest radiograph of a horse prior to thoracic drainage. A fluid line is visible (arrows) and structures in the ventral region of the thorax are obscured due to the presence of the pleural effusion.

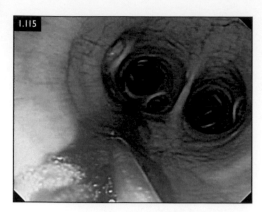

FIG. 1.115 Bronchoscopic view of the carina in a horse with pleuropneumonia secondary to rupture of a pulmonary abscess. It was possible to localise the abscess to the right lung by viewing serosanguineous discharge coming from the right mainstem bronchus. Aspiration of this discharge was performed using a catheter passed through the biopsy channel of the bronchoscope, allowing for culture and antimicrobial susceptibility testing.

- o facilitate optimal response to systemic antimicrobial therapy.
- o alleviate clinical signs associated with fluid accumulation.
- o drainage can be performed using:
  - ◆ cannula, large-bore intravenous catheter, or indwelling chest tube.
  - ◆ depends on the character and volume of the pleural fluid.
  - ◆ single event thoracocentesis.
  - ◆ indwelling chest tubes with a one-way valve to permit ongoing drainage.
- o intravenous fluid therapy is indicated if large volumes of pleural fluid are to be removed or if signs of endotoxaemia or dehydration are evident.
- o very cellular or flocculant pleural fluid:
  - ◆ pleural lavage by infusing a sterile physiological fluid solution through the chest tube.
  - ◆ then free-flow drainage by gravity.
  - ◆ alternatively, fluids can be infused through a separate tube placed dorsally in the thorax and allowed to drain through a ventral chest drain.
- • NSAIDs (following restoration of hydration) to control pain and inflammation.

- • more severe pain may be managed by butorphanol, morphine, or fentanyl.
- • common complications:
  - o laminitis.
  - o thrombophlebitis for horses with indwelling intravenous catheters.
- • chronic cases, thoracostomy with or without rib resection, may be performed:
  - o facilitates large-volume lavage and increased drainage of purulent material.
  - o **care must be taken to ensure that:**
    - ◆ lung has adhered to the body wall.
    - ◆ or that the normal fenestrations of the mediastinum are closed.
    - ◆ otherwise, bilateral pneumothorax will occur during the procedure.
- • prolonged rest and good nutritional support are essential to a satisfactory recovery.

Prognosis

- • survival and return to previous athletic function are largely dictated by the severity and duration of the disease.
- • survival is usually good if early diagnosis and aggressive treatment are provided.
- • typically, poorer prognosis for long-term survival in horses with:
  - o fibrinous loculation and abscess formation (Fig. 1.116).
  - o extensive pulmonary necrosis evident on ultrasonography.

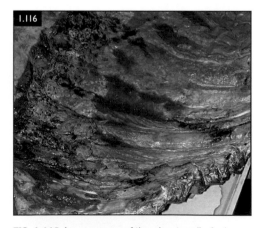

FIG. 1.116 Appearance of the chest wall of a horse with pleuropneumonia as seen at necropsy. A thick layer of fibrin ('fibrin peel') is present covering the parietal pleura.

Pneuntocystis jiroveci (formerly *P. carinii*)

Definition/overview

- unicellular eukaryote (classified as a fungus) which is a respiratory tract commensal.
- causes interstitial pneumonia in foals between 6 and 12 weeks of age:
  - immunocompromised foals (foals with SCID).
  - foals with other causes of pneumonia, especially *R. equi*.
  - rarely causes pneumonia in older foals or adult horses, where affected individuals are immunocompromised.
- difficult to diagnose because the organism cannot be cultured.
- *P. jiroveci* cysts can be identified within macrophages from BAL samples:
  - special stains such as Calcofluor white stain and Grocott–Gomori methenamine silver stain can be helpful in achieving a diagnosis.
- prognosis for affected foals is poor, but treatment with trimethoprim–sulphonamide combinations may be effective.

Mediastinal abscessation

Definition/overview

- uncommon.
- may develop from:
  - translocation of bacteria via the bloodstream into mediastinal lymph nodes during pleuropneumonia.
  - extension of infection from a neck or chest wound, or rupture of oesophagus.
- metastatic *Streptococcus equi* and *Rbodococcus equi* infection (bastard strangles).
- clinical signs vary with the inciting cause:
  - concurrent pleuropneumonia/severe wounds may obscure signs of the abscess.
  - abscessation as the primary problem:
    - weight loss, inappetence, and intermittent fever are common.
    - tracheal compression may result in progressive inspiratory impairment.
    - laryngeal dysfunction may occur from damage to the recurrent laryngeal nerve.
    - advanced cranial mediastinal masses may have jugular distension.
- diagnosis:
  - chronic inflammatory haematological changes.
  - deviation of the trachea or mainstem bronchi observed endoscopically.
  - transthoracic ultrasonography may reveal pleural effusion (frequently present):
    - thoracic inlet ultrasonography may detect a mediastinal mass (Fig. 1.117).
    - ultrasound-guided thoracocentesis samples.
  - thoracic radiography is useful in identifying a mediastinal mass:
    - thoracocentesis prior to radiography optimises detection of thoracic masses.
  - CT useful to confirm location and associated structures of abscesses in foals.
- sporadic reports of successful resolution when treated by long-term antimicrobial administration:
  - surgical drainage of the abscess improves the response to antibiotic therapy.
  - difficult and generally limited to those at the thoracic inlet.

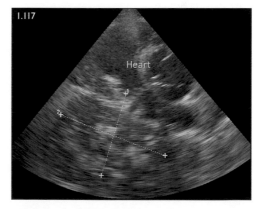

FIG. 1.117 Cranial mediastinal mass in an adult horse. Thoracic ultrasonography revealed the presence of a circular mixed echogenicity 12 × 16 cm thoracic mass cranial to the heart.

- variable prognosis depending on the location of the abscess within the mediastinum, but overall prognosis is guarded.

Glanders and melioidosis

Definition/overview

- glanders (farcy) is one of the most serious contagious diseases of Equidae.
- infection with *Burkbolderia mallei*.
- eradicated from many parts of the world, but it is endemic in:
  - Middle East, Africa, India, SE Asia, China, and Mongolia.
  - absent in the USA and the UK, where it is a notifiable disease.
  - most countries have strict import regulations (testing and/or quarantine).
- glanders is a significant zoonosis in endemically infected countries.
- melioidosis is a similar disease caused by the related bacterium *B. pseudomallei* and occurs in the Far East and northern Australia.

Clinical presentation

- glanders and melioidosis are generally chronic diseases:
  - insidious onset and slowly progressive respiratory disease:
    - ◆ typical URT infection clinical signs – nasal discharge and lymphadenopathy.
    - ◆ often with nasal mucosal ulceration.
  - mild, chronic and debilitating disease may continue for several months.
  - more acute disease then develops:
    - ◆ due to abscessation and ulceration along the URT and in the lungs.
    - ◆ possibly triggered by stress or intercurrent illness.
    - ◆ pyrexia, depression, coughing, and weight loss.
  - ◆ clinical signs of pneumonia (tachypnoea and dyspnoea).
  - ◆ death.
- disease in donkeys and mules is usually acute, with rapid death from pneumonia.
- cutaneous ulcerative lesions ('farcy') also develop along the limbs:
  - especially the medial thigh and hock.
  - discharge a yellow-brown pus containing granules.
  - often marked lymphatic cording.

Differential diagnosis

- other causes of URT and LRT infectious disease should be considered.

Diagnosis

- initial clinical signs are non-specific:
  - horses may appear relatively healthy during the chronic form of the disease.
- acute forms, with LRT signs, nasal ulceration, and skin ulceration over the medial hindlimbs, are more characteristic.
- post-mortem examination reveals variable sized abscesses:
  - containing brown/yellow granular pus.
  - throughout the respiratory tract
  - other organs, including the liver and spleen.
  - isolation of the organism confirms the diagnosis.

Management

- glanders and melioidosis respond poorly to treatment and the prognosis is poor.
- intradermal skin test using bacterial antigen (Mallein test) is used to identify carriers or horses that have been exposed to the organism and have antibody.
- disease is a zoonosis and infection control precautions must be followed when handling tissues that might be infected.
- further information is available from various governmental sources.

OBSTRUCTIVE CONDITIONS

- equine asthma syndrome has been used to incorporate two inflammatory conditions of the airways of adult horses, with distinct phenotypes:
  - IAD:
  - ◆ milder form that occurs in younger horses.
  - heaves, or recurrent airway obstruction (RAO), is the more severe form.

Inflammatory airway disease (IAD)

Definition/overview

- IAD, or non-septic IAD, is an inflammatory process of the lower airways that causes pulmonary dysfunction and reduced exercise tolerance in affected horses.

Aetiology/pathophysiology

- multiple inciting agents have been proposed as causes for the small-airway inflammation in young horses with IAD, including:
  - recent viral or bacterial infection.
  - exposure to environmental irritants (e.g. dusts, noxious gases) or sources of endotoxin.
  - pulmonary haemorrhage.
- exact pathophysiology of this condition remains unknown:
  - most likely multifactorial in nature.

Clinical presentation

- reduced athletic performance and/ or prolonged time for recovery from exercise are frequently the only presenting signs.
- nasal discharge may be present, ranging from serous to mucopurulent.
- coughing may be observed during exercise or at the time of feeding.
- clinical signs of respiratory difficulty are absent at rest.

Differential diagnoses

- other common causes of reduced performance, particularly:
  - musculoskeletal abnormalities.
  - cardiac dysfunction.
  - neurological disorders.
  - other respiratory diseases:
    - upper airway obstruction viral infection.
    - bronchopneumonia.
    - EIPH   ◆ lungworm.
    - neoplasia.

Diagnosis

- auscultation of the thorax during use of a rebreathing bag may reveal:
  - presence of increased bronchial tones, wheezes, and/or crackles.
  - movement of secretions during tracheal auscultation.
  - absence of these signs does not preclude a diagnosis of IAD.
- no abnormalities may be detected with a thorough physical examination.
- radiography no diagnostic use to confirm IAD:
  - may help to exclude diagnoses of bronchopneumonia or pulmonary abscessation.
- bronchoscopy is useful to assess:
  - airway hyperreactivity, hyperaemia, oedema, and bronchoconstriction.
  - evaluate the presence and nature of any airway secretions (Fig. 1.118).
- BAL is the test of choice to diagnose IAD:
  - cytology required to determine the type(s) of leucocyte contributing to airway inflammation.
  - IAD characterised by elevations in the percentage of eosinophils, mast cells, and/or neutrophils in the differential cell count (Figs. 1.119–1.121).
  - cytological assessment of fluid obtained by tracheal aspiration is not an adequate substitution for BAL.
- Pulmonary function testing can confirm IAD where BAL results are equivocal:
  - open plethysmography with histamine bronchoprovocation.

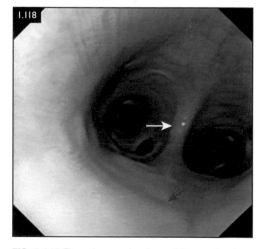

FIG. 1.118 Bronchoscopic view of the carina in a horse with IAD. Mucus is visible at the tracheal puddle (red arrow), and the carina is blunted due to oedema (white arrow).

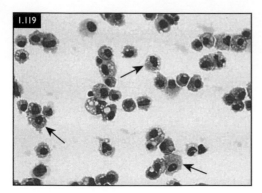

FIG. 1.119 Cytology of BAL fluid from a normal horse. Pulmonary alveolar macrophages are the predominant cell type (arrows).

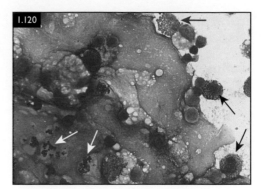

FIG. 1.120 Cytology of BAL fluid from a horse with IAD. Leucocytes are seen trapped in mucus. Mast cells (black arrows), an eosinophil (red arrow), and granules from globular leucocytes (white arrows) are present.

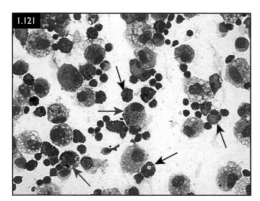

FIG. 1.121 Cytology of BAL fluid from a horse with IAD. Multiple eosinophils are present (black arrows). Pulmonary alveolar macrophages containing eosinophilic granules in phagosomes are also visible (red arrows).

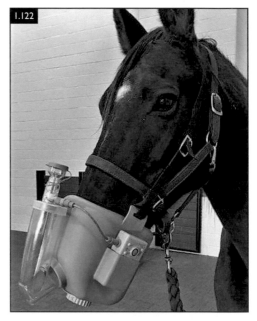

FIG. 1.122 The Flexineb® portable equine nebuliser system for the delivery of inhaled medications.

Management

- adequate rest of affected horses and environmental modification to significantly reduce exposure to respirable particles are key to recovery from IAD (Table 1.3).
- medical therapy:
  - inhalation therapy with mast cell stabilisers (Fig. 1.122) and/or corticosteroids depending on the type(s) of cell identified on the BAL differential count.
  - oral and parenteral corticosteroids may be used instead to reduce cost:
    - require a higher overall dose to be administered to the animal.
    - present the possibility of side effects.
  - bronchodilators may be useful prior to light exercise (Table 1.4):
    - should be avoided when the animal is housed indoors.
  - low-dose interferon-alpha has improved the outcome in recent studies.

1

> **TABLE 1.3** Environmental modification options for management of inflammatory airway disease and heaves
>
> - Feed only good-quality hay using bales that are visibly free from any dusts or moulds when the bale is broken open. Do not feed horses using round bales
> - Soak hay by fully immersing it in water for at least 15 minutes prior to feeding. Change the water used to soak the hay daily to prevent accumulation of endotoxins and microbes
> - Feed hay on the ground. Do not use a haynet or elevated manger
> - As an alternative to hay, feed 'dust-free' options such as haylage, hay cubes, or complete pelleted rations
> - Concentrates are usually an insignificant source of dust. Adding molasses to concentrates and grains may reduce the respirable dust
> - Optimise ventilation by providing continuous pasture turnout (24 hours/day or as much as possible)
> - Ensure appropriate ventilation of the stable
> - For any period that affected horses must be indoors, house them in a stall with ventilation to the outside of the barn (e.g. window, end of aisle near door)
> - Do not stable affected horses next to hay or straw storage or arenas. Ideally, hay or straw will be stored in a different building
> - Avoid straw or sawdust as types of bedding. Use shredded paper, large wood shavings, peanut kernels, or peat moss instead. Stalls adjacent to heaves-affected horses should be managed similarly
> - Affected horses should not be indoors during 'dusty' periods such as mucking and bedding of stalls or sweeping. A light misting of bedding with water, before returning the horse to the stall, may also be helpful
> - Regular cleaning and disinfecting of stables is recommended to prevent the persistence of dust and infectious agents in the environment

Prognosis

- long-term impact of IAD on athletic performance of affected animals is uncertain:
  - pathophysiology of IAD is currently poorly understood.
  - some animals respond fully to treatment and return to a normal level of performance.
  - others will show variable response to treatment and may deteriorate over time.

Heaves

Definition/overview

- episodic condition characterised by obstruction of the lower airways in response to inhaled allergens in the environment.
- referred to as severe equine asthma, RAO, and formerly as chronic obstructive pulmonary disease (COPD).

Aetiology/pathophysiology

- obstruction is a consequence of bronchoconstriction and airway septal thickening from inflammatory cell infiltrate and oedema:
  - blockage of the airway lumen by mucus and inflammatory cells.
- animals have airway hyperresponsiveness to inhaled antigens (aeroallergens):
  - multiple agents in the environment may act as allergens.
  - moulds and dusts in improperly baled hay are most frequently implicated.
  - not known whether heaves is a sequela to IAD in some horses.
  - genetic propensity to develop heaves has been suggested.

Clinical presentation

- differentiated from horses with IAD by the presence of respiratory difficulty at rest.
- seasonal pattern of heaves exacerbation is often reported:
  - clinical signs during exacerbation frequently include:
    - expiratory dyspnoea accompanied by a visible 'heave line' as the external abdominal oblique muscles are used to facilitate expiration.
- nasal discharge is serous to mucopurulent.

TABLE 1.4 Common drugs used for the treatment of IAD and heaves

DRUG	DOSE	ROUTE*	COMMENTS
Bronchodilators			
Albuterol	0.8–2 µg/kg q1–3h	Inhalation: MDI	Rapid onset of duration of activity with short duration of effect (0.5–3 hours)
Ipratropium bromide	0.5–1 µg/kg q6h	Inhalation: MDI	Rapid onset of action with moderately long-lasting effect (4–6 hours). No known side effects
Salmeterol	63–210 µg q8h	Inhalation: MDI	Rapid onset of action with long-lasting effect (6–8 hours)
Fenoterol	1–2 mg	Inhalation: MDI	Rapid onset of action
Clenbuterol	0.8–3.2 µg/kg q12h	p/o Inhalation: nebulised	Also increases the rate of muco-ciliary clearance. Side effects include sweating, trembling, tachycardia, and excitement
	0.8 µg/kg q12h	i/v or i/m	
Aminophylline	5–10 mg/kg q8–12h	p/o or i/v	Therapeutic plasma concentrations vary among horses and margin of safety is very narrow. May cause excitement. Dilute i/v dose in 1 litre of saline and administer over 30–60 minutes while monitoring animal for signs of toxicity
Corticosteroids			
Dexamethasone	0.04–0.1 mg/kg q24h (0.2 mg/kg q24h for p/o)	i/v, i/m, or p/o	Increased dosage required for oral administration due to limited bioavailability with oral dosing
Dexamethasone 21-isonicotinate	0.04–0.06 mg/kg q3d	i/m	Depot form of dexamethasone
Prednisolone	1.1–2.2 mg/kg q24h	p/o	Good GI absorption
Isoflupredone acetate	10–14 mg q24h	i/m	Repeated administration has induced significant hypokalaemia in other species.
Triamcinolone acetonide	0.09 mg/kg once	i/m	Depot drug with prolonged effect after single dose (e.g. 3–5 weeks)
Beclomethasone dipropionate	1–8 µg/kg q12h	Inhalation: MDI	Minimal systemic effects due to low dose plus delivery by inhalation. Actual dose depends on delivery system used
Fluticasone propionate	1–6 µg/kg q12h	Inhalation: MDI	Minimal systemic effects due to low dose plus delivery by inhalation
Ciclesodine prodrug activated in lungs and binds to glucocorticoid receptors	2744 µg q12h for 5 days, followed by 4116 µg q24h for 5 days	ASERVO® EQUIHALER®	No statistically significant decrease in serum cortisol

Cromogens			
Sodium cromoglycate	80–200 mg q12–24h	Inhalation: nebulised	Mast cell stabiliser. Prophylactic use only
Nedocromil sodium	24 mg q12h	Inhalation: MDI	Mast cell stabiliser. Prophylactic use only
Other			
Interferon-alpha	50–150 U q24h for 5 d	Oral	Reduced airway inflammation in horses with IAD

*Inhaled drugs must be administered using an equine delivery device/mask in combination with a metered dose inhaler (MDI) or nebulisation system.

- intermittent to paroxysmal coughing may be observed.
- flaring of the nostrils may be seen.
- severe cases may have:
  - depression.
  - lack of interest in feed due to difficulty breathing.
  - rocking of the animal as it breathes.
  - wheeze or tracheal rattles may be audible at the nares during expiration.

Differential diagnoses

- pulmonary infections (viral or bacterial), interstitial pneumonia, and pulmonary neoplasia may have a similar presentation:
  - heaves cases typically afebrile with normal fibrinogen and SAA.
  - in contrast to infectious causes of respiratory disease.

Diagnosis

- clinical history:
  - may suggest a seasonal pattern of occurrence, corresponding with:
    - ♦ increased indoor housing during periods of poor weather (winter months).
  - lack of improvement in response to antibiotic treatment.
- thoracic auscultation using a rebreathing bag is indicated in all cases (Fig. 1.123):
  - **except animals demonstrating signs of dyspnoea or respiratory distress.**
  - frequently, crackles and wheezes are identified over the lower airways.
  - movement of secretions within the trachea.
- percussion may reveal an expanded caudodorsal margin to the lung field:

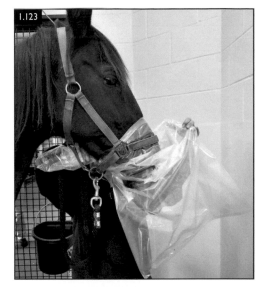

FIG. 1.123 Placement of a rebreathing bag. The handler is taking care to prevent the bag from obstructing the nostrils of the horse.

  - due to hyperinflation of the lungs consequent to air-trapping.
  - differentiate from a caecal gas cap when percussing the right abdomen.
- thoracic radiographic changes are not specific for heaves:
  - may include an increased interstitial and/or bronchial pattern.
  - helpful to exclude bronchopneumonia as a differential diagnosis.
- bronchoscopy is useful to assess:
  - airway hyperreactivity, hyperaemia, oedema, and bronchoconstriction.
  - evaluate the presence and nature of any airway secretions (Fig. 1.124).

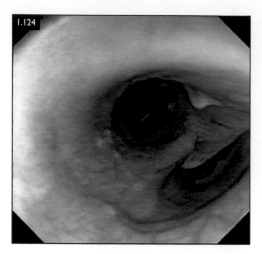

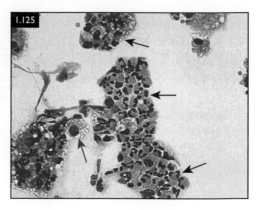

FIG. 1.125 Cytology of BAL fluid from a horse with heaves during exacerbation of clinical signs. Well-preserved neutrophils (black arrows) are the predominant cell type. Pulmonary alveolar macrophages are also visible (red arrow).

FIG. 1.124 Bronchoscopic view of the carina in a horse with heaves during severe exacerbation of clinical signs. The carina is markedly blunted due to oedema, and flecks of mucus are visible. Airways are hyperresponsive, resulting in excessive coughing and constriction of the airways in response to passage of the bronchoscope.

- BAL is the test of choice to diagnose heaves:
  - transendoscopically or blindly using a flexible cuffed nasotracheal catheter passed into the bronchi.
  - cytological assessment to determine:
    - type(s) of leucocyte contributing to the airway inflammation (Fig. 1.125).
    - elevation in percentage of neutrophils (>25%) in differential cell count during episodes of clinical exacerbation of heaves.
    - elevated percentages of mast cells and eosinophils may also be observed.
- administration of N-butylscopolammonium bromide (0.3 mg/kg i/v once):
  - short-acting bronchodilatory effects.
  - may assist in the diagnosis, as horses with pneumonia do not typically respond to bronchodilators.

Management

- clinical cure is not generally possible in horses with heaves:
  - treatment is aimed at achieving and maintaining remission from clinical signs.

  - best achieved through persistent and aggressive environmental management to reduce exposure to inhaled allergens (Table 1.3).
  - hay should be good quality with minimal dust and moulds present:
    - preferably changed to haylage or a pelleted complete feed.
  - continuous pasture turnout is recommended to optimise ventilation.
  - effort should be made to avoid dusty activities if housed indoors for any period:
    - during cleaning and bedding of stalls, feeding hay, and sweeping.
  - stall should not be located near to an arena or hay storage facility:
    - overhead hay storage is particularly detrimental.
  - bedding should be wood shavings or peat moss rather than straw or sawdust.
- alleviation of lung inflammation through therapy with corticosteroids:
  - oral (e.g. prednisolone):
    - **should be avoided as poorly absorbed.**
    - active metabolite is not reliably produced in many horses.
  - parenteral (e.g. isoflupredone, dexamethasone).
  - inhalation (e.g. beclomethasone, fluticasone, ciclesonide) (Table 1.4):
    - severely affected animals will require initial therapy with

systemically administered corticosteroids before inhaled corticosteroids are considered.
  ○ tapered course of corticosteroid administration over 2–4 weeks is commonly required.
- during episodes of heaves exacerbation, rescue therapy may be required in animals demonstrating dyspnoea or respiratory distress:
  ○ best achieved through bronchodilation with rapid-acting drugs such as beta-2 adrenergics (e.g. albuterol, levalbuterol, salbutamol, clenbuterol).
  ○ followed by longer-acting bronchodilation (e.g. salmeterol).
  ○ chronic use of beta-agonist medications such as clenbuterol leads to tolerance or desensitisation to the drug (limit use to 2 weeks).
- omega-3 polyunsaturated fatty acid supplement containing docosahexaenoic acid (1.5–3 g) and a low-dust diet for 2 months improved clinical signs in one study.
- use of skin allergen testing or serum antibody testing to direct allergen desensitisation treatment has been used:
  ○ no controlled studies evaluating this treatment and efficacy is unknown.

Prognosis

- heaves is generally a lifelong disease in affected horses:
  ○ progression in severity of signs and development of chronic airway remodelling occurs in animals with unregulated airway inflammation.
- prognosis for achieving and maintaining remission from clinical signs is variable:
  ○ highly dependent on owner's ability to institute aggressive management changes to reduce exposure to inhaled allergens all year round.

Summer pasture-associated obstructive pulmonary disease

Definition/overview

- recurrent disease of adult horses that are kept on pasture.

- most common in the warm and humid months of June to September in the south-eastern USA and in the UK.
- animals gradually recover during the winter and spring months but may experience a return of clinical signs the following summer.

Aetiology/pathophysiology

- pathophysiology of airway inflammation in this condition is poorly understood.
  ○ presumed to represent an inflammatory response to environmental allergens that are encountered at pasture.
  ○ airway hyperresponsiveness has been linked to increased bronchial smooth-muscle sensitivity to 5-hydroxytryptamine in affected horses.

Clinical presentation

- similar to heaves.
- signs may include:
  ○ nasal discharge ○ nostril flaring.
  ○ coughing.
  ○ tachypnoea laboured expiratory effort.
  ○ expanded lung field on chest percussion.
  ○ crackles and wheezes throughout the lung fields on thoracic auscultation.

Differential diagnoses

- heaves and viral or bacterial pneumonia are the most common differential diagnoses.

Diagnosis

- clinical signs and history of seasonality are suggestive.
- thoracic radiography can be useful:
  ○ interstitial pattern is present.
  ○ pulmonary overinflation in chronic cases (Fig. 1.126).
- increased mucus is evident in the upper airways on bronchoscopy but not diagnostic.
- BAL and cytology of the fluid should be performed:
  ○ increased cell count with an increase in non-degenerative neutrophils is diagnostic.

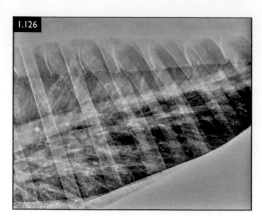

FIG. 1.126 Thoracic radiographs of a horse with equine asthma. Findings include a diffuse interstitial pattern and mild concavity of the diaphragm due to hyperinflation.

Management

- management is critical:
  - indoor housing, in a barn with minimal dust, during the summer months.
- drug therapy as described for heaves is an important adjunctive measure (Table 1.4):
  - response may be limited if environmental modification is not feasible.
- cases refractory to medical and local environmental management may benefit from relocation to a different climate.

Prognosis

- resolution of the disease is poor.
- careful environmental and medical management may induce remission of clinical signs.

PARASITIC CONDITIONS

Lungworm

Definition/overview

- *Dictyocaulus arnfieldi* causes parasitic pneumonia in horses:
  - donkeys and foals are the patent hosts:
    - ♦ infection in donkeys is usually subclinical.
  - infection is usually non-patent in the horse.
- presence of adult worms and late-stage larvae in the bronchi and bronchioles causes clinical signs:
  - signs closely resemble those of RAO.
- successfully treated with anthelminthics.

Aetiology/pathophysiology

- *D. arnfieldi* is a nematode and has a typical lifecycle with a migratory larval phase.
- donkeys and foals with patent infections shed onto pasture:
  - eggs containing first-stage (L1) larvae.
  - hatched L1 larvae mature to infective L3 stage within days.
- L3 larvae ingested and mature into migratory L4 larvae:
  - enter mesenteric lymphatics, then the circulation via the thoracic duct.
  - reach the lung haematogenously.
  - migrate into the alveoli and develop into L5 and then adults in the airway.
  - bronchi and especially bronchioles.
- donkeys and foals, but not usually adult horses, develop patent infections:
  - adult female worms lay eggs containing L1 larvae.
  - coughed into the pharynx and swallowed.
  - eggs containing L1 larvae may be passed in faeces.
  - or eggs may hatch in the gut, releasing L1 larvae into the faeces.

Clinical presentation

- usually no obvious clinical signs in donkeys.
- foals show few, if any, clinical signs.
- adult horses, the clinical disease closely resembles heaves:
  - affected horses are bright.
  - present with a history of coughing and decreased exercise capacity.
  - may be moderate tachypnoea and dyspnoea at rest.

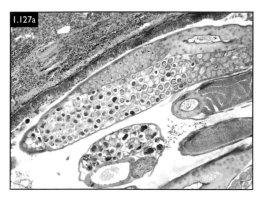 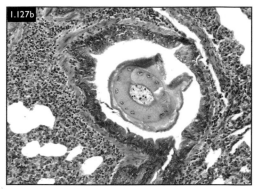

FIGS. 1.127 Adult *Dictyocaulus* worms in the (a) bronchus (10x magnification) and (b) bronchiole (20x magnification). Images courtesy of K. Sakamoto.

- ○ wheezes and crackles are audible on lung auscultation.

Differential diagnosis

- other causes of pulmonary disease should be considered, especially:
  - ○ heaves and primary eosinophilic pulmonary disease.

Diagnosis

- clinical signs are not diagnostic:
  - ○ heaves-like disease in one or more horses in a group at pasture in the late summer that have been grazing with donkeys should raise suspicion.
- donkeys and foals only:
  - ○ faecal examination using the modified Baermann technique will reveal larvae.
  - ○ not useful in adult horses as patent infections are not established.
- horses:
  - ○ airway lavage samples reveal eosinophilia with L5 larvae and/or adult nematodes (Fig. 1.127).
  - ○ **note airway eosinophilia is not pathognomonic for pulmonary parasitism.**

Management

- successfully treated with a variety of anthelminthics including:
  - ○ benzimidazoles, ivermectin, and moxidectin:
    - ♦ benzimidazoles are given for 5 consecutive days.
    - ♦ single doses of ivermectin and moxidectin are highly effective.

- regular anthelminthic treatment of donkeys will control shedding of eggs and L1 larvae and reduce pasture contamination.
- picking up droppings and sweeping also help to reduce pasture contamination.

Prognosis

- good.

Parascaris equorum

Definition/overview

- *Parascaris equorum* causes parasitic pneumonia in foals and yearlings:
  - ○ typically, towards the end of their first summer at pasture.
- adult parasites live in the small intestine.
- clinical signs are caused by larvae migrating through the lung.
- immunity develops after infection:
  - ○ disease is uncommon in foals older than 12–18 months.
- treated successfully with anthelmintics.
- prognosis is good.

Aetiology/pathophysiology

- *P. equorum* is a large ascarid (roundworm).
- adults live in the small intestine and lay eggs containing L1 larvae.
- shed onto pasture in faeces:
  - ○ quickly mature (<2 weeks) into the infective L2 larvae inside the egg.
  - ○ single infected foal can shed millions of eggs each day.

- o foals become infected by ingestion of L2 larvae within eggs from the pasture.
- o L2 larvae migrate through the small intestinal wall.
- o via the hepatic portal vein reach and migrate through the liver as L3 larvae.
- reach the lungs via the heart and pulmonary artery within 2 weeks of infection:
  - o migrate through alveolar capillary walls into the airway.
  - o coughed up into the pharynx and swallowed.
- within small intestine, larvae develop into L4 larvae and then adult worms.
- prepatent period is between 3 and 4 months.

Clinical presentation

- foals between 6 and 12 months old are most affected:
  - o typically, towards the end of their first summer at pasture.
  - o sometimes referred to as 'summer colds'.
  - o affected foals may have poor body composition.
- clinical signs referable to the respiratory tract include:
  - o nasal discharge, coughing, tachypnoea, and dyspnoea.
  - o crackling and wheezing on auscultation of the lung field.
  - o modest pyrexia and weight loss.
  - o heavy infections of adult parasites can cause death due to small intestinal obstruction and rupture.

Differential diagnosis

- variety of causes of pneumonia (bacterial, viral) in foals and yearlings may have a similar presentation.

Diagnosis

- outbreak of pulmonary disease in foals at pasture is highly suggestive of *P. equorum* infection.
- secondary bacterial pneumonia can occur.
- confirmation by faecal egg counts and demonstration of thick-walled ascarid eggs.

Management

- treated using any of the available anthelmintics including:
  - o benzimidazoles, ivermectin, and moxidectin.
- faecal egg count reduction testing of foals should be carried out regularly to detect resistance to macrocyclic lactones (ivermectin, moxidectin):
  - o reports in multiple countries of resistance to these anthelmintics.
  - o early treatment with pyrantel or benzimidazoles may limit development of high burdens in the intestinal tract that predispose to ascarid impactions.

Prognosis

- good for most cases:
  - o death from small intestinal rupture in very heavily infected foals can occur.
- solid immunity develops on recovery from infection:
  - o infections in animals older than 12 months are unusual.

MISCELLANEOUS CONDITIONS

Aspiration pneumonia

Definition/overview

- aspiration is a potential cause of serious pneumonia.
- occurs in adult horses and foals for a variety of reasons.

Aetiology/pathophysiology

- many potential causes of aspiration:
  - o neonatal foals, aspiration of milk may occur because of:
    - ◆ congenital abnormalities.
    - ◆ weakness secondary to other illness.
    - ◆ improper supplemental (bottle or nasogastric tube) feeding.
  - o adult horses:
    - ◆ inadvertent drenching or passing a nasogastric tube into the lungs:

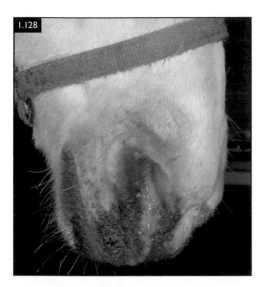

FIG. 1.128 Oesophageal obstruction in a horse subsequent to improper soaking of beet pulp prior to feeding. Feed material is visible at the nares of the horse.

- – depositing fluids, pharmaceutical products, or other substances into the lower airways is a common cause.
  - ♦ aspiration of saliva and feed material is a common complication of oesophageal obstruction (choke) and can occur during GA.
  - ♦ dysphagia from any cause may also predispose to aspiration.
- quantity and composition of the aspirated fluid/material:

- o largely dictates the clinical signs, progression of disease, and outcome:
  - ♦ large quantities of fluids are aspirated, animals may die acutely.
  - ♦ more frequently, they develop pneumonia, which can progress to:
    - – lung consolidation.
    - – pleuropneumonia.
    - – gangrenous pneumonia.
    - – and/or pulmonary abscessation.

Clinical presentation

- acute clinical signs, following aspiration, are similar to other forms of pneumonia:
  - o tachypnoea, cough, anxiety, and increased lung sounds.
  - o shortly after aspiration, a raspy, fluid-like sound may be heard during respiration.
  - o ingesta may be observed at the nostrils (Fig. 1.128).

Differential diagnoses

- viral or bacterial pneumonia, including pleuropneumonia, should be considered.

Diagnosis

- history and physical examination are suggestive:
  - o particularly recent oesophageal obstruction or nasogastric intubation.
- thoracic radiography is a useful tool (Fig. 1.129):
  - o ventral consolidation is common due to gravitational flow of aspirated material.

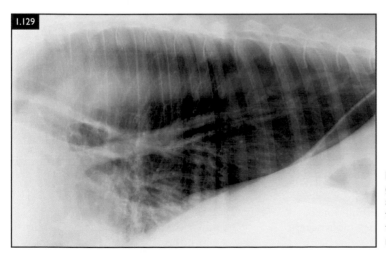

FIG. 1.129 Thoracic radiograph of the horse in 1.128 showing ventral consolidation due to pneumonia from aspiration of feed material into the lungs.

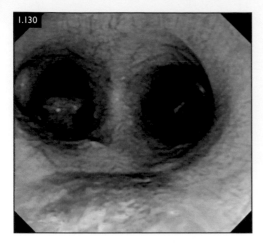

FIG. 1.130 Bronchoscopic examination at the carina of the horse in Fig. 1.128 revealed feed material within the trachea down to the level of the tracheal puddle.

- without respiratory distress:
  - bronchoscopy to visualise fluid/food debris within the trachea (Fig. 1.130).
- cytological examination of tracheal or bronchial aspirates may reveal:
  - extra- and intracellular bacteria or foreign material such as mineral oil.
- reason for aspiration must be explored:
  - clinical examination to identify primary causes and direct subsequent testing.

Management

- broad-spectrum antimicrobial administration to target both Gram-positive and Gram-negative, as well as anaerobic, bacteria is indicated.
- NSAIDs are beneficial to control lung inflammation.
- specific measures to address the cause of, and prevent further, aspiration are required.

Prognosis

- variable, depending on the severity of the pneumonia, the inciting cause, and the ability to prevent ongoing aspiration.
- volume and nature of the aspirated material or fluid, type(s) of bacteria introduced into the lung, and time of initiation of treatment may influence the outcome.

Granulomatous pneumonia

Definition/overview

- uncommon, multisystemic granulomatous disease that resembles sarcoidosis in humans.
- no seasonal, breed, age, or sex predispositions have been identified.

Aetiology/pathophysiology

- currently, recognised causes include:
  - fungal, bacterial, and/or parasitic agents.
  - silicate pneumoconiosis.
  - neoplasia.
- cause cannot be identified in many cases.
- pathophysiology is poorly understood:
  - presumed to involve an abnormal host immune response to chronic exposure to an antigen.

Clinical presentation

- chronic signs of weight loss, anorexia, depression, and fever are common.
- skin lesions are frequently present.
- progressive respiratory signs including exercise intolerance, tachypnoea, cough, nasal discharge, and abnormal lung sounds.
- clinical signs do not respond to antibiotic therapy and NSAIDs.

Differential diagnoses

- fungal, parasitic, or bacterial pneumonia and pulmonary neoplasia.

Diagnosis

- disease caused by silicate pneumoconiosis or coccidioidomycosis:
  - geographical origin of the horse from an endemic area may be suggestive.
- haematological testing is indicated in all cases:
  - evidence of a chronic inflammatory process:
    - anaemia, neutrophilia, hyperfibrinogenaemia, and increased globulins.
- thoracic radiographs are important (Fig. 1.131):
  - miliary or nodular interstitial pattern may be present throughout the lung.

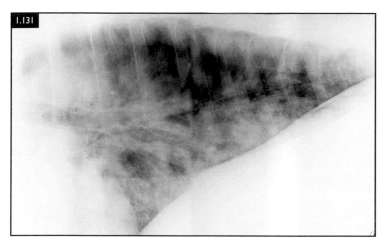

FIG. 1.131 Thoracic radiograph of a horse with granulomatous pneumonia. Multifocal opacities are visible throughout the lung field.

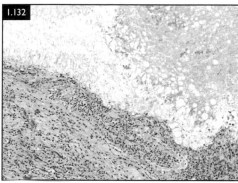

FIG. 1.132 *Aspergillus* granuloma in the lungs of a horse with fungal pneumonia (20× magnification). (Image courtesy Kaori Sakamoto)

- tracheal aspirate and BAL cytology are non-specific:
  - mild suppurative inflammation may be present.
- lung biopsy is required for diagnosis:
  - sampling of the nodular masses optimised by ultrasound-guided lung biopsy.
  - histopathology reveals:
    - non-caseating granulomas affiliated with bronchi/bronchioles (Fig. 1.132).
    - intracellular crystalline material may be observed in silicosis.
- elucidate other causes:
  - serum immunodiffusion testing for antibodies against *Coccidioides immitis*.
  - selective histopathological staining of lung tissue for fungal and mycobacterial agents.

  - bacterial and fungal culture of tracheal aspirate or BAL fluids.

Management

- adequate target therapy cannot be prescribed since the cause remains unknown.
- corticosteroids are widely used, but there is no information supporting their efficacy.

Prognosis

- poor because of the lack of a proven treatment.
- affected horses are commonly euthanased because of progressive and severe debilitation associated with the disease.

Smoke inhalation

Definition/overview

- clinical syndrome resulting from inhalation of harmful gases, vapours, and/or particulate matter contained in smoke, usually originating from barn fires (Fig. 1.133).

Aetiology/pathophysiology

- insult to the respiratory tract (especially URT) by:
  - direct thermal injury and inhalation of toxic chemicals.
  - causing lung injury directly or indirectly:
    - through activation of an inflammatory response.

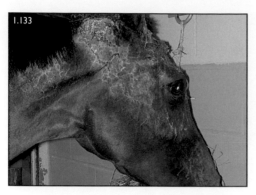

FIG. 1.133 External skin burns subsequent to a barn fire. Smoke inhalation resulted in marked damage to the respiratory epithelium, causing respiratory distress in this horse from excessive debris within the trachea and bronchi.

◆ low oxygen delivery to the lung due to combustion processes.
- pulmonary dysfunction occurs initially through exposure to a high concentration of carbon monoxide:
  ○ combines with haemoglobin to form carboxyhaemoglobin, resulting in hypoxaemia.
  ○ hypoxaemia may be exacerbated if concurrent bronchoconstriction in the lower airways occurs in response to the irritating effects of noxious gases.
  ○ pulmonary dysfunction may subsequently progress due to:
    ◆ pulmonary oedema formation due to lung inflammation.
    ◆ airway obstruction from the accumulation of inflammatory and necrotic cells in the airways.
    ◆ extensive destruction of airway epithelium impairs host respiratory immune defences, predisposing to secondary bronchopneumonia.

Clinical presentation

- clinical signs will depend on the degree of exposure and the types of gas inhaled:
  ○ animals may be mildly affected or clinically normal after smoke inhalation, with severe disease developing 12–24 hours later.
  ○ severely affected animals may show signs of hypoxaemia, depression, disorientation, and ataxia.

  ○ tachypnoea, dyspnoea, and respiratory stridor may occur.
  ○ crackles, wheezes, or decreased air movement may be obvious:
    ◆ initial chest auscultation.
    ◆ may take 12–24 hours to develop.
- nasal discharge is common due to oedema or inflammatory exudate in the upper airway.

Diagnosis

- history and physical examination are usually diagnostic:
  ○ presence of external thermal injuries is confirmatory.
- blood gas analysis should be performed if available:
  ○ venous concentration of carboxyhaemoglobin above 10% is consistent with carbon monoxide toxicity.
- horses without signs of significant respiratory distress:
  ○ thoracic radiographs, bronchoscopy, and cytological evaluation of tracheal aspirate or BAL fluid.

Management

- tracheotomy may be required:
  ○ upper airway obstruction resulting from severe oedema and inflammation.
  ○ remove pseudomembranes from the trachea to facilitate ventilation of the lung.
- humidified oxygen support by nasal insufflation or via a transtracheal catheter is recommended to displace carbon monoxide from haemoglobin.
- bronchodilators may be indicated in cases of severe bronchoconstriction.
- diuretics and NSAIDs usually required:
  ○ control pulmonary oedema, inflammation, and pain.
- **use of corticosteroids is controversial and usually avoided** (may predispose to infections).
- some cases may require the use of analgesics such as fentanyl, morphine, or ketamine.
- supportive therapy is commonly indicated including:

- o   intravenous fluids, plasma transfusion, or parenteral nutrition supplementation.
- o   high-risk patients or confirmed bacterial infections should be treated with appropriate antimicrobials.

Prognosis

- variable:
  - o   prolonged exposure to gases and extensive/severe thermal injuries – poor prognosis.
  - o   onset of clinical signs may be delayed, and close monitoring is indicated in any animal that has been exposed to smoke.

Pneumothorax

Definition/overview

- accumulation of air or gas in the pleural space causing partial or total collapse of the lung.
- uncommon in horses and usually occurs due to trauma.
- usually, bilateral due to the fenestrations in the mediastinum of horses.

Aetiology/pathophysiology

- air enters the pleural cavity and may result from:
  - o   open chest wound, rib fracture or blunt trauma to the thorax.
  - o   defect in the lung parenchyma allowing communication between the airways and pleural space:
    - ♦   rupture of an emphysematous vesicle on the surface of the lung.
    - ♦   pneumonia cases may develop bronchopleural fistulas.
  - o   barotrauma.
  - o   thoracic procedures (e.g. surgery or lung biopsy) may result in pneumothorax.
  - o   spontaneously without evident cause.
- Simple pneumothorax:
  - o   intrapleural pressure less than or equal to atmospheric pressure:
    - ♦   air may enter and exit the chest cavity freely with each breath.
    - ♦   insufficient negative pressure is generated within the chest cavity to expand the lungs for ventilation.

- Tension pneumothorax:
  - o   respiratory embarrassment escalates more rapidly.
  - o   continued influx of air into the chest cavity while no exit of air is possible.
  - o   intrapleural pressure quickly exceeds atmospheric pressure and causes life-threatening compression of the lungs.

Clinical presentation

- clinical signs may range from:
  - o   mild increase in respiratory rate and sweating.
  - o   tachypnoea, dyspnoea, and cyanosis.
- oral mucous membrane colour is often abnormal:
  - o   range widely in appearance from pale to congested, toxic, or cyanotic.
  - o   depends on degree of pneumothorax and underlying cause.
- chest auscultation:
  - o   lung sounds are absent in the dorsal lung field.
- percussion may reveal hyperresonance over the affected area.
- subcutaneous emphysema, may obscure auscultation and percussion findings.

Differential diagnoses

- Diaphragmatic hernia and pleural effusion may produce similar signs.

Diagnosis

- history, evidence of trauma to the thoracic cavity, or the presence of subcutaneous emphysema is suggestive.
- thoracic radiographs are important:
  - o   air within the pleural space compresses the lung ventrally.
  - o   absence of pulmonary vasculature over the caudodorsal lung field.
  - o   sharp lung border in the dorsal and caudal regions (Fig. 1.134).
- ultrasonographic examination:
  - o   middle and dorsal areas of the thorax may reveal air artefact images.
  - o   combined with inability to identify a sliding motion between the visceral and parietal pleura.

Management

- treatment of the underlying disease or cause should be addressed.

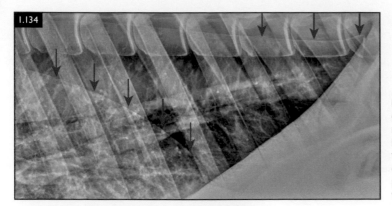

FIG. 1.134 Thoracic radiograph of bilateral pneumothorax in an adult horse. Arrows indicate two distinct crura of the dorsal lung lobes, displaced ventrally by air within the pleural space.

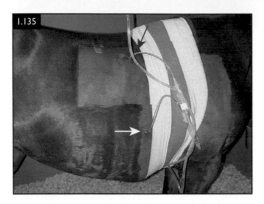

FIG. 1.135 Two indwelling chest drains were placed in this horse to remove air (dorsal drain, red arrow) and pleural effusion (ventral drain, white arrow). Negative pressure was applied to the dorsal drain using a suction apparatus. Heimlich valves were attached to both drains for unidirectional movement of gas and fluid, preventing further pneumothorax from the presence of the drains.

- simple pneumothorax cases can recover with confinement and rest:
  - intranasal oxygen insufflation can be administered with hypoxaemia.
- removal of free air from the pleural cavity may be required in more severely affected cases (Fig. 1.135):
  - air suction of the thoracic cavity performed in upper mid-thorax between ribs.
  - ultrasonography will assist by revealing areas where air is present.
  - overlying skin is surgically prepared.
  - site desensitised with local anaesthetic.
  - full-thickness skin stab incision.
  - teat cannula or small-bore thoracic tube inserted into the pleural space.
  - suction equipment if available is attached and gentle suction is applied.
  - alternatively, a three-way stopcock tube system can be used:
    - repeated aspiration of air using a large syringe.
  - all the air is removed from the chest cavity:
    - allows reinflation of the lung.
    - cannula/tube removed, and skin incision sutured closed.

Prognosis

- commonly dictated by the underlying cause:
  - cases secondary to pleuropneumonia have a poorer prognosis compared with other causes of pneumothorax.

Chylothorax

Definition/overview

- accumulation of chyle in the pleural cavity is infrequently reported in horses.
- chylous fluid is generally odourless and milky and opalescent in appearance.
- most case reports are in foals.

Aetiology/pathophysiology

- cause could not be determined in the majority of foals diagnosed with chylothorax.

Clinical presentation

- clinical signs reported in foals include:
  - tachypnoea, dyspnoea and coughing.
  - lethargy and pyrexia.
  - muffled lung sounds on auscultation.

Differential diagnoses

- pleuropneumonia, haemothorax, hydrothorax, and diaphragmatic hernia.

Diagnosis

- fluid line is evident on chest percussion, with lung sounds decreased in ventral lung fields.
- thoracic ultrasonography is useful to detect fluid in the pleural cavity and to guide thoracocentesis:
  - physical appearance of the fluid is suggestive.
  - important to distinguish between true chyle and pseudochyle (Fig. 1.136):
    - chyle fluid:
      - does not clear on centrifugation.
      - chylomicron globules seen under microscopic examination:
        - special staining with Sudan III or IV, or oil red 0.
      - triglyceride levels usually increased in chyle compared with serum.
      - cytological analysis is variable:
        - generally, chyle is rich in lymphocytes.
        - chronic cases, non-degenerate neutrophils may predominate.

Management

- limited information is available in horses.
- foals have been successfully managed with supportive care, broad-spectrum antimicrobials, thoracic drainage, and dietary management.
- surgical management has not been reported in horses.

Prognosis

- chances of long-term survival are not known due to the limited number of cases.
- successful medical treatment has been reported in foals.

Haemothorax

Definition/overview

- blood accumulation in the pleural cavity may result from:
  - trauma to the pleural or pulmonary vessels.
  - rupture of a large thoracic blood vessel (Fig. 1.137).
  - other causes include:
    - haemangiosarcoma or other neoplasia.
    - coagulopathy.
    - iatrogenic haemothorax after thoracotomy or lung biopsy.
- unilateral or bilateral haemothorax depending on:
  - cause of the haemorrhage.
  - whether the mediastinum is intact.
- pneumothorax may also occur in some cases of traumatic haemothorax.

Clinical presentation

- clinical signs may be variable, depending on the cause:

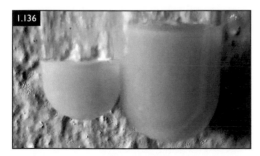

FIG. 1.136 Chylous pleural effusion from a horse. Chyle can have a milky white to light pink appearance, depending upon the degree of haemorrhage present in the sample. (Photo courtesy K. Christie).

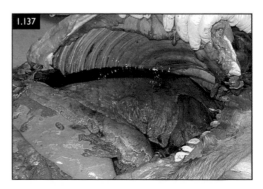

FIG. 1.137 Haemothorax in a foal that occurred as a result of rib fracture from external trauma.

- signs of tachypnoea, distress, pain, and shallow respiration following rib fracture.
- sudden death from severe haemorrhage, in cases of rupture of a large vessel.
- may develop anaemia and hypoproteinaemia if more gradual haemorrhage into the thoracic cavity.

Differential diagnoses

- other fluids in the thoracic cavity such as pleuropneumonia or hydrothorax may produce similar signs.

Diagnosis

- clinical examination is non-specific:
  - decreased lung sounds ventrally.
  - muffled heart sounds that radiate over a wide area.
  - percussion may detect ventral areas of dullness:
    - ♦ procedure may be painful, especially in cases of thoracic trauma.
- thoracic ultrasonography method of choice to detect fluid within the chest cavity:
  - rib ultrasonography may identify defects consistent with a fracture.
  - haemothorax should appear homogeneous with no flocculation.
- thoracocentesis:
  - cytology, packed cell volume (PCV), and total protein concentration.
  - indicated if no diagnosis of haemothorax on ultrasonography.
  - risk of iatrogenic infection.
  - aspirated fluid should be submitted for culture with thoracic trauma.
- thoracic radiographs useful for identifying an underlying cause, such as rib fracture.

Management

- underlying cause should be addressed (i.e. fractured ribs stabilised if possible).
- **chest drainage is controversial** and should only be performed to:
  - alleviate distress in cases with respiratory compromise, resulting from:
    - ♦ excessive fluid accumulation.
    - ♦ presence of infection.

- many cases are treated successfully without drainage.
- drainage is generally not recommended if haemothorax is due to clotting disorders.
- supportive medical therapy, including:
  - intranasal oxygen supplementation.
  - analgesics.
  - intravenous fluids, or whole blood or plasma transfusions:
    - ♦ administration of fluids performed gradually to prevent systemic hypertension exacerbating haemorrhage in the acute period of treatment.
- trauma cases with penetration into the thoracic cavity:
  - broad-spectrum antimicrobial administration is recommended.

Prognosis

- variable and depends largely on the underlying problem.
- uncomplicated thoracic trauma may respond to medical therapy.
- cases that develop secondary pleuritis carry a worse prognosis.
- poor in cases of haemothorax secondary to neoplasia or clotting disorders.

Hydrothorax

Definition/overview

- accumulation of serous fluid in the pleural cavity:
  - usually secondary to infectious causes such as AHS.
  - non-infectious causes include multicentric lymphoma, congestive heart failure, or hypoproteinemia.

Clinical presentation

- clinical signs reflect:
  - volume of fluid accumulation.
  - underlying disease process.
- range from mild to severe and include dyspnoea and cyanosis.

Differential diagnoses

- Pleuropneumonia, haemothorax, and chylothorax may present similarly.

Diagnosis

- physical findings may include:
  - dyspnoea and absent lung sounds ventrally.
  - dullness on percussion over the lower areas of the thorax.
- thoracic ultrasonography is method of choice to detect fluid within the chest cavity:
  - fluid should appear clear and homogeneous, with no flocculation.
- thoracocentesis for cytology, PCV, and total protein concentration is indicated:
  - accompanied by a risk of iatrogenic infection.
- thoracic radiographs may be helpful to identify an underlying cause, such as neoplasia.

Management

- underlying cause should be addressed if possible.
- drainage of the chest is controversial:
  - only performed to alleviate distress in cases with respiratory compromise.

Prognosis

- condition itself is not fatal, but the underlying disease dictates the prognosis.

Exercise-induced pulmonary haemorrhage (EIPH)

Definition/overview

- presence of blood in the airways after exercise.
- bursts of intense exercise are commonly associated with EIPH:
  - affected animals include sprint-racing horses worldwide.
  - majority of racing horses experience some degree of EIPH during exercise:
    - concern to the racing industry due to:
      - financial implications from decreased performance.
      - lost training days.
      - necessity for pre-race medication under some racing authorities.
      - banning of horses from racing in some jurisdictions.
  - other high-performance equine athletes may also be affected:
    - barrel-racing.
    - cutting.
    - reining.
    - roping.
    - polo ponies.
    - cross-country or 3-day-eventing horses.
    - showjumpers.
    - hunter-jumpers.
    - steeplechasers.
    - draught horses.

Aetiology/pathophysiology

- cause of condition is currently unknown – number of theories have been proposed:
  - stress failure of pulmonary capillaries because of high transmural pressure generated during exercise:
    - fails to explain caudodorsal location within lung where haemorrhage first seen.
    - pattern of progression that occurs with EIPH.
  - locomotory forces generated by the forelimb during galloping are responsible for damaging the lung:
    - explains site of initiation, nature of the lesion, and pattern of progression.
- commonly accompanied by airway inflammation, as detected by BAL:
  - role of inflammation in the pathogenesis is unknown.
- increased upper airway resistance, from nasal, pharyngeal or laryngeal dysfunction, can exacerbate EIPH.
- possible that the cause of EIPH is multifactorial in origin.

Clinical presentation

- main clinical sign is the presence of blood within the airways:
  - majority of affected horses do not demonstrate epistaxis:
    - blood is often coughed up and swallowed.
  - may be slow to return to a resting respiratory rate after exercise:
    - accompanied by prolonged peripheral vasodilation and sweating.
- poor performance may occur in some horses.

Differential diagnoses

- other causes of epistaxis include:
  - guttural pouch mycosis.
  - ethmoidal haematoma.
  - pneumonia or pleuropneumonia.
  - haemangiosarcoma.
  - atrial fibrillation.
- uncommon causes of lung bleeding, include:
  - lung abscess, neoplasia, or foreign body.

Diagnosis

- epistaxis only seen in a small percentage of EIPH horses after exercise.
- diagnosed by endoscopic visualisation of blood in the trachea post-exercise (Fig. 1.138):
  - examination is recommended 90 minutes after exercise to increase detection of haemorrhage from the distal airways in mild cases (Fig. 1.139).
- haemosiderin in alveolar macrophages (haemosiderophages) can be detected in BAL fluid (Fig. 1.140) and confirms previous lung haemorrhage:
  - not possible to estimate the time or severity of haemorrhage.
- radiography, ultrasonography, and nuclear scintigraphy have limited diagnostic value in the evaluation of EIPH, and their interpretation is difficult.

Management

- furosemide is widely used to manage EIPH during exercise, especially in the Thoroughbred racing industry:
  - 0.5–1 mg/kg administered i/v 4 hours before strenuous exercise:
    - reduces severity and incidence of EIPH.
    - associated with improved racing outcomes.
  - **use is prohibited in some racing jurisdictions.**
  - may reduce the severity of haemorrhage in some horses but does not prevent bleeding completely.

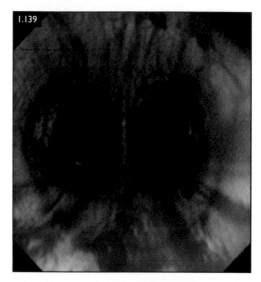

FIG. 1.139 Haemorrhage noted in the trachea of a horse with EIPH, immediately post-exercise.

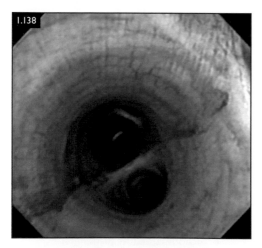

FIG. 1.138 Bronchoscopic view of the carina in a horse with mild pulmonary haemorrhage as seen 30 minutes after intense exercise. A small trace of blood is visible from the right mainstem bronchus.

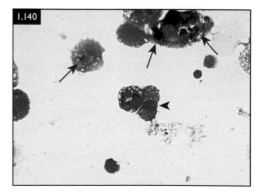

FIG. 1.140 Cytology of BAL fluid from a horse with previous pulmonary haemorrhage. Haemosiderin is visible as dark pigment within pulmonary alveolar macrophages (arrows). A mast cell (arrowhead) is also present in this sample.

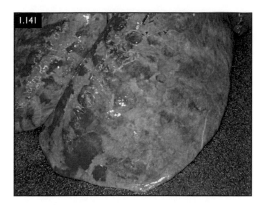

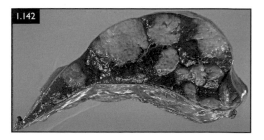

FIGS. 1.141, 1.142 Lung tumours. Note the multifocal white, roughened patches (1.141), that correspond to variably sized tumours within the lung parenchyma, seen in section (1.142).

- several additional treatments are used but their efficacy in treating and/or preventing EIPH is unknown:
  - bronchodilators, broad-spectrum antimicrobials, and corticosteroids may improve general pulmonary health.
  - commercially available nasal strips have been shown to reduce upper airway inspiratory resistance and reduce the severity of EIPH during intense exercise.
  - use of hyperbaric oxygen therapy in affected horses is an emerging treatment:
    - ♦ currently scientific evaluation of this treatment is lacking.

Prognosis
- majority of horses with mild EIPH, the prognosis for performance is unaffected.
- more severely affected animals, it can be performance-limiting:
  - poor understanding of the pathogenesis, progression, and appropriate treatment of this condition makes the prognosis uncertain in such animals.

Lower respiratory tract neoplasia

Definition/overview
(Figs. 1.141, 1.142)
- primary pulmonary neoplasia is reported infrequently in horses and include:
  - pulmonary lymphosarcoma.
  - granular cell tumour.
  - pulmonary and bronchogenic carcinoma.
  - bronchogenic SCC.
  - pulmonary chondrosarcoma.
  - bronchial myxoma.
  - affected animals are generally mature horses (>7 years of age).
- metastatic pulmonary neoplasia is uncommon in the horse (more frequent than primary lung tumours) and includes:
  - haemangiosarcoma.
  - squamous cell carcinoma.
  - adenocarcinoma.
  - fibrosarcoma   o   hepatoblastoma.
  - chondrosarcoma.
  - undifferentiated sarcomas or carcinomas.
  - lung metastatic tumours have been reported in animals as young as 3 months old.

Clinical presentation
- clinical signs are non-specific, but may include:
  - depression   o   exercise intolerance.
  - weight loss.
  - fever, which can be intermittent.
  - other signs such as cough, epistaxis, or dyspnoea.
- pleural effusion is common, especially in some metastatic tumours.

Diagnosis
- cytological examination of tracheobronchial aspirates, BAL fluid, or pleural fluid may help to identify lung neoplasia.
- thoracic radiographs usually identify:
  - presence of one or multiple soft tissue opacities (Fig. 1.143).

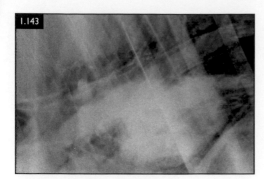

FIG. 1.143 Thoracic radiograph of a horse with a granular cell tumour. A discrete oval opacity is present in the dorsal lung field.

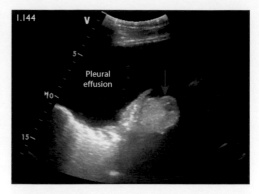

FIG. 1.144 Ultrasound image of a horse with thoracic metastatic neoplasia. Hypoechoic pleural fluid surrounds the poorly aerated tip of a lung lobe. A mixed echogenicity circular mass is confluent with the pleural surface of the lung.

- o may suggest the presence of pleural effusion.
- thoracic ultrasonography will confirm the presence of:
  - o pleural fluid.
  - o irregular lung surface or architecture for masses located at the lung surface (Fig. 1.144).
  - o ultrasound-guided biopsy of thoracic or pulmonary masses:
    - ♦ diagnosis by histology/ histochemistry, and/or immunohistochemistry.

Prognosis

- generally poor, although it may depend on the type of tumour.
- clinical signs and subsequent diagnosis are often delayed:
  - o lesions are frequently advanced.
  - o animal has developed systemic complications.

Acute bronchointerstitial pneumonia of foals

Definition/overview

- rare condition in foals less than 10 months of age, which are affected by the acute onset of severe interstitial lung disease.
- respiratory distress is apparent, and the disease progresses rapidly.
- prognosis is poor, although foals surviving past the first 7–10 days are likely to recover.

Aetiology/pathophysiology

- cause is unknown:
  - o viral aetiology has been postulated based on:
    - ♦ characteristic histological lesions.
    - ♦ marked inflammatory infiltrates in the interstitium.
    - ♦ presence of multinucleated syncytial cells in some foals.

Clinical presentation

- acute onset of respiratory distress:
  - o marked tachypnoea.
  - o increased respiratory effort with nasal flare, and extended head and neck.
- foals are often febrile.
- auscultation of lung fields reveals reduced air movement with crackles and wheezes, apparent in areas where sufficient air movement remains.
- cough and nasal discharge are variably present.

Differential diagnosis

- includes bacterial pneumonia or pleuropneumonia, fungal pneumonia, and *Pneumocystis jiroveci* infection of immunocompromised foals.

Diagnosis

- laboratory findings include:
  - o neutrophilia, with or without a left shift, and elevated fibrinogen.

- blood gas analysis reveals hypoxaemia.
  - azotaemia may reflect dehydration secondary to reduced intake of fluids.
- thoracic ultrasonography characterised by diffuse irregularities of the pleural surface:
  - comet tails (Fig. 1.145).
- thoracic radiographs reveal:
  - prominent diffuse bronchointerstitial pattern which may coalesce into a diffuse nodular pattern (Fig. 1.146).
  - foals with underlying or secondary bacterial pneumonia can develop an alveolar pattern, typically in the ventral lung fields.
- tracheobronchial aspiration should be performed if the foal is stable enough:
  - cytological inflammation can be septic or non-septic.
  - bacterial culture may isolate a variety of bacteria including *S. zooepidemicus*, *R. equi*, or Gram-negative organisms.

Treatment

- foals most often require hospitalisation in a controlled climate, and provision of humidified intranasal oxygen.
- NSAIDs are recommended.
- systemic corticosteroids are used to reduce inflammation.
- bronchodilators, administered via inhalation, may be beneficial in some foals.
- address any underlying infections.

Prognosis

- poor for foals unless rapid and aggressive therapy is instituted.
- foals that survive the first week of medical treatment have a favourable prognosis.

Equine interstitial pneumonia (EIP)

Definition/overview

- group of lung disorders in adult horses characterised by diffuse interstitial tissue and alveolar wall inflammation.
- progressively reduced oxygen transfer from air to blood ultimately leads to respiratory distress due to hypoxaemia.
- broad category of pulmonary disease has several reported causes including:

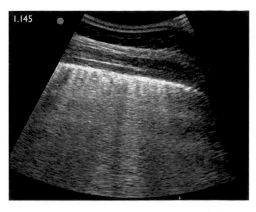

FIG. 1.145 Thoracic ultrasound from a foal with interstitial pneumonia. Diffuse comet tails (B-lines) are present in all lung fields.

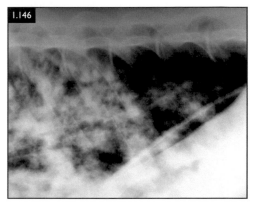

FIG. 1.146 Thoracic radiographs from a foal with interstitial pneumonia. A diffuse bronchointerstitial pattern coalesces into a diffuse nodular pattern.

  - hypersensitivity pneumonitis, toxic plant ingestion, and exposure to various infectious agents.
  - definitive cause not identified for many cases.
- subset of EIP is equine multinodular pulmonary fibrosis (EMPF):
  - viral aetiology has been suggested but has not been established.
  - EHV-2 and EHV-5 isolated from the lungs of affected animals at a higher rate than reported for normal horses.

Clinical presentation

- most common clinical signs are progressive weight loss and tachypnoea:
  - does not respond to antimicrobial therapy.

- o increased respiratory effort is present.
- o many horses present with a cough, and fever is commonly present with EMPF.
- laboratory findings are non-specific.

Differential diagnosis

- heaves, bacterial pneumonia or pleuropneumonia, fungal pneumonia, or neoplasia.

Diagnosis

- thoracic radiographs:
  - o horses with EIP will reveal a diffuse interstitial pattern.
  - o horses with EMPF:

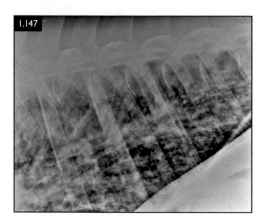

FIG. 1.147 Thoracic radiograph of the caudodorsal lung fields from an adult horse with EMPF. A diffuse interstitial pattern with coalescing patchy nodules is present.

- ◆ multiple nodular opacities commonly noted throughout all lung fields (Fig. 1.147).
- thoracic ultrasonography:
  - o EMPF cases reveal diffuse pleural roughening and multiple discrete nodules.
- tracheobronchial aspiration with culture, and BAL, are recommended to rule out infectious and non-infectious causes.
- detection of EHV-5 by PCR in BAL fluid of horses with pulmonary nodules is supportive of a diagnosis of EMPF.
- lung biopsy with histopathology is the most definitive means of diagnosing EIP:
  - o **considerable risk associated with the procedure.**

Treatment

- systemic corticosteroids are commonly used to limit inflammation and prevent further fibrosis.
- cases of EMPF, when EHV-2 and EHV-5 are identified:
  - o antiviral agents have been used (intravenous acyclovir or valcyclovir).

Prognosis

- cases commonly remain undiagnosed until the disease is advanced:
  - o prognosis is guarded to poor.
- recovery has been reported in a few horses with presumptive EMPF that were diagnosed and treated with corticosteroids and antiviral agents, early in the course of disease.

The Upper Gastrointestinal Tract

THE ORAL CAVITY

Introduction

Normal dentition and age-related changes

- horses have 24 deciduous teeth.
- Triadan system of dental nomenclature is used (Fig. 2.1).
- no deciduous molars.
- 1st premolar termed the 'wolf tooth' is variably present.
- each tooth is composed of an exposed clinical crown and a larger reserve crown:
  - latter is embedded in the bony alveolus.
- attrition at the occlusal surface occurs at 2–3 mm/year.

- equine teeth are composed of a laminate of three mineralised tissues:
  - enamel, dentine and cementum.
  - arranged around the dental pulp:
    - contains the nervous and vascular supply to the tooth.

Incisors

- simple rooted or brachydont teeth.
- each mandible and incisive bone contain three incisors:
  - close apposition to each other arranged in an approximate semicircle.
- opposing incisors meet closely to enable close cropping of grass.
- occlusal surface has a conical indentation – when worn appears as a ring of enamel:

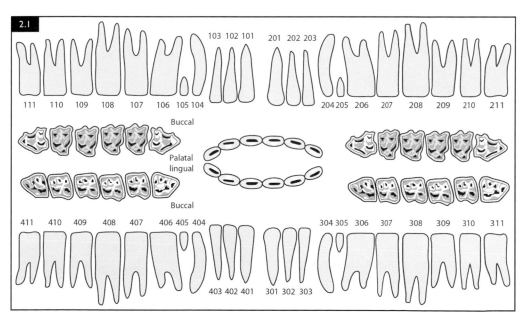

FIG. 2.1 Diagram showing Triadan dental nomenclature for Equidae.

DOI: 10.1201/9781003427711-2

- o infundibulum (*dental cup*) which varies with age.
- progressive attrition reveals the brown-stained secondary dentine:
  - o labial to the infundibulum.
  - o associated with the pulp cavity (*dental star*).

Canine teeth

- present in the male, and occasionally female.
- erupt between '03 and '06 teeth in the interdental space.
- lower canine is more rostral.
- brachydont teeth and sustain no occlusal attrition.
- reserve crown is sickle shaped and extends caudally towards the apex.

Premolars/molars

- 1st premolars (*wolf teeth*) are often rudimentary with a short reserve crown.
- found variably from middle of interdental space to closely apposed rostral to the second premolar.
- present in most horses and historically removed routinely often without evidence.
- remaining premolars and three molars (*cheek teeth*) differ between mandibular and maxillary arcades.
- **Maxillary** (Fig. 2.2):
  - o middle of the occlusal surface lie two crescent-shaped enamel infundibula:
    - ♦ lined with infundibular cement making them variable in appearance.
  - o ongoing attrition reveals dark areas of secondary dentine which overlies a pulp horn:
    - ♦ five on the '07–'10 teeth.
  - o first ('06) and sixth ('11) cheek teeth typically have an additional pulp horn at the rostral and caudal aspect, respectively.
  - o apices of '06, '07 and the rostral root of the '08 typically lie in the maxillary bone.
  - o remaining roots of '08 and all of '09 are closely associated with the rostral maxillary sinus.
  - o alveoli surrounding the apices of '10 and '11 lie in the caudal maxillary sinus.

- o position of the septum dividing rostral and caudal maxillary sinus can vary:
  - ♦ roots of '09 can lie in the caudal compartment in some horses.
- **Mandibular** (Fig. 2.3):
  - o no infundibula.
  - o '06 has six pulp horns.
  - o next four teeth in the mandibular arcade have five pulp horns.
  - o '11 has six pulp horns, and sometimes seven.
  - o apices of the mandibular cheek teeth lie in the mandible:
    - ♦ aligned in an approximately straight line.
- maxillary arcade is 23–30% wider than the mandibular arcade (*anisognathism*).

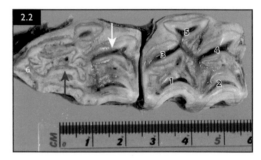

FIG. 2.2 Occlusal view of right maxillary dentition, teeth 106 and 107 showing occlusal secondary dentine (white arrow) overlying pulp horns (labelled 1–6) and infundibular enamel (red arrow).

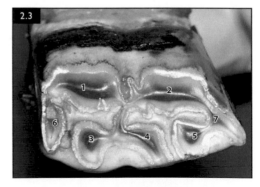

FIG. 2.3 Occlusal view of mandibular tooth 411 showing absence of infundibula and enamel, peripheral cement, primary and secondary dentine, overlying pulp horns numbered 1–7.

Age-related changes in the appearance of teeth with eruption and ageing

- eruption ages of equine teeth in the Thoroughbred are shown in Table 2.1.
- breed and individual variability.
- ageing by dentition has become obsolete for official records in many countries.
- physiological remodelling of ventral mandibular cortex in 2–3-year-old horses and ponies:
  - observed and palpated as bilaterally symmetrical, bony, non-painful swellings (*bumps*) overlying the apices of the '07s and '08s.
- similar corresponding swellings from maxillary modelling are less obvious due to the overlying muscles.

- both maxillary and mandibular swellings resolve with maturity.

Dental examination of the horse

- routine dental care involves:
  - regular dental examination.
  - correction of any dental lesions causing pain.
  - treatment of any pathology of dental structures and soft tissues.
  - aim is to restore normal occlusion and enable normal mastication.
- checklist for routine examination is listed below:
  - assess body condition.
  - observe while eating forage.
  - palpation:

TABLE 2.1 Eruption ages of equine teeth			
TOOTH	**TRIADAN NUMBER**	**ERUPTION AGE**	**IN WEAR**
Deciduous incisors			
Central	501	3 days	
Middle	502	3 weeks	
Corner	503	3 months	
Deciduous premolars			
1st cheek tooth	506	birth	
2nd cheek tooth	507	birth	
3rd cheek tooth	508	birth	
Permanent incisors			
Central	101 (2, 3, 401)	2.5 years	
Middle	102	3.5 years	
Corner	103	4.5 years	
Canines	104	5 years	
Permanent premolars			
1st premolar (wolf tooth)	105	2–2.5 years	
2nd premolar (1st cheek tooth)	106	2–2.5 years	2.5–3 years
3rd premolar (2nd cheek tooth)	107	3–3.5 years	3.5–4 years
4th premolar (3rd cheek tooth)	108	4 years	4.5 years
1st molar (4th cheek tooth)	109	1–1.5 years	1.5–2 years
2nd molar (5th cheek tooth)	110	2–2.5 years	2.5–3 years
3rd molar (6th cheek tooth)	111	3–3.5 years (later in miniature breeds)	3.5–4 years

- ◆ temporomandibular joints and temporal muscles.
- ◆ buccal molar arcades through cheeks.
- ◆ submandibular lymph nodes.
- ○ lateral movement of the mandible to check excursion (Fig. 2.4).
- ○ sedation allows for safer and more thorough examination:
  - ◆ alpha-2 antagonists combined with opiate partial agonists at standard doses.
  - ◆ support head on head-stand or suspended halter.

- ○ examination of the incisors on their lingual and occlusal aspects.
- ○ palpation of the bars of the mouth in the diastema.
- ○ application of gag (e.g. Hausmann's) (Fig. 2.5):
  - ◆ thorough visual examination of all four molar arcades:
    - – bright light source is essential.
    - – speculum or head-mounted.
  - ◆ digital palpation of each tooth if safe to do so:
    - – count the teeth to detect supernumerary teeth (Fig. 2.6).
- ○ detailed examination of occlusal surfaces of caudal cheek teeth can be performed using a dental mirror or oroscope (Fig. 2.7).
- ○ recording of observations and intended treatments.

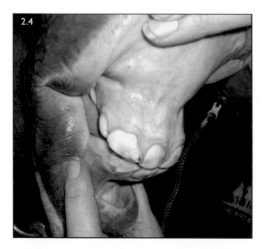

FIG. 2.4 Examination of the gums, soft tissues and 'lateral excursion' test.

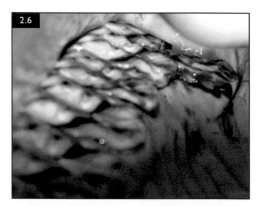

FIG. 2.6 Supernumerary distomolar in upper left (Triadan 2-) arcade.

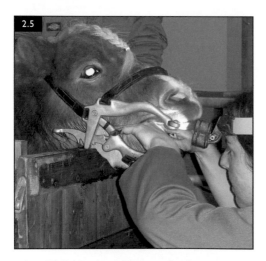

FIG. 2.5 Examination of the mouth of a pony using a Hauseman's speculum.

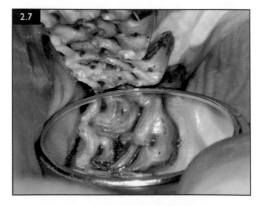

FIG. 2.7 Occlusal view using a dental mirror of a caries in an upper equine cheek tooth.

- perform dental treatments on molar arcades.
- remove gag.
- perform incisor treatments after removal of speculum.
- elevation of cheek to visualise buccal aspect of maxillary arcade.

Dental imaging
Radiography
- allows examination of the dental apices and surrounding alveolar bone.
- most portable machines have sufficient kV to obtain diagnostic images.
- portable and wireless digital systems have greatly increased the ease of image capture, the resolution of the images and image manipulation.
- sedation is essential to reduce head movement.
- support the head on a headstand, stool or hay bale.
- radiolucent rope halter avoids artefacts.
- adequate radiation protection and monitoring is mandatory:
  - lead gowns, thyroid shield and gloves/ sleeves.
  - always use cassette holders mounted on handles or suspended from a stand.
- primary beam should always be collimated to minimise exposure of any assistants.
- **Views:**
  - laterolateral (Fig. 2.8) projection:
    - sinus contents – cheek teeth superimposed.
  - lateral 30° dorsolateral oblique (L30°D-LO) (Fig. 2.9):
    - separates apices of maxillary cheek teeth allowing individual assessment.
  - lateral 45° ventrolateral oblique (L45°V-LO) (Fig. 2.10):
    - apices of the mandibular teeth.
  - dorsoventral (Fig. 2.11).
  - ventrodorsal or dorsoventral intraoral projections (Fig. 2.12):
    - apices of the incisors.
    - use plate protection.

Scintigraphy
- complements radiography.
- useful for diagnosis of suspected dental apical disease at an early stage.

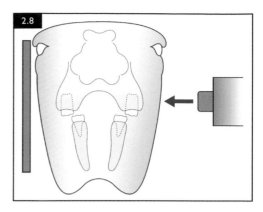

FIG. 2.8 Laterolateral projection.

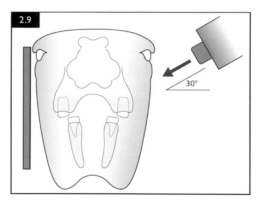

FIG. 2.9 Lateral 30° dorsolateral oblique projection.

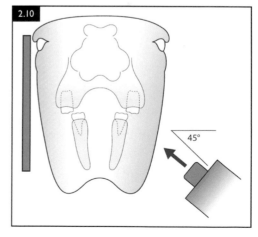

FIG. 2.10 Lateral 45° ventrolateral oblique projection.

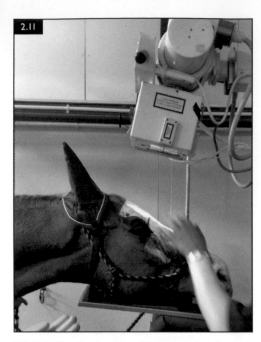

FIG. 2.11 Positioning for a dorsoventral radiograph using a gantry-mounted X-ray generator. Note the radiograph was taken after the hands were removed from the field of radiation.

Computed tomography (CT)
(Figs. 2.13, 2.14)

- standing sedated horses.
- detailed three-dimensional reconstruction.
- greater contrast, avoids superimposition, and increased sensitivity.

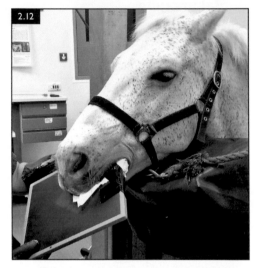

FIG. 2.12 Intraoral dorsoventral view of a horse's incisors using a computed radiography cassette.

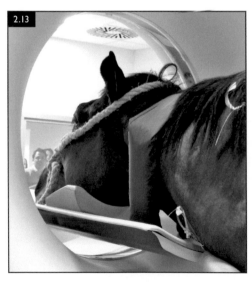

FIG. 2.13 A horse undergoing CT of the head while under standing sedation.

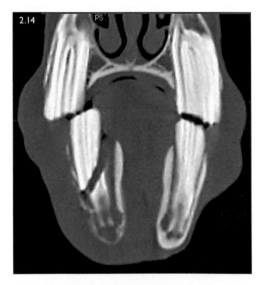

FIG. 2.14 transverse reconstruction of a horse with a fractured mandible involving a mandibular tooth.

DISEASES OF THE TEETH AND ORAL CAVITY

Conditions associated with development and eruption of teeth

- often detected in younger horses up to 4 years of age:
  - teeth erupting with deciduous dentition replaced by permanent dentition.
- anatomical abnormalities consequent to developmental abnormalities may have secondary consequences in older horses.

Cemental hypoplasia

Definition/overview

- developmental abnormalities in the infundibular cement:
  - predispose the tooth to degenerative diseases affecting the deeper layers.

Aetiology/pathophysiology

- cementum laid down in incisor and maxillary infundibula prior to eruption.
- seen in maxillary cheek teeth:
  - cementosis is frequently incomplete but may appear normal from occlusal view.
  - cemental defect only appears after several years of wear as occlusal caries.
  - 109 and 209 appear most affected.
- mandibular occlusal caries is rare (absence of infundibula).
- peripheral cemental hypoplasia is diagnosed in mandibular and maxillary teeth:
  - often observed in conjunction with periodontal disease.

Clinical presentation

- infundibular pocket on occlusal surface of maxillary cheek teeth:
  - may become packed with food.
  - discolouration indicates caries of the cementum.
  - described as infundibular necrosis and cemental caries.
- teeth with cemental hypoplasia are more predisposed to caries (Fig. 2.15):
  - penetrates deeper through the enamel into the dentine.

- predisposes to weakness and fracturing of the tooth through the infundibula.
- deep caries can occasionally extend apically resulting in pulpitis.

Differential diagnosis

- hypoplasia is diagnosed when it leads to caries of the occlusal infundibula.

Diagnosis

- careful oral examination demonstrates friable cementum and pitting:
  - use of dental probes (Fig. 2.16):
    - ◆ confirms depth of the defect.
  - oral endoscopy (Fig. 2.17).
  - CT can reveal cemental hypoplasia apically that is not exposed occlusally.

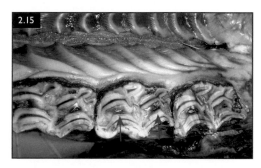

FIG. 2.15 A post-mortem specimen showing caries (grade 2) of maxillary infundibula (arrows).

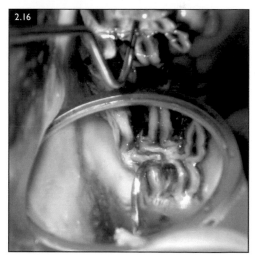

FIG. 2.16 Using a probe and mirror to clear a packed infundibular defect.

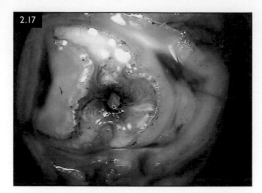

FIG. 2.17 Occlusal oroscopic view of an infundibulum showing grade 1 caries (within physiologically normal limits).

Management

- may be clinically insignificant but can predispose to caries.
- teeth with advanced caries usually require removal by:
  - extraction, repulsion or buccotomy.
- debridement and restoration of carious infundibula may delay progression to tooth fracture.

Oligodontia/hypodontia

Definition/overview

- Oligodontia is the loss or absence of multiple teeth in an arcade or row.
- Hypodontia is a subnormal number of teeth in a row (absence of an individual tooth).

Aetiology/pathophysiology

- occasionally observed and most acquired cases result from:
  - acquired tooth loss following periodontal disease in aged horses.
  - interventional exodontia.
  - after trauma in younger animals:
    - acquired incisor oligodontia in the young horse.
    - injury to developing permanent secondary dentition prior to eruption.
- following loss of a tooth, migration of the adjacent teeth occurs:
  - can result in complete obliteration of the interproximal space.

- shortening of overall length of the arcade.
- developmental hypodontia occurs in certain breeds:
  - quite common where conspicuous overcrowding of teeth:
  - Shetland ponies and Welsh Section A ponies.

Clinical presentation

- presents as a malocclusion subsequent to uneven wear due to the absence of a tooth.
- secondary dental disorders, including periodontitis, can ensue.

Diagnosis

- careful oral examination in conjunction with oral endoscopy (to count the teeth):
  - loss of a cheek tooth in a mature horse frequently leads to:
    - digitally palpable space between the remaining teeth.
    - invagination of the empty alveolus with fibrous tissue/bone/oral epithelium.
  - super-eruption of opposing tooth can occur in the opposing arcade.
- radiography may be useful especially if delayed dental eruption is observed.

Management

- more frequent reduction of overgrowths in the super-erupting and adjacent teeth may be required – every 4–6 months.
- developmental hypodontia may be clinically insignificant:
  - malocclusion is likely unless it is symmetrical.

Polydontia (hyperdontia)

Definition/overview

- extra (supernumerary) dentition in the arcade exceeding the normal dental formula.
- consequence of retained deciduous dentition or developmental poly- or hyperdontia.

Aetiology/pathophysiology

- retained deciduous incisors are a common finding during routine dental examinations:

- during normal eruption, permanent incisors emerge on palatal and labial aspects of deciduous counterparts:
  - ♦ latter are shed due to the emergence of the permanent dentition.
  - occasionally, after the permanent incisors erupt the temporary incisors are left displaced labially and retaining the gingival attachments (Fig. 2.18).
- temporary premolars are commonly retained in young horses:
  - due to compression in a rostrocaudal direction along the arcade.
  - results in failure of the deciduous teeth or 'caps' to be shed.
  - most commonly the deciduous 07s and 08s are retained.
  - accumulation of ingesta underneath the shell-like caps can exaggerate the mild periodontitis associated with normal eruption, resulting in painful gingivitis.
- some breeds such as the Welsh Section A:
  - obstruction of the eruption pathway due to permanent premolar impaction.
  - leads to retained deciduous premolars.
- permanent hyper-/polydontia occurs most commonly in the maxillary arcade:
  - bilateral symmetrical supernumerary distomolars are sometimes observed (see Fig. 2.6).
  - incisor polydontia and hyperdontia of the mandibular teeth also occur.
  - permanent hyperdontia can lead to maleruptions, impactions and periodontal disease:
    - ♦ some cases can remain asymptomatic until an advanced age (Fig. 2.19).

Clinical presentation

- deciduous teeth may resemble the erupting teeth on the occlusal view:
  - labial aspect of the incisor tooth appears much smaller.
  - gingiva appearing to expose less clinical crown.
- retention of deciduous premolars common finding in racing Thoroughbreds:
  - reluctance to perform is sometimes attributed to retention.
- permanent hyper- or polydontia can be noted incidentally on an oral examination or due to clinical signs associated with secondary consequences.

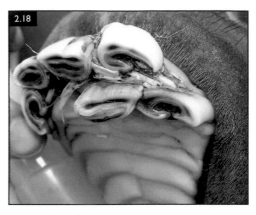

FIG. 2.18 Misaligned supernumerary incisors.

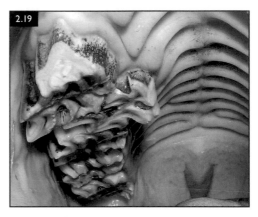

FIG. 2.19 Orthograde view of a supernumerary maxillary molar with areas of reduced wear causing sharp 'overgrowths'.

Diagnosis

- thorough oral examination should reveal retained deciduous dentition without gingival attachments.
- supernumerary teeth are often overlooked on an oral examination and can be diagnosed incidentally when radiographs are viewed.

Management/prognosis

- retained deciduous incisors:
  - sedation and local analgesia.
  - periodontal attachments are separated with a flat or curved elevator.
  - tooth extracted easily using a small single-handed dental cap extractor.
  - excellent prognosis.

- deciduous premolar caps:
  - premature extraction may expose the occlusal surface of the permanent dentition before maturation of the cementum.
    - ♦ potentially an increased risk of caries.
  - removal of retained caps may be indicated but only if:
    - ♦ division between the temporary and permanent dentition can be palpated on the buccal/palatal aspect of the tooth.
    - ♦ under sedation using cap extraction forceps.
    - ♦ **beware palatine artery with maxillary caps:**
      - **– rotate in ventromedial direction.**
- permanent supernumerary dentition:
  - can be asymptomatic and exodontia may be contraindicated.
  - clinically significant cases, dental removal is indicated:
    - ♦ complicated by impaction and overcrowding by additional teeth.

Brachygnathia and prognathia

Definition/overview

- relative asymmetric growth rate between rostral mandible and incisive bone:
  - overshot (Class 2 malocclusion) (Fig. 2.20).

  - undershot incisive bone (Class 3 malocclusion) (Fig. 2.21).

Aetiology/pathophysiology

- Brachygnathism or parrot mouth (Class 2 malocclusion) is a common disorder:
  - incisive bone overgrows the rostral mandible causing a malocclusion.
  - maxillary incisors lie rostral to the mandibular ones:
    - ♦ no occlusion or partial occlusion in milder cases.
  - heritability is unclear but low:
    - ♦ autosomal dominant with low penetration and multifactorial.
- Prognathism or sow mouth (Class 3 malocclusion) is a rare condition:
  - incisive bone grows less rapidly than the mandible resulting in 'underbite'.
  - more common in Shetlands and miniatures.

Clinical presentation

- suckling may be impaired in young foals.
- grazing may be impaired where there is no incisor occlusion (termed severe 'overjet'):
  - most horses compensate sufficiently for a satisfactory weight gain.
- usually diagnosed in foals.
- cosmetic appearance may be prejudicial to a show career.
- occlusion of the cheek teeth is usually not affected and normal mastication is possible.

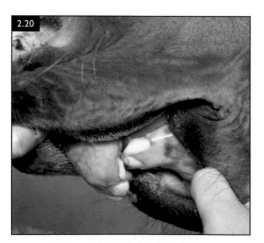

FIG. 2.20 Class 2 malocclusion described as parrot mouth or overbite.

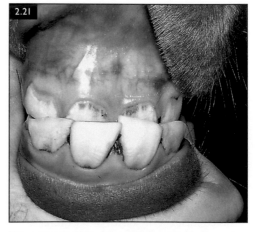

FIG. 2.21 Class 3 malocclusion with the lower jaw undershot and overgrowth of the lower incisors.

Differential diagnosis

- trauma to the rostral mandible and wry nose.

Diagnosis

- clinical oral examination and radiography (Fig. 2.22).
- occasionally, the deviation occurs caudal to the interdental space and CT can be helpful to reveal caudal malocclusions.

Management

- mild cases may be clinically insignificant or improve spontaneously.
- severe cases will require orthodontic correction:
  - maximum benefit is derived by early correction (from 1 to 3 months of age) while growth of the bone is rapid.
  - weight loss may occur post-surgery and attentive nursing is necessary to ensure food ingestion is maintained.
  - growth rate of the bones slows after 9–12 months limiting degree of correction.
- careful attention to incisor alignment may be necessary during the animal's life to prevent lesions on the mandibular gingiva from the impingement of the upper incisors.

Campylorrhinus lateralis (Wry nose)

Definition/overview

- major congenital deformity of the face (Fig. 2.23).

Aetiology/pathophysiology

- due to an asymmetric dysplasia of the incisive bone and maxilla on one side:
  - lateral deviation of the nostrils to the affected side.
  - can involve the nasal septum and maxillary and palatine bones.
- no breed predisposition although Arab foals appear overrepresented.
- heritability is unproven.
- suggested that fetal malpositioning may be a contributing factor.

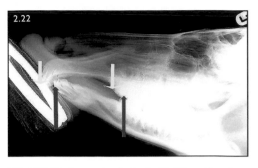

FIG. 2.22 Radiograph of a foal with Class 2 malocclusion resulting from mandibular brachygnathism (yellow arrows, upper jaw; red arrows, lower jaw).

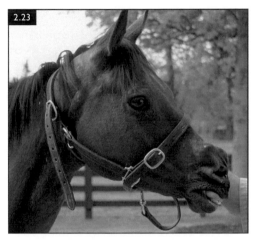

FIG. 2.23 A Thoroughbred mare with wry nose, which, unusually, has been reared and used for breeding. Such animals do not appear consistently to produce offspring with the same defect.

Clinical presentation

- immediately identifiable at birth by clinical examination and may result in:
  - severe airflow obstruction.
  - incisor and premolar malocclusions and difficulty in feeding.
- examine foal for other congenital abnormalities, including axial and appendicular deformities.

Differential diagnosis

- Brachygnathism and trauma.

Diagnosis

- clinical appearance and radiography.

- CT demonstrates the extent of the lesions most thoroughly to enable rational decisions on the foal's viability.

Management

- major reconstructive surgery has been reported.
- many neonates are euthanased when the deformity is identified.

Heterotropic polydontia (Dentigerous cysts)

Definition/overview

- anatomically inappropriate dental tissue.

Aetiology/pathophysiology

- well-recognised lesion involving the presence of ectopic dental tissue containing rudimentary enamel and other dental elements.
- abnormality can present at any age and is often coincidental with the age of eruption of the teeth (usually less than 3 years).
- cyst is lined by stratified squamous epithelium and goblet cells:
  - secrete a seromucinous fluid.
  - commonly discharges through a duct onto the skin.
- degree of development and organisation of the dental elements varies:
  - minimal mineralisation of the cyst.
  - partially molarised, rudimentary teeth.
- lesion is derived from the first branchial arch, which is displaced into the temporal region.

Clinical presentation

- present as non-painful swellings over the temporal bone.
- characteristically have a duct discharging mucoid or mucopurulent exudates from an orifice at the base or edge of the pinna (Figs. 2.24, 2.25).

Differential diagnosis

- discharging sinus tracts, sequestra, and skull fractures.

Diagnosis

- position of the cyst can make radiography awkward:

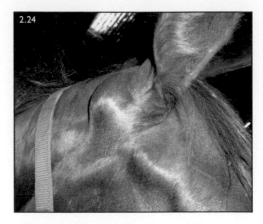

FIG. 2.24 Dentigerous cysts can present as swellings at the base of the pinna.

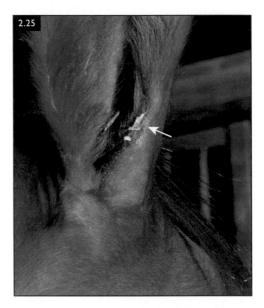

FIG. 2.25 The tract discharging from the base of the pinna in this horse (arrow) is typical in cases of dentigerous cyst.

  - lesion-orientated oblique projections complement the standard views.
- ultrasonography can be useful.
- CT scans are very useful to reveal the extent, size, anatomical associations, and depth of the lesion:
  - invaluable when considering or planning treatment.

Management

- surgical excision of the lesion including its entire cystic lining is effective in symptomatic cases.
- recurrence is rare following complete removal of the cyst lining.
- redevelopment of a secretory and discharging epithelial-lined sinus tract can occur if remnants remain.

Rudimentary teeth ('wolf teeth')

Definition/overview

- presence of vestigial brachydont 1st premolars (Fig. 2.26).

Aetiology/pathophysiology

- 1st upper premolar (105, 205) commonly present in both male and female horses:
  ○ vestigial 'wolf teeth' are present in an estimated 20–60% of horses.
  ○ usually in contact with 106 and 206 but rarely in occlusion.
  ○ occasionally, molarised 105s and 205s are present (Fig. 2.27).
- traditional practice has been to remove the wolf teeth:
  ○ reduced performance and bit sensitivity have been attributed to discomfort associated with the impingement of the bit over the wolf teeth.
  ○ little/no supportive evidence in most cases of normally situated vestigial wolf teeth.
  ○ recent practice of excessive rasping of the buccorostral aspects of the 106 and 206 to create 'bit seats' is said to be impaired by the presence of wolf teeth:
    ♦ scientific merit of this practice is unclear and may not justify extraction of wolf teeth.
  ○ appropriate to extract the whole vestigial tooth where:
    ♦ teeth are mandibular.
    ♦ prominent.
    ♦ erupting in a rostral or buccal position.
    ♦ clear indication of pain over an unerupted tooth.
    ♦ bit impingement.
- entrapment of the buccal mucosa between the bit and the wolf tooth or rostrolateral

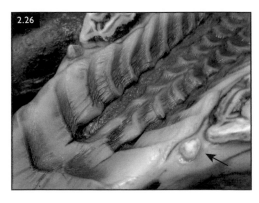

FIG. 2.26 Specimen showing a normally positioned wolf tooth (Triadan 205, arrow).

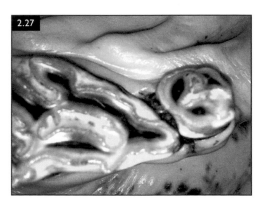

FIG. 2.27 Wolf teeth occasionally can be large and molarised with multiple pulp horns.

aspect of the 2nd premolar can result in discomfort:
  ○ consequently, a lack of responsiveness on the bridle is attributed to the presence of the wolf tooth, whether implicated or not.

Clinical presentation/diagnosis

- palpation and visual examination of the rostral arcade will reveal the presence of erupted or subgingival wolf teeth.
- radiography is advised in abnormally situated or extremely large teeth.

Management

- wolf tooth removal is easily accomplished in the field:
  ○ sedation of the horse using an alpha-2 agonists.

- o local analgesia of the tooth is advised using:
  - ♦ infraorbital nerve block.
  - ♦ local subgingival infiltration of mepivacaine.
  - ♦ topical application of cinchocaine to the gingival mucosa.
- o gingiva is elevated from all around the tooth using:
  - ♦ circular Burgess-type elevator or small curve-bladed periodontal elevator.
- o aberrantly placed teeth or very large wolf teeth should be radiographed to assess:
  - ♦ size and placement of the apical portion before attempts at extraction.
  - ♦ very large molarised wolf teeth may require extensive periodontal separation before sufficiently loose to extract.
- o once periodontal elevation is completed the tooth can be extracted using a small pair of incisor or specialised wolf tooth extractors.
- o subgingival wolf teeth can be exposed by a small incision in the overlying gingival mucosa:
  - ♦ periodontal attachments carefully loosened using an osteotome pointing caudally between the rostrally angled tooth and the hard palate (Fig. 2.28).
  - ♦ alveolus can be packed with gel foam/gauze to prevent food impaction, although this is rarely necessary.
  - ♦ failure to loosen the periodontium sufficiently can result in fracture of the tooth.
  - ♦ remaining sharp fragments should be elevated and removed to enable healing of the alveolus.
  - ♦ subgingival apical fragments rarely cause clinical signs:
    - – loose fragments may be removed after several days.
    - – usually migrate to a more superficial position.
- o mandibular lower 1st premolars (Triadan 305, 405) are rare:
  - ♦ can usually be palpated on the ventral mandible rostral to the first cheek tooth (Fig. 2.29).

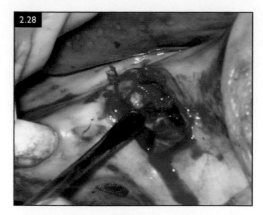

FIG. 2.28 After elevation of the gingiva, the periodontium is separated with luxators.

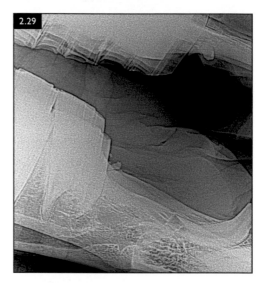

FIG. 2.29 A laterolateral radiograph of the cranial part of the mouth demonstrating wolf teeth within both the upper and lower jaws.

- ♦ commonly small but vary in size and position.
- ♦ more likely to be associated with discomfort with the bit.
- ♦ noteworthy observation during pre-purchase examinations.
- ♦ technique for removal is as described previously.

Maleruption

Definition/overview

- misalignment of teeth within an arcade due to asymmetric or delayed eruption.

Aetiology/pathophysiology

- eruption of permanent cheek teeth to replace the primary dentition is a carefully coordinated sequence of events.
- disturbances leading to:
  - alteration of the position of the permanent tooth buds.
  - anatomical variations and relative shortening of the maxilla or mandible.
- can result in impaction of the erupting tooth and consequent disease processes:
  - displacement during eruption, with subsequent misalignment of the tooth arcade.
  - predispose to apical compression with resultant hypoxic ischaemia.

Clinical presentation

- maleruption resulting in misalignment is commonly bilateral.
- careful inspection for early signs of misalignment should be performed at each dental examination:
  - consequences of misalignment are malocclusion with the opposing arcade:
    - ◆ development of focal overgrowths and diastema (gaps), between the adjacent teeth in the row.
    - ◆ loss of the close association between adjacent teeth.
    - ◆ enables accumulation of food adjacent to the gingival sulcus.
    - ◆ destructive bacteria in periodontal pockets.
    - ◆ causes gingivitis, gingival recession and peripheral cemental caries.
  - painful, with affected horses often exhibiting signs including:
    - ◆ slow eating and quidding (oral dysphagia).
    - ◆ chronic cases, development of periodontitis.

Diagnosis

- oral examination will reveal maleruptions, misalignment, and consequences.
- radiography may be indicated to demonstrate:
  - secondary consequences such as impacted teeth (Fig. 2.30).
  - deep periodontal disease or caries.

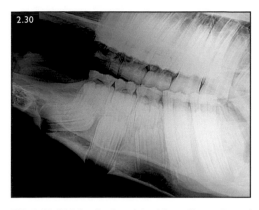

FIG. 2.30 306 is displaced in this radiograph and its maleruption could impede the normal eruption of 307.

Management

- treatment of the secondary consequence is often indicated.
- extraction of individual malerupted teeth may be part of the management.

Acquired dental disease

Diastema leading to periodontitis

Definition/overview

- diastema is an inappropriate space between two teeth of the same type:
  - pathological in Equidae if it results in food retention and periodontitis.
- diastemata often occur in multiple sites, especially between the mandibular cheek teeth.
- periodontitis is inflammation of the periodontal tissues, including the periodontium, +/– gingivitis.

Aetiology/pathophysiology

- primary periodontitis is rare in the horse.
- plaque accumulation has not been identified as a major factor in this species.
- extensive periodontitis usually accompanies the presence of diastemata:
  - possibly due to misalignment or age-related loss of mesiodistal compression.
  - allows the development of periodontal food pockets.

- ○ allows pathogenic bacteria to accumulate in the gingival sulcus:
  - ♦ results in gingivitis and periodontitis (Figs. 2.31–2.33).

Clinical presentation

- clinical history may include:
  - ○ slow eating, spilling food, and difficulty with mastication of long-fibre diets.
  - ○ weight loss.

Diagnosis

- oral examination, including use of a dental mirror:

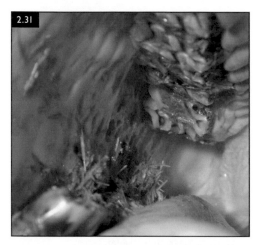

FIG. 2.31 Food entrapped between the teeth on an oral examination signals periodontal disease.

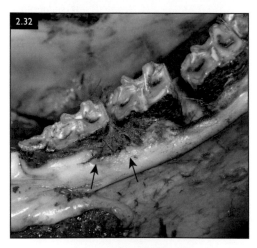

FIG. 2.32 A valve diastema with occlusal contact, and packed food trapped at the gingival margin causing inflammation (arrows).

- ○ identify food trapped in periodontal pockets.
  - ○ common in aged horses:
    - ♦ reduced areas of periodontal attachment and short reserve crowns.
    - ♦ physiological reduction in the mesiodistal compression.
  - ○ chronic cases may have multiple teeth which are loose on palpation.
- advanced cases reveal chronic sclerosis of the dental alveolus on radiography or CT.

Management

- aim of therapy is to:
  - ○ reduce periodontal food accumulation.
  - ○ treat alveolar periodontitis.
  - ○ remove any dental overgrowths and transverse ridges:
    - ♦ allowing normal occlusion and mastication.
  - ○ remove grossly loose teeth that have no periodontal attachments.
- treatment of widespread periodontitis associated with diastemata is variably successful:
  - ○ effective long-term management is usually possible:
    - ♦ focused lavage of the interdentium after removal of gross food accumulation.
    - ♦ followed by debridement of the periodontal pockets with:
      - – water, descaling or air abrasion devices (Fig. 2.34).

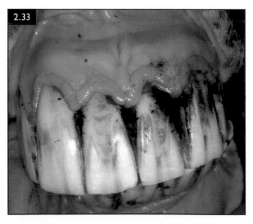

FIG. 2.33 Diastema and resulting gum recession with incisor periodontitis.

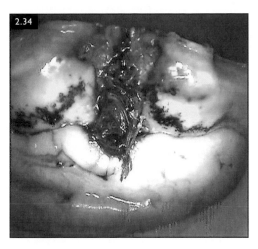

FIG. 2.34 Gingival recession due to periodontitis underneath the putrefying food.

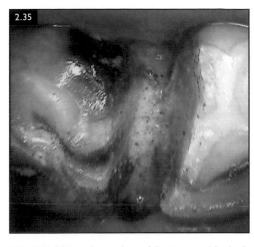

FIG. 2.35 After odontoplasty (diastema widening), entrapped food is removed allowing debridement of the periodontal lesions.

♦ followed by widening of the diastema to enable food release.
♦ temporary stenting of the periodontal pockets with acrylic materials may give an improvement in clinical signs (Figs. 2.35, 2.36).
- treatment augmented with systemic antibiotics and antiseptic mouthwash solutions.
- diastema due to focal misalignment or maleruption:
  ○ dental removal may be effective in relieving the diastema.
- feeding of reduced long-fibre food.
- above treatments often result in clinical improvement:
  ○ recurrence is highly probable.
  ○ constant management is the usual outcome rather than any clinical cure.

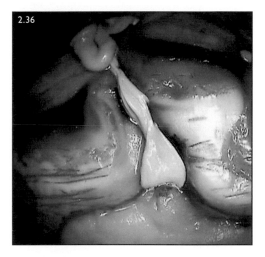

FIG. 2.36 Once the diastema is debrided, food re-entry can be impeded by temporary stenting using polyvinyl siloxane.

Dental pulpitis

Definition/overview
- infection of the apical pulp of the tooth, which manifests as localised pulpitis with ensuing caries.
- incisors, canines, and cheek teeth can be affected.
- other terms: apical infections, apical necrosis, and tooth root abscessation.

Aetiology/pathophysiology
- bacterial contamination of the dentinopulp complex, leading to inflammation.
- oedema of the pulp in the dental pulp cavity results in:
  ○ congestion and irreversible ischaemic necrosis of the pulp.
  ○ results in suppuration, causing a periapical coronitis:

♦ some cases a gingival, submandibular or facial discharging tract.
- caudal maxillary teeth tend to suppurate into the sinus leading to a maxillary sinusitis.
- dental apical infections are the most common endodontic lesion of equine teeth (Fig. 2.37):
  ○ incisors and canines are infrequently affected.
  ○ cheek tooth pulpitis is observed in all types of horses.
  ○ most common at 3–5 years of age for mandibular teeth:
    ♦ 307, 308, 407, and 408 are the most affected in the lower jaw.
  ○ 2–7 years of age for maxillary cheek teeth:
    ♦ 108, 109, 208, and 209 are the most affected in the upper jaw.
- aetiology of dental apical infections is unclear, and they may be slightly different in maxillary and mandibular teeth.
- suggested possible pathways include:
  ○ anachoretic (blood-borne) inoculation of the pulp.
  ○ infundibular cemental hypoplasia may predispose to apical infection.
  ○ bacterial contamination after penetration of the porous dentine on the occlusal surface, or subsequent to fissure fractures.
  ○ congenital enamel defects predisposing to structural weakness and resulting fractures may allow pulp infection.
- probably painful initially, but many chronic cases are apparently non-painful.

Clinical presentation

- unilateral maxillary and mandibular swellings are typical (Fig. 2.38):
  ○ ipsilateral submandibular lymphadenopathy.
- apical infections can abscessate:
  ○ discharge through tracts in the thin ventral mandible for affected lower teeth.
  ○ maxillary infections rarely discharge through the maxillary bone:
    ♦ except after aspiration or trephination over the swelling is attempted.
- caudal (Triadan 08–11) maxillary apical infections frequently discharge into the maxillary sinuses:
  ○ sinus empyema.
  ○ rostral maxillary, caudal maxillary or ventral conchal sinuses.
  ○ depending on which tooth and dental roots are involved.
  ○ usually present with a malodorous unilateral nasal discharge.

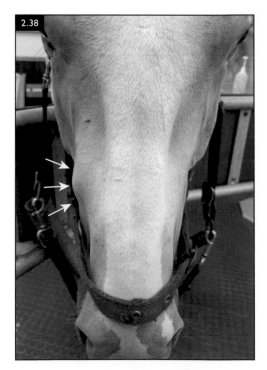

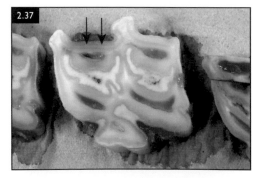

FIG. 2.37 This section of an extracted tooth shows four vital pulp horns with one single necrotic pulp (arrows).

FIG. 2.38 A unilateral maxillary swelling typical of apical pulpitis of the maxillary premolars (arrows).

- rare to have more than a single tooth involved.
- suppuration is usually localised to a single dental root:
  - necrosis of multiple root pulps may occur due to pulp communication.

Differential diagnosis

- mandibular fractures, dental cysts, primary maxillary sinusitis (if nasal discharge present) and traumatic lesions.

Diagnosis

- complete oral and dental examination:
  - occlusal exploration with a probe will reveal dentinal occlusal fissures in over 50% of cases:
    - considered significant, especially in conjunction with diagnostic imaging changes (Fig. 2.39).
  - gross caries and pathological dental fracture can be observed in some cases.
- diagnosis confirmed radiographically or by CT (Figs. 2.40, 2.41):
  - multiple radiographic projections in the standing sedated horse including:
    - lateral, lateral 30° dorsolateral and dorsoventral views.
  - radiographic changes associated with dental apical infections include:
    - presence of a radiolucency of the affected apex.
    - often surrounded by region of radiopaque sclerotic bone (chronic cases).
    - subtle indications of infection of the apex include:
      - loss of definition and widening of the periodontal space.
      - loss of the lamina dura denta.
    - occasionally in chronic infection, a granular radiopacity is observed ('coral pattern' or dental rhinitis) in the nasal cavity:
      - dystrophic mineralisation in the nasal conchae.
  - dorsoventral projections are useful for imaging periodontal remodelling on:
    - buccal aspects of the maxillary cheek teeth.
    - lingual aspects of the mandibular teeth.

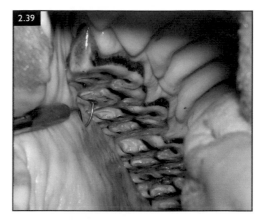

FIG. 2.39 A fissure in the secondary dentine raises suspicion of exposure of the underlying pulp.

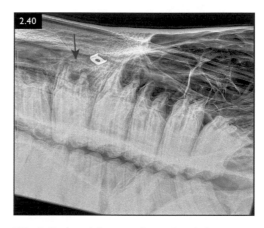

FIG. 2.40 An oblique radiograph of the upper molars on the right side. Note the distorted caudal root of 108 with surrounding maxillary bone lysis (arrow).

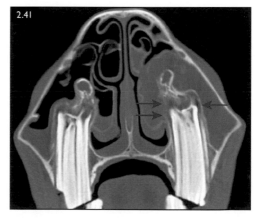

FIG. 2.41 Transverse CT reconstruction showing maxillary 09s with buccal fractures and apical pulpitis of 109 (arrows).

- comparison with the contralateral tooth may help detect subtle apical changes.
- chronic cases of mandibular apical infections with a discharging tract:
  - ♦ additional radiographs after placing a radiopaque marker into the tract.
  - ♦ help identify the tooth and root involved (Fig. 2.42).
- sinus empyema may reveal fluid lines on erect lateral radiographs.
- radiographs are neither very sensitive nor specific in detecting early dental apical disease.
- additional ancillary techniques such as CT are more sensitive:
  - ♦ practised routinely in standing horses.
  - ♦ desirable if endodontic treatments are to be considered.
- scintigraphy has been shown to be sensitive for detecting dental apical infections:
  - ♦ poor specificity of scintigraphy does not enable lesions to be distinguished from localised primary sinus empyema.

Management

- young horses with wider apical foraminae:
  - long-term (2–4 weeks) antibiotic therapy using broad-spectrum antimicrobials:
    - ♦ trimethoprim–sulphadiazine and/or metronidazole administered p/o.
    - ♦ can result in clinical remission.

- older horses with narrow apical foramina:
  - only a transient clinical improvement in response to antibiotics:
    - ♦ nidus of infected necrotic pulp remains in the pulp cavity.
- apical curettage and drainage of mandibular apical infections:
  - outcome has been variable.
- endodontic root canal filling for cheek teeth apical infections has been reported:
  - limited success but improving with:
    - ♦ better diagnosis.
    - ♦ earlier intervention/imaging.
    - ♦ increased technical skill.
  - salvage of the tooth is attractive as exodontia has consequences.
- many cases, the infected tooth will require removal by:
  - oral extraction, repulsion or lateral alveolar buccotomy (Figs. 2.43, 2.44).

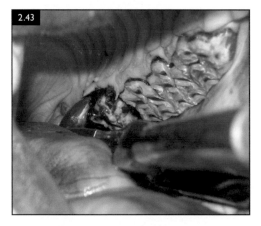

FIG. 2.43 Diseased teeth can be extracted orally with the horse sedated and using local analgesia techniques.

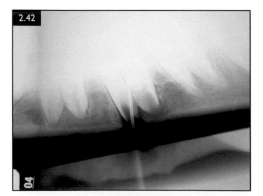

FIG. 2.42 Lateral 45° oblique radiograph of the ventral mandible of a 7-year-old horse showing a radiopaque probe placed in a draining mandibular tract, which is demarcating the infected root of the apex of cheek tooth 208.

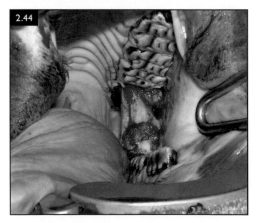

FIG. 2.44 The tooth is extracted along its eruption pathway with minimal damage to the alveolus.

Dental caries

Definition/overview

- consequence of the action of cariogenic bacteria on mineralised dental tissues in the presence of a carbohydrate substrate.
- known as tooth decay in humans.

Aetiology/pathogenesis

- occurs in the infundibula of incisors and maxillary teeth and peripherally on the buccal cementum.
- sites are prone to chronic contact with impacted food.
- diet may affect the pH in the local environment.
- epidemiology of equine cariogenic bacteria is not well understood:
  - presence of a biofilm (plaque) less prominent role than in brachydont teeth.
  - variations in infundibular morphology, presence of concurrent dysmastication or periodontitis are probable risk factors, along with feeding lower pH foods.

Clinical presentation

- affected teeth may be asymptomatic.
- sequential demineralisation of peripheral and occlusal cementum, progressing into enamel and eventually into dentine (Fig. 2.45).

- graded according to a modified Honma scale.
- structural weakening occurs once enamel is affected:
  - can lead to dental fracture under normal masticatory forces.
- penetration into the dentine, which is porous, can result in pulpitis.
- rate of progression is highly variable:
  - advanced grade 3 caries (involving dentine) is clinically significant.

Diagnosis

- detailed oral examination:
  - occlusal and peripheral dental observation:
    - signs of pitting, discolouration, and demineralisation of dental tissues.
  - oroscopic examination will reveal greater detail of any damage:
    - particularly if used in combination with a fissure probe (Fig. 2.46).

Differential diagnoses

- dental fracture.
- normal wear patterns.

Management

- indications for management are currently poorly defined.
- grade 3 caries that involves discolouration of dentine probably structurally significant.

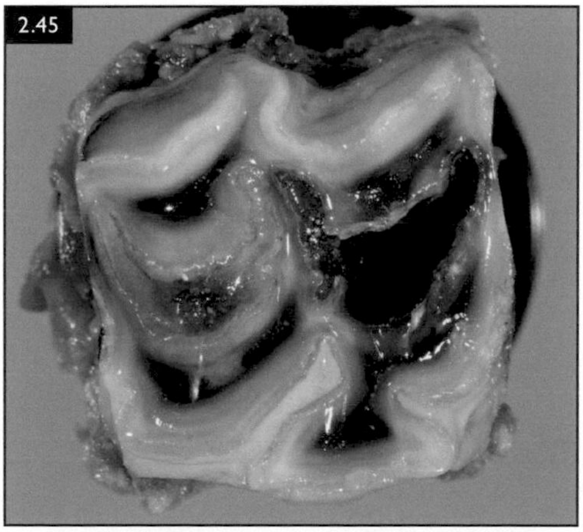

FIG. 2.45 This tooth has grade 3 infundibular caries that can structurally weaken the tooth, leading to parasagittal fracture.

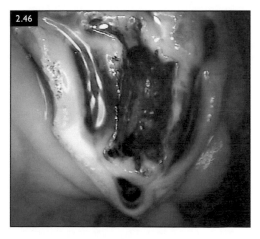

FIG. 2.46 Oroscopic view of a tooth afflicted with grade 2 infundibular cemental caries.

- argument for treating grade 2 lesions:
  - prevent progression leading to pathological dental fractures:
  - debridement of diseased tissues using high-speed burrs, files, and abrasion:
  - combined with full etch and bonding with restoration dental composites.
  - efficacy in the long term is currently unproven.
- teeth with peripheral caries may benefit from debridement:
  - dietary management and concurrent treatment of periodontitis.

Dental fracture

Definition

- fracture involving a tooth.

Aetiology

- trauma:
  - involve transverse fractures to incisors or avulsion injuries involving the rostral mandible or incisive bones.
- pathological fractures of teeth predisposed by:
  - affliction with overgrowths, caries or pulpitis.
- simple fractures involving peripheral cementum and enamel may be clinically asymptomatic.
- complex fractures involve dentine or pulp chambers.
- cheek tooth compound fractures usually occur in a plane coalescing two pulp horns or two infundibula with subsequent pulpitis.
- pathologicial dental fractures occur commonly in the maxillary cheek teeth:
  - 109 and 209 are most involved (Fig. 2.47).

Clinical presentation

- compound fractures are painful initially.
- incisor fractures will often present with bleeding from the lips.
- chronic cheek tooth fracture:
  - displacement of fragments leading to mucosal trauma.
  - often painful and associated with mucosal ulceration.
- many latent dental fractures are detected on routine examinations:
  - clinical signs may have been overlooked.

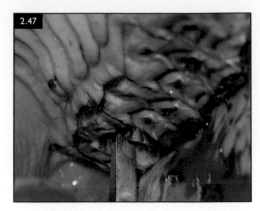

FIG. 2.47 Fractured teeth can be challenging to remove and are not always identified early.

Diagnosis

- detailed oral examination including oroscopic.
- radiography.
- CT.

Differential diagnosis

- Supernumerary teeth.

Treatment

Incisor fractures

- often the result of external trauma, such as kicks and avulsion forces.
- usually transverse and expose the pulp cavity (Fig. 2.48).

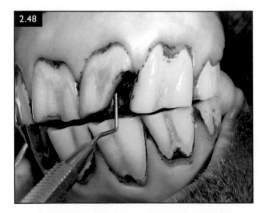

FIG. 2.48 Incisor fractures often expose the pulp and can be very sensitive.

- first aid of exposed pulps can involve application of calcium hydroxide paste (within 48 h of the fracture).
- fractured teeth can be extracted, or restoration attempted.

Cheek teeth fractures

- almost invariably pathological fractures of teeth with pulpitis, caries or excessive overgrowths.
- treatment depends on the fracture plane and the consequences of the fracture:
  - simple buccal slab fractures that occur in mandibular and maxillary teeth:
    - removal of the fragment.
    - leave the remainder of the tooth *in situ* but reduce it from occlusion.
    - provided pulp exposure has not occurred, horses can remain asymptomatic for many years.
- complex fractures are more common in maxillary teeth:
  - consequence of:
    - advanced caries when fracture occurs coalescing infundibula.
    - after pulpitis when fracture planes coalesce pulp canals.
  - fractured teeth are brittle and often associated with paranasal sinus disease.
  - can be problematic to remove as they fragment during extraction:
    - removal is challenging whatever technique is used (Figs. 2.49, 2.50).
    - outcome failures are common:
      - presence of dental fragments or non-vital alveolar sequestra.
      - both can lead to oroantral fistula formation.

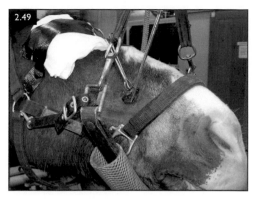

FIG. 2.49 Repulsion of root fragments can be achieved in the conscious horse with precise diagnostic imaging, nerve blocks and instrumentation.

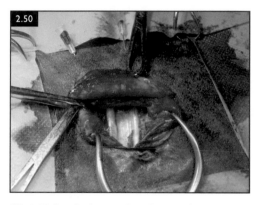

FIG. 2.50 Surgical extraction via a corticotomy and lateral buccotomy is technically challenging but yields good results.

DENTAL DISEASES ASSOCIATED WITH WEAR

Abnormalities of incisor wear

- incisors rarely sustain wear abnormalities alone.
- full lateral movement of the mandible results in:
  - occlusion of the molar arcades.
  - eventual separation of the incisors by about half the width of one incisor.
- extreme overgrowths of an incisor may prevent normal movement (uncommon).
- concave or convex occlusal angle when the incisors are closed is seen in older horses.
- slanted occlusal angle is usually indicative of abnormalities of the cheek teeth:
  - causing a unilateral masticatory action resulting in imbalanced wear.

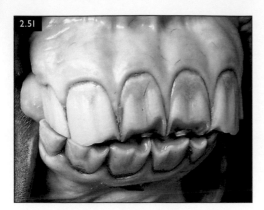

FIG. 2.51 Increased wear of the incisors of a horse that crib bites.

- correct any cheek tooth abnormalities before correcting any incisor asymmetry.
- stereotypical behavioural problems including crib biting will lead to:
  - accelerated wear of the incisor tables.
  - appearance of a prematurely ageing horse (Fig. 2.51).

Abnormalities of wear of the cheek teeth

Focal dental overgrowths, dental points, shear mouth

Definition/overview

- normal mastication:
  - mandible is lowered and then raised in a dorsal movement.
  - circumducting from buccal to lingual.
  - brings the mandibular teeth into occlusion in an axial direction.
  - occlusal surfaces shear over each other in a grinding action.
  - referred to as the 'power stroke'.
  - driven by the powerful masseter and pterygoid muscle groups.
  - anisognathism in the equine mouth:
    - only one molar arcade is in occlusion during each masticatory stroke.
- temporomandibular joint permits free lateral and a degree of rostrocaudal movement.
- as horse lowers its head into a grazing position, the mandible drops and moves rostrally and normal occlusion would be expected at this point.

Aetiology/pathophysiology

- range of lateral mandibular movement appears to be wider when chewing grass or forage than concentrate processed feeds.
- rotary chewing action leads to the angled occlusal surface (10–30° to the horizontal):
  - increased wear on:
    - palatal aspect of maxillary arcade.
    - buccal aspect of mandibular arcade.
- factors that limit lateral jaw movement can result in:
  - exaggeration of the angle of the occlusal surface.
  - causes dysmastication and uneven wear over the tooth.
  - ultimately leads to development of focal overgrowths (due to reduced attrition):
    - lingual aspects of the mandibular teeth.
    - buccal aspects of the maxillary teeth (Fig. 2.52).

Clinical presentation

- focal overgrowths develop sharp enamel points:
  - impinge on soft tissue causing masticatory pain and ulceration.
  - overgrowths of the lateral, buccal aspect of maxillary teeth can become particularly prominent.

Diagnosis

- overgrowths detected by extraoral and intraoral digital palpation during thorough routine examinations:
  - particularly prevalent on the 10s and 11s.

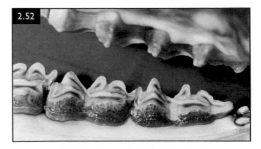

FIG. 2.52 Overgrowths on the buccal and lingual aspect of the cheek teeth.

- using a mirror or oroscope reveals mucosal trauma and extent of overgrowth.
- continuing development of overgrowths can result in occlusal angles approaching 45°:
  - termed 'shear mouth' (Fig. 2.53).
  - exaggerated overgrowths physically prevent lateral masticatory movement:
    - result in a scissor-like action, leading to further exacerbation of the problem.

Management

- removal of overgrowths is a fundamental part of routine dental prophylaxis.
- correction of severe shear mouth may be a long-term project:
  - gradual reduction of overgrowths over a period (6 months) in several treatments.
- correction of focal overgrowths is achieved using a variety of instruments:
  - rasps (different handle types) fitted with blades made from chipped or solid tungsten carbide.
  - electrically and battery-operated diamond-coated burrs with water cooling are the most efficient instruments.
  - reduce the possibility of iatrogenic damage when performing corrections by:

- good patient restraint with sedation of the horse.
- use of water cooling to avoid overheating the tooth.
- precise visual control.

Rostral and caudal overgrowths ('hooks, beaks, ramps')

Definition/overview

- prominent overgrowths on the rostral and caudal aspects of the arcade resulting from uneven wear.

Aetiology/pathophysiology

- focal dental overgrowths at the rostral and caudal aspects of either the maxillary or mandibular arcades can result from several mechanisms.
- anisometria of the maxillary and mandibular arcades can lead to the development of a rostral overgrowth (hook) on the 106 and 206, or on the 311 or 411 (Fig. 2.54):
  - probably due to a relatively caudal displacement of the mandible during mastication resulting in incomplete occlusion.
  - domesticated horses that are fed with the head raised may be more susceptible.
- caudal overgrowths may cause trauma to the tongue and other soft tissues.

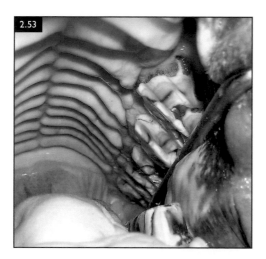

FIG. 2.53 Extreme dysmastication can lead to extreme occlusal angles termed shear mouth.

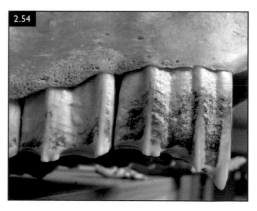

FIG. 2.54 Rostral maxillary overgrowths (hooks) such as on this specimen are the consequence of malocclusion.

Clinical presentation and diagnosis

- hooks may present as:
  - masticatory disorders, oral pain, hypersalivation, and equitation problems.
- careful oral examination and palpation will demonstrate such overgrowths:
  - caudal mandibular overgrowths can remain undetected on cursory visual examinations of the mouth.
- rostral overgrowths can contribute to equitation problems when ridden:
  - pain caused by entrapment of gingival mucosa between bits and the sharp buccal/rostral overgrowth.

Management

- removal of overgrowths using hand rasps (Figs. 2.55, 2.56) and mechanical grinding instruments:
  - enables more precise correction of the overgrowths.

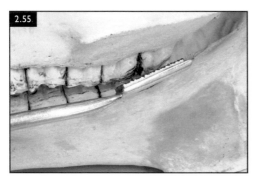

FIG. 2.55 An up-angled low-profile dental rasp is required to reduce sharp overgrowths on buccal maxillary 10s and 11s.

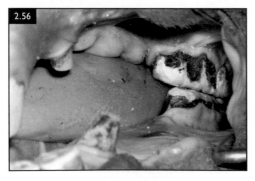

FIG. 2.56 Post-rasping, the periphery of the tooth is smooth to prevent mucosal trauma, but peripheral cement is intact at the gingival margin.

- reduced risk of pulpal exposure.
- used with care to avoid overheating the teeth.

Excessive transverse ridges (ETRs)

Definition/overview

- presence of exaggerated ridges in a buccopalato or buccolingual direction:
  - focally prominent and may be associated with:
    - ♦ reduced masticatory movement.
    - ♦ impaction of food into diastema on the opposite arcade.

Aetiology/pathophysiology

- transverse elevations on occlusal surfaces of teeth are a normal consequence of mastication:
  - usually present on the surface of equine teeth in normal wear.
  - elevations on mandibular teeth interdigitate with troughs on maxillary teeth.
  - combined with different rates of wear of dental tissues, enhances the efficiency of mastication.
- horses with impaired mastication:
  - exaggerated transverse ridges may restrict rostrocaudal mandibular movement.
  - manifest as poor tolerance of the bit and reduced performance.
- normal transverse ridges do not significantly restrict movement or the bit.
- ETRs also develop opposite the diastema created after exodontia.

Diagnosis

- ETRs are easily detected on oral examination with digital palpation.

Management

- removal of the ETRs to free up movement is attributed with improved performance:
  - reduced using a powered burr.
- removal of ridges in asymptomatic horses during routine examinations is not justified.

Step mouth and wave mouth

Definition/overview

- severely uneven mastication resulting in severe 'steps' in the occlusal surface of the arcade (step mouth).
- undulation of the occlusal surface in a rostral to caudal direction (wave mouth) (Fig. 2.57).

Aetiology/pathophysiology

- abnormal masticatory movement can result in:
  - area of the arcade undergoing attrition at an increased rate relative to others.
  - occlusal surface that undulates:
    - ♦ longer and shorter clinical crowns in adjacent areas.
  - maxillary and mandibular arcade undulations complement each other when the arcades come into occlusion.
  - common in aged horses that have suffered chronic reduced masticatory movements.
- Step mouth is a consequence of local oligodontia or displacements:
  - allowing super-eruption or drastically reduced attrition on a single tooth.
  - develop a crown that is prominent (>1 cm) to the remainder of the arcade.

Clinical features and diagnosis

- severe step and wave mouth:
  - consequence or cause of additional masticatory disorders.
  - can be associated with oral pain.

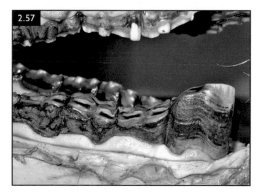

FIG. 2.57 This cadaver specimen shows a wave profile of the upper arcade and a step at the caudal mandibular molar.

- oral examination and careful digital palpation will reveal their presence.

Management

- correction of wave mouth is possible until dental eruption ceases (about 20 years old).
- once normal mastication is restored, tendency for the condition to recur is reduced.
- gradual correction (maintain occlusion and masticatory efficiency) is advisable in severe cases.
- preservation of viable functional dental tissues is desirable in aged horses.
- dietary changes to less abrasive sources of fibre are helpful.
- step mouth corrected gradually using a diamond-coated, water-cooled mechanical burr:
  - reduce the prominent tooth to arcade level and the remainder into occlusion.
  - pulp may extend to within a few mm of the occlusal surfaces.
  - correction of large (>1 cm) steps carried out gradually with repeated treatments.

Geriatric (>20 years of age) dental disease

- increasing prevalence of periodontitis, severe caries and oligodontia, with age.
- require their dentition to be carefully maintained to retain body condition.
- dietary manipulation can compensate for loss of masticatory effectiveness:
  - geriatric diets and oil supplementation.
  - avoiding long-fibre roughage.

Equine odontoclastic tooth resorption and hypercementosis (EOTRH)

Definition/overview

- syndrome afflicting incisors and canines of geriatric (>15 years of age) horses.
- results in destruction of the reserve crown with severe painful gingivitis (Fig. 2.58).

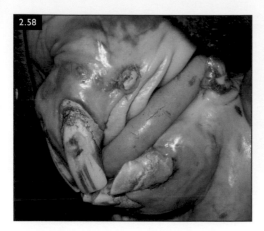

FIG. 2.58 Resorption of the reserve crown subgingivally followed by reactive hypercementosis are features of EOTRH.

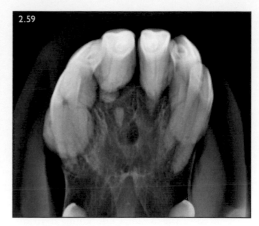

FIG. 2.59 EOTRH is diagnosed radiographically using intraoral projections.

Aetiology/pathophysiology

- cause of EOTRH is unclear but mechanical and immune factors are possible.
- osteolytic demineralisation of the cementum and dentine of the reserve crown and alveolar bone is observed.
- may be accompanied by a severe chronic gingivitis and periodontitis.
- subsequently hypercementosis around the affected teeth.

Clinical signs and diagnosis

- oral pain, gingivitis and hypersalivation.
- palpable digital loosening of the teeth and usually elicits pain.
- diagnosis based on clinical signs and radiography.
- typical radiological changes include (Fig. 2.59):
  - hypercementosis subgingivally.
  - lytic demineralisation of the reserve crowns.
  - apical lysis of enamel and dentine.

Differential diagnosis

- periodontitis.

Management

- removal of the affected tooth is the only effective treatment.
- exodontia of all incisors has resulted in clinical remission in some cases (Fig. 2.60).

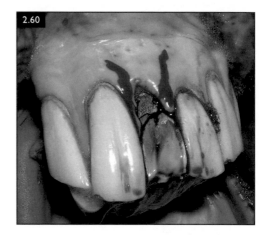

FIG. 2.60 A mucoperiosteal flap is created to expose the reserve crown of incisors prior to their extraction.

Disease of canine teeth

- canine teeth have no role in prehension and mastication of food:
  - less commonly involved in dental disease than masticatory teeth.
- found predominantly in male horses.
- can be fractured after bit contact or iatrogenically:
  - can lead to pulp exposure, subsequent necrosis, and possible abscessation.
  - some fractures are clinically obscure while others can be extremely painful.
  - all require careful appraisal.

- rasping of canines was considered a valid and useful procedure in the absence of any supporting clinical data:
  - iatrogenic canine pulp exposure can ensue from inappropriate treatments.
  - radiographs reveal changes to the endodontium and periodontium of the caudal roots in the incisive bone.
- calculus accumulation on the canines is common in older male horses:
  - normally asymptomatic, but in severe cases gingivitis and gingival recession.
  - removal of excess calculus with a dental elevator is easily accomplished in the standing horse during routine dental examinations.
- canine teeth in geriatric horses are occasionally affected by EOTRH and should be included in radiographic screening for this disease.
- canine teeth with pulpitis but an intact crown can be considered for endodontic therapy and restoration.
- canine teeth not suitable for salvage can be removed with the horse under sedation and regional and local analgesia:
  - non-compliant horses or those requiring multiple exodontia procedures may require general anaesthesia.

Treatment of common pathologies

- terms such as 'balancing, equilibration, performance floating and bit seating' are often used when promoting dental treatments:
  - **inaccurate, misleading, and unnecessary.**
- little evidence that removal of non-pathological dental tissue is of any benefit to the horse.
- removing sharp foci traumatising soft tissues and causing soft tissue pain or impeding mastication is useful:
  - masticatory wear in a normally eating horse will produce surfaces and edges that are reasonably angular and hence efficient for chewing.
  - bridle sidepieces may exert pressure over these edges resulting in mucosal trauma in harnessed and performing horses.

- stabled horses fed a high proportion of non-grazed food probably perform less masticatory movement than grazing animals:
  - some compensation for this lack of occlusal wear may be beneficial.
- careful appraisal both visually/digitally of any overgrown prominences should occur before any reductive treatments.
- prone to develop overgrowths 'enamel points':
  - buccal aspects of maxillary cheek teeth.
  - lingual aspects of mandibular dentition.
- overgrowths or hooks can develop on:
  - caudal mandibular molars.
  - rostral maxillary premolars.
- rasping to prevent the development of hooks and points is prophylactically sensible:
  - manual instruments or rotary or reciprocating powered tools.
  - latter are ever increasing in efficiency, popularity, and usage.
  - models with small heads, water cooling and a variety of contact angles are useful.
  - **powered tools, if used incorrectly, are capable of excessive rasping and pulpar and sensitive dentine exposure:**
    - short periods of contact and frequent checking on progress are essential to avoid problems.
  - generally, used with much greater safety, less stress to the horse, and more precision if the animal is **sedated**.
  - rasping should, ideally, be done under **visual control**.
  - manual instruments are safe and effective in less restrained horses but can lead to repetitive strain injuries to the veterinarian.
  - use of headstands and mirrors is increasingly popular to aid with the precision of dental rasping.
- teeth with exposed pulps, gingival tracts, caries or dental fracture should be appraised radiographically:
  - treatments based on tooth viability and their impact on the patient.
- record all findings and treatments on a dental chart plus:
  - plan for re-examination or follow-up treatment.

NON-DENTAL DISEASE OF THE ORAL CAVITY

Cleft palate (palatoschiasis)

Definition

- congenital defect resulting in an incomplete symphysis:
  - can affect the upper lip and hard palate.
  - most commonly involves the caudal portion of the soft palate (Fig. 2.61).

Aetiology/pathogenesis

- defect is the result of failure of the lateral palatine processes to fuse.
- normally occurs at approximately day 47 of gestation.
- heritability has not been established in horses.

Clinical presentation

- primary cleft palate affects the upper lip and rostral hard palate:
  - presents as sagittal facial deformity with incomplete aponeurosis of the upper lip.
  - usually evident during an examination at birth or once the foal commences to suck.
- more commonly only the soft palate is affected, and this is not evident externally.

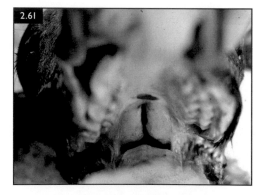

FIG. 2.61 This post-mortem picture shows a cleft soft palate in a 2-week-old Thoroughbred foal that presented with bilateral nasal discharge of milk soon after starting to suck from the mother.

- foals with a cleft palate present with nasal reflux during feeding:
  - milk entering the oral cavity passes into the nasal cavity.
  - exits via the nares bilaterally during sucking.
- foals can swallow but aspiration may occur in the first few days.
- complications result from the dysphagia and can include:
  - failure of passive transfer of gamma-globulins from colostrum.
  - dehydration and hypoglycaemia.
  - aspiration pneumonia.

Diagnosis

- oral and digital examination of the hard and soft palate will reveal a defect:
  - upper lip and rostral palate will be affected in primary cases.
  - soft palate defects in a sagittal plane which vary from:
    - ♦ approximately 1 cm to the whole caudal portion of the soft palate.
- confirmed by nasal or oral endoscopy.
- full investigation includes tracheoscopy and standing thoracic radiography:
  - confirm the presence of food aspiration and pneumonia.

Management

- surgical repair of palatal defects has been described:
  - limited number of cases.
  - prognosis for attainment of athletic ability is guarded.
  - repair as early as possible.
  - repair of lesions of the soft palate is more successful than those involving the hard palate.
  - complications are common.
  - foals of low value are euthanased without treatment in most cases.

Mouth: Lacerations/wounds and foreign bodies

Definition

- acquired traumatic lesions of the oral cavity.

Aetiology/pathogenesis

- ingestion of sharp foreign bodies.
- entrapment of loose soft tissue structures.
- rostral mandible and incisive bone fractures (Fig. 2.62).
- laceration of the mouth and tongue (Fig. 2.63).
- occur sporadically and result in painful lesions.
- may be complicated by loss of vascularity or embedded foreign material.

- lip lacerations are common in young horses:
  - result of becoming hooked on sharp objects and rearing to escape (Figs. 2.64, 2.65).

Clinical presentation

- traumatic mouth wounds involving foreign bodies or sharp dental overgrowths:
  - may bleed profusely initially.

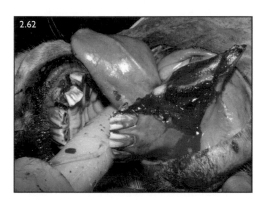

FIG. 2.62 A severe laceration of the oral mucosa associated with a mandibular fracture and avulsion of lower incisors.

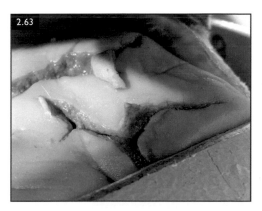

FIG. 2.63 Lacerations of the tongue on sharp objects are extremely painful initially but heal well spontaneously in most cases.

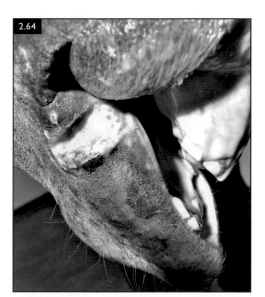

FIG. 2.64 A laceration to the right lower lip of a few days' duration. This could easily be freshened up and repaired at this stage.

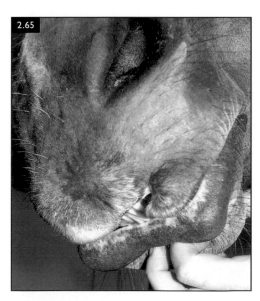

FIG. 2.65 An old wound of the upper lip that has been allowed to heal by secondary intention and which has distorted the outline and affected function.

- ○ rapidly cease discharging and normally heal spontaneously in 3–10 days.
- foreign material in the wound will delay healing, or lead to formation of a sinus tract communicating with the foreign body:
  - ○ eventually abscessation may occur.
  - ○ present with painful soft tissue swelling in the oral cavity:
    - ♦ particularly in the intermandibular space.
    - ♦ may be palpable externally.
  - ○ foetid discharges may exude from sinus tracts.
  - ○ halitosis, hypersalivation, and pain when masticating.
- abscessation involving the tongue can be extremely painful and is difficult to diagnose.
- regional lymph nodes, including the submandibulars, may be enlarged.
- lacerations or ulceration (Fig. 2.66) of the tongue may be associated with reluctance to accept the bit or pain when ridden on the bridle.

Differential diagnosis

- painful swellings in the oral cavity must be distinguished from abscesses caused by systemic diseases such as *Streptococcus equi* var. *equi*.

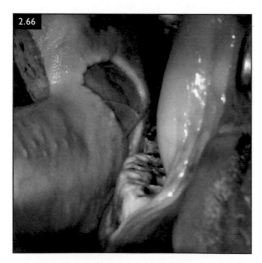

FIG. 2.66 Severe ulceration of the tongue can ensue where sharp dental prominences and dysmastication are present.

- discharging tracts from the gingiva can also be associated with mandibular fractures and occasionally sequestra in the interdental spaces due to bit trauma.

Diagnosis

- most lacerations are clearly visible on a thorough oral examination and only minimal further investigation is necessary.
- tongue lacerations are more difficult due to the high mobility of the tongue and the difficulty of examination when it is injured.
- injuries with chronically discharging tracts should be assessed by radiography:
  - ○ rule out the presence of sequestra or fractures.
- ultrasonography useful to image the intermandibular soft tissues and mandibular cortices.
- CT is useful to reveal deeper lying structures, especially osseous.

Management

- most oral lacerations heal spontaneously with minimal intervention:
  - ○ tetanus prophylaxis and broad-spectrum antibiotics.
- damage to salivary ducts can be associated with a chronic salivary fistula, which may granulate eventually.
- semi-liquidised diets can enable animals with severe oral pain to eat.
- severe lacerations can be repaired in multiple layers, to accelerate healing.
- tongue lacerations involving almost full-thickness transection may require surgical debridement, and repair in multiple layers, under general anaesthesia, with a reasonable prognosis (Figs. 2.67, 2.68).
- loss of the rostral portion of the tongue can adversely affect the ability of the horse to accommodate a normal bitted bridle.

Stomatitis

Definition

- inflammation of the soft tissues of the oral cavity.

Aetiology/pathogenesis

- uncommon condition in horses.

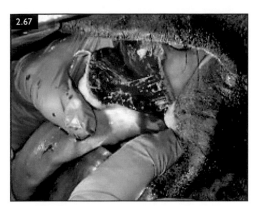

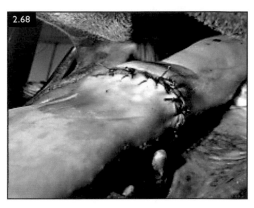

FIGS. 2.67, 2.68 A severe laceration of the dorsal middle part of the tongue preop (2.67) and after repair consisting of a multiple layer muscle closure and initial coaptation of the mucosa with vertical mattress non-absorbable sutures (2.68). The mucosa was subsequently closed with a fine simple continuous non-absorbable suture to seal it from excess contamination.

- usually associated with inflammation secondary to other disease processes:
  - viral stomatitis may affect the dorsum of the tongue and the lips and is usually self-limiting in adult horses.
  - migrating *Gastrophilus* larvae in the oral mucosa may cause a painful stomatitis.
  - ingestion of caustic chemicals, severe periodontal disease secondary to food impaction in the interdontium, and trauma.

Clinical presentation
- increased salivation may be observed.
- raised vesicles on the lips or tongue.
- gingival reddening or haemorrhage.
- ulceration of the tongue and lips.
- reluctance to masticate.

Differential diagnosis
- inflammatory disease of the oral cavity may be confused with:
  - neoplastic conditions such as squamous cell carcinoma.
- presence of the primary cause (e.g. dental disease) must be identified.

Diagnosis
- clinical findings.
- confirmed by:
  - oral endoscopy.

- radiography to eliminate the presence of dental apical disease.
- biopsy of any lesions suspected to be neoplastic.

Management
- treatment of any inciting cause, such as dental overgrowths, diastema or caries.
- symptomatic treatments:
  - broad-spectrum antibiotics, soft diets, and mouthwashes.

Lampus

Definition
- swollen soft tissues covering the hard palate resulting in loss of occlusion of the incisors.

Aetiology/pathogenesis
- hyperaemia and swelling of the gingiva on the ventral aspect of the hard palate:
  - observed in young horses shedding their deciduous incisors.
  - typically, when grazing coarse forage.
  - considered to be a normal physiological condition in a percentage of young horses and not requiring treatment.

Differential diagnosis
- older horses may develop oedema of the hard palate associated with certain

abrasive or spikey leaves that is similar in appearance to the juvenile condition.

Management

- no pathological lesions identified with this condition and there is no treatment required.
- swellings invariably recede spontaneously and without any negative consequences.
- slight oedema or loose palatal gingival mucosa may ensue in a few cases.
- non-steroidal anti-inflammatory drugs (NSAIDs) may be useful if the condition is sufficiently painful to impede eating.

Fractures of the rostral skull

Definition/overview

- fractures of this region are not uncommon:
  - mandible is the most frequently fractured bone in the head.
- many rostral skull injuries initially appear dramatic:
  - profuse haemorrhage and distortion of the bones.
  - most carry a good prognosis for full recovery.

Aetiology/pathophysiology

- kick trauma.
- self-induced trauma (feeders, gates etc.)
- collisions or falls.
- rostral mandible predisposed due to shape and narrowing at interdental space:
  - often bilateral.
- rostral mandibular and premaxilla fractures are often:
  - displaced, open and heavily contaminated (Figure 2.69).
- fractures may only involve alveolar bone and/or teeth (Figure 2.70).
- horizontal/vertical ramus and maxilla fractures are much less common.

Clinical presentation

- vary with severity of injury:
  - few or no signs with incisive fractures of the mandible.
  - caudal based fractures may cause:
    - ptyalism ♦ dysphagia.
    - halitosis (food impaction).
- maxillary fractures may have concurrent nasal and/or frontal fractures.
- haemorrhage from the mouth.

Differential diagnosis

- other causes of dysphagia:
  - soft tissue trauma of the mouth and tongue.
  - dental disease.

Diagnostic techniques

- full clinical examination should include:
  - palpation of the rostral skull – abnormal movement or crepitus.
  - examine the incisors, canines and inside of muzzle:
    - fractured or avulsed teeth.
    - misaligned incisors.

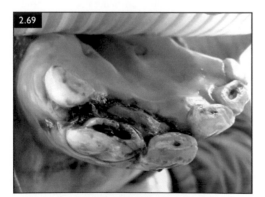

FIG. 2.69 An avulsion fracture of the 401 and 402 teeth, with contamination and a large haematoma within in the fracture gap.

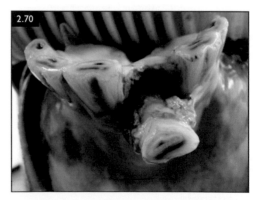

FIG. 2.70 A traumatic fracture of a 301 tooth with exposure of the pulp tissues, but no evidence of collateral damage to the adjacent teeth or the mandibular bone.

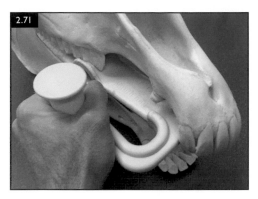

FIG. 2.71 A cheek tooth gag placed between two opposing cheek teeth arcades.

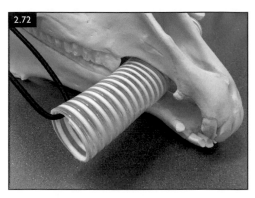

FIG. 2.72 A tube gag placed in the interdental space between the incisors and cheek teeth to allow safe examination and access to the occlusal surfaces of the incisors.

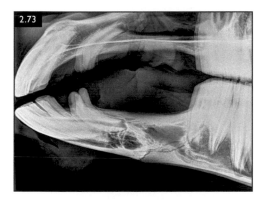

FIG. 2.73 Laterolateral radiograph of a unilateral mandibular fracture within the 404 and 406 interdental space, with extension of the fracture line into the apices of the 406 tooth.

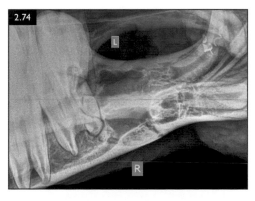

FIG. 2.74 Laterolateral oblique radiograph of the same fracture shown in 2.73.

- ♦ fracture in the interdental space.
- ♦ bilateral or unilateral.
- ♦ wounds ♦ haemorrhage.
- ♦ food contamination.
- ○ caudal mouth lesions may require mirrors or rigid endoscope to assess.
- ○ place a cheek tooth or tube gag to examine rostral oral cavity (Figs. 2.71 and 2.72).
- ○ avoid an oral speculum with incisor plates in rostral fracture cases.
- ○ determine any concomitant fractures e.g. nasal or frontal bone fractures.
- • neurological and cranial nerve examination prudent in all cases of head trauma:
  - ○ deficits are rare in cranial lesions.

- • **radiography usually confirms the diagnosis:**
  - ○ patient adequately sedated and head supported:
    - ♦ laterolateral (Fig. 2.73).
    - ♦ laterolateral oblique (Fig. 2.74).
    - ♦ dorsoventral views (Fig. 2.75).
    - ♦ intraoral mandible and maxilla (Fig. 2.76):
      - – use a plate protection device or radiolucent speculum *in situ*.
- • CT examination (Fig. 2.77):
  - ○ standing sedation.
  - ○ caudal fractures.
  - ○ temporomandibular joint.
  - ○ hyoid apparatus.

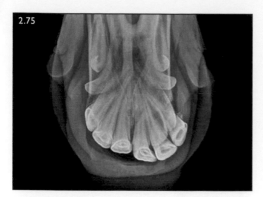

FIG. 2.75 Dorsoventral radiograph of the rostral skull of a horse with a maxillary bone fracture, showing the superimposition of the mandibular structures.

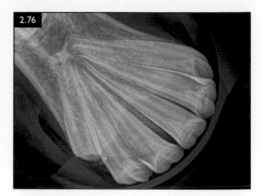

FIG. 2.76 Intraoral radiograph of a mandibular incisor arcade with a fractured crown of the tooth 303. The radiograph was taken using a radiolucent bit plate attached to a conventional oral speculum.

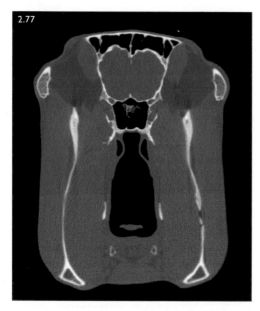

FIG. 2.77 CT cross-sectional reconstruction of a fracture of the vertical ramus of the right mandible.

Management

- minor injuries may heal spontaneously following wound lavage and debridement.
- single tooth avulsed with minimal soft tissue attachment:
  - removal may be indicated.
- preserve deciduous teeth if possible.
- fractures confined to the tooth alone may warrant:
  - endodontic debridement and restoration of tooth or extraction.

- most displaced osseous fractures benefit from reduction and fixation:
  - cerclage wiring between remaining incisor teeth can be used for:
    - fractures of the incisive region of maxilla (Figs. 2.78 and 2.79).
    - rostral mandible fractures.
    - avulsion of incisors.
  - usually standing, sedated horse with perineural local anaesthesia.
  - wires can also pass:
    - around canine teeth (notch on caudal aspect of crown).
    - through interdental spaces between the '06 and '07 cheek teeth.
    - through hole drilled in the mandible in the interdental space:
      - wrapping around a cortex screw positioned in a similar location.
  - alignment of incisor occlusal surfaces used to assess fracture reduction.
- viability of any teeth involved in the fracture may be unknown at time of repair:
  - should always remain *in situ* – remove later if necessary.
- postoperatively horses can be fed forages spread loosely on the ground.
- may be able to return to ridden work using a bit before removal of wires:
  - depending on the position of the intraoral wires.

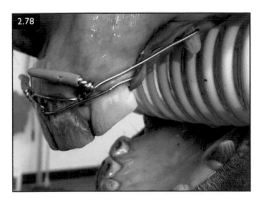

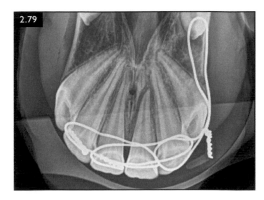

FIGS. 2.78, 2.79 (2.78) Cerclage wire fixation of a maxillary fracture using intraoral wires placed in the incisor interdental spaces and in the groove cut in the caudal aspect of the canine. (2.79) Radiographic view of the repaired maxillary bone fracture shown in 2.78 prior to intraoral wire removal.

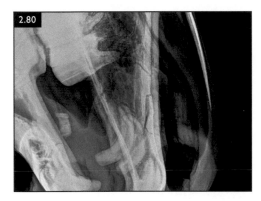

FIG. 2.80 Slightly oblique laterolateral radiograph of a horse with a bilateral fracture of the maxilla and incisive bones. (Photo courtesy Mark Grant)

- o wires usually removed about 6 weeks later.
- unilateral fractures of interdental space are often treated conservatively:
  - o usually stabilized by contralateral mandible or maxilla.
- bilateral maxillary fractures may also involve trauma to:
  - o nasal septum, nasal process, facial bones and hard palate (Fig. 2.80).
  - o often heal conservatively.
- bilateral mandibular fractures involving the interdental space are often completely unstable and demand fixation using a variety of techniques:
  - o tension-band wires between incisors and cheek teeth.

- o U-shaped frames held by wires around the teeth.
- o external fixation frames using pins through the mandible.
- o Pin-less external fixation devices.
- o often a combination of one or more of the above.
- o usually performed under general anesthesia:
  - ♦ sedation/local anaesthesia used in some cases with some techniques.
- internal fixation using bone plates is uncommon:
  - o caudal fractures that are restricting mastication.
  - o most caudal fractures of horizontal and vertical rami heal conservatively.

Fractures of the cranium and face

Definition/overview
- fractures of the cranium are rare:
  - o may have serious consequences due to concurrent neurological trauma.
- two types of cranial fracture are seen more regularly:
  - o basilar skull fractures.
  - o dorsal or dorsolateral cranial fractures.
- facial fractures (nasal and frontal bones) are relatively common:
  - o may appear dramatic due to profuse haemorrhage and facial distortion.
  - o not usually life threatening.
- fractures in either region can be closed or open.

Aetiology/pathophysiology

- Basilar skull fractures usually caused by a backward fall.
- dorsal cranial fractures usually a consequence of a head-on collision.
- Facial fractures usually involve nasal and/or frontal +/– maxilla or lacrimal bones:
  - direct trauma.
  - falling forwards, kicks, or rearing and striking a solid object above the head.

Clinical presentation

- facial and cranial fractures often present as emergencies.
- neurological signs in cranial fractures caused by accompanying brain damage:
  - may increase in severity as pressure from oedema and subarachnoid haemorrhage grows, and can include:
    - recumbency
    - depression.
    - ataxia
    - head tilt.
    - nystagmus.
    - cranial nerve deficits.
  - altered cardiac and respiratory function:
    - irregular breathing, with periods of apnoea (poor prognosis).
  - CNS exposed – CSF leaking from wound or ear canal.
- epistaxis:
  - nasal passage and paranasal sinus trauma:
    - may lead to chronic sinusitis.
  - tearing of the *rectus capitis* muscles.
- poll or the dorsal cranium trauma:
  - avulsion of the nuchal ligament origin.
  - fracture of the basisphenoid or basihyoid bones.
- facial fractures may have obvious signs of external trauma (Figure 2.81):
  - may communicate with the nasal passages or paranasal sinuses.
  - overlying swelling due to oedema and trapped air.
  - facial asymmetry and, in the longer term, deformity.
  - wounds may or may not be present.
  - crepitus and subcutaneous emphysema on palpation.
  - distortion/partial blockage of the upper airway leading to respiratory stridor.
  - damage to the nasolacrimal duct leading to epiphora.

Differential diagnosis

- neurological signs similar to acute-onset vestibular disease and inflammatory disease of the CNS.
- facial swelling and epistaxis may be due only to soft tissue trauma.

Diagnostic techniques

- Radiography (Fig. 2.82):
  - several, often lesion-oriented oblique, views may be needed.
  - signs suggestive of basilar skull fractures include:
    - fluid opacity (blood) in the guttural pouches.
    - ventral deviation of the dorsal pharyngeal wall.
    - irregular bone opacities ventral to the skull base.
- Computed tomography (CT):
  - more comprehensive and detailed assessment of damage (Fig. 2.83).
- Ultrasonography:

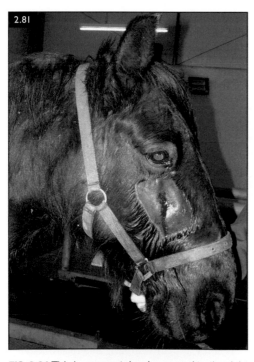

FIG. 2.81 This horse sustained a wound to the right side of the skull. Note the depression centred over the maxillary region. Radiography revealed a slightly displaced fracture of the facial crest.

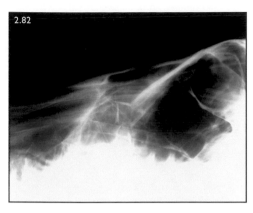

FIG. 2.82 Lateral radiograph of the maxilla of a horse that sustained a blow to the head and which clearly shows a ventrally displaced fracture of the frontal bone into the paranasal sinuses.

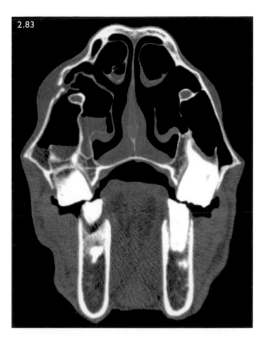

FIG. 2.83 CT cross-sectional reconstruction showing a depression fracture of the left maxillary bone.

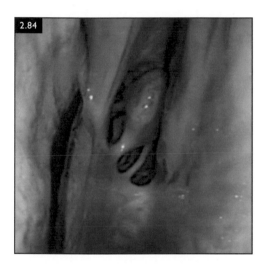

FIG. 2.84 Endoscopic photograph of the sinus drainage angle showing haemorrhage emanating from the sinuses.

- osseous nasal and paranasal lesions, especially when non-displaced.
- Endoscopy:
  - airway stenosis or blood from sinus drainage angle (Fig. 2.84).
  - bilateral guttural pouch endoscopy confirms presence of:
    - blood ◆ *Rectus capitus* tears.
    - Stylohyoid bone fracture.

Management

- examination immediately after a fall or collision rapid assessment for:
  - significant concomitant injuries.
  - signs of neurological and respiratory debilitation.
  - provide first aid immediately and this may include:
    - sedation.
    - anti-inflammatory medication – steroids and/or NSAIDs.
    - emergency tracheostomy may be required.
    - stabilise an ataxic horse prior to transport:
      - prolonged recumbency associated with a poor prognosis.
- many small, non-displaced facial fractures will heal spontaneously:
  - risk of the previously mentioned complications.
- larger displaced fragments:
  - surgical correction indicated where cosmetic appearance is important.
- wounds should be lavaged and debrided.
- fragments can be wire-sutured together once elevated into position.
- periosteum should be preserved and sutured over defect if possible.

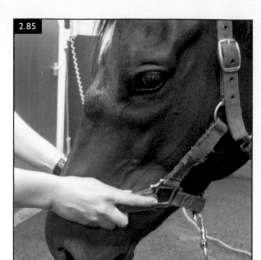

FIG. 2.85 Extensive new reaction along the suture lines of adjacent bones of the head, both in the midline and underneath the left eye.

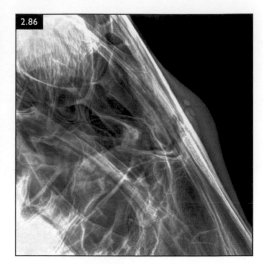

FIG. 2.86 Lateral radiograph of the head of a horse showing the osseous changes associated with a mature suture periostitis.

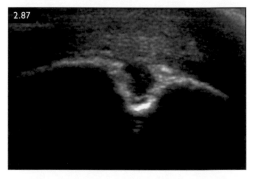

FIG. 2.87 Ultrasonogram of a mature suture periostitis.

- suture skin over the defect if possible:
  - transposition flaps of periosteum and skin for larger defects.
- lavage the sinuses using an indwelling catheter:
  - if haemorrhage is present or evidence of contamination.

Nasofrontal suture periostitis

Definition/overview

- bony swelling at joint between the frontal and nasal bones (Fig. 2.85).
- usually idiopathic but often thought to be trauma related:
  - may follow recent head trauma or paranasal sinus surgery.
- normally non-painful, focal, often linear, swelling of the head:
  - occasionally associated draining tracts.

Diagnosis

- clinical appearance is characteristic.
- radiographic and ultrasonographic examination useful (Figs. 2.86 and 2.87):
  - may have appearance of a healing fracture.

Management

- conservative management with anti-inflammatories.
- antibiotics where draining tracts are present have been used.
- complete resolution of the swelling is rare - usually considered a cosmetic blemish.

Temporomandibular joint disease (TMJ)

Definition/overview

- uncommon
- occasional case reports of osteoarthritis, septic arthritis and luxation.

Aetiology/pathophysiology

- OA of the TMJ is associated with chronic and severe dental abnormalities:
  - cause or effect is often undetermined.
- luxation of the joint is caused by trauma.

Clinical presentation

- often diagnosed at advanced stage.
- marked problems when feeding:
  - slow feeding o quidding.
  - food pouching in cheeks.
  - weight loss o dental abnormalities.
  - mouth soft tissue trauma.
- masseter muscle atrophy is common:
  - reduced movement of mandible.
  - damage to the mandibular branch of CN VII medial to temporal condyle.
- head shaking, head tilts and behavioural changes.
- concomitant signs of wounds, fractures and draining tracts in luxation cases.

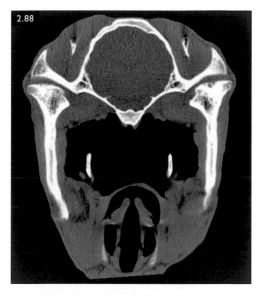

FIG. 2.88 Cross-sectional CT image of bilateral osseous changes to the mandibular condyles of the temporomandibular joint.

Differential diagnosis

- dental abnormalities for other reasons.
- other causes of dysphagia.

Diagnosis

- pain on palpation of the joint, especially where there is sepsis.
- diagnostic local analgesia of the joints where pain or quidding are present.
- oral examination:
  - reduced range of movement of mandible.
  - resentment to opening of mouth.
  - dental abnormalities.
  - soft tissue trauma in mouth – cheeks and tongue.
- **Radiography:**
  - number of views are described but only lateral aspect readily visualised.
  - bone proliferation and local bone lysis associated with OA.
- **Ultrasonography:**
  - exam meniscus, joint capsule, supporting ligaments and articular cartilage.
  - only lateral aspect of the joint and structures are visualised.
- **Scintigraphy:**
  - useful in conjunction with radiography for osseous lesions.

- **Computed tomography (CT):** (Fig. 2.88)
  - three-dimensional imaging of entire joint.
  - standing facilities available.
- **Magnetic resonance imaging (MRI):**
  - three-dimensional imaging of entire joint.
  - more detailed soft tissue information.
  - less commonly available and requires general anaesthesia.

Management

- treat any concurrent dental disease.
- intra-articular corticosteroids provide some relief from signs of OA:
  - only likely to be temporary.
- arthroscopic debridement of meniscal borders and removal of osteochondral fragments is described but of limited use.
- replacement of luxated joint in recent cases.
- septic cases can be treated successfully with a combination of antibiotics, local debridement and intra-articular lavage.
- mandibular condylectomy for unresponsive and chronic cases.

Diseases of the hyoid apparatus

Definition

- hyoid apparatus is the trapeze-like arrangement of bones that suspend the larynx and tongue from the base of the skull.
- bones comprise paired ketarohyoid, epihyoid, stylohyoid, and thyrohyoid bones joined by a single basihyoid and the linguohyoid, into which the base of the tongue inserts.
- injuries affecting the hyoid apparatus include:
  - fracture of the hyoid apparatus.
  - temporohyoid osteopathy (see page 67, Book 1).
- primary fractures of the hyoid apparatus are extremely rare:
  - reported occasionally following severe trauma to the ventral aspect of the head.
  - basihyoid bone fracture has been reported after laryngeal tie-forward surgery.
  - pathological fracture of the stylohyoid bones is suspected in cases with temporohyoid osteopathy.

ORAL NEOPLASIA

Introduction

- tumours affecting the oral cavity can be of dental, osseous or soft tissue origin.
- relatively rare compared with other species.
- oral tumours are often detected incidentally during a routine oral or dental examination:
  - often at an advanced stage.
  - limiting options for treatment.
  - rendering a guarded prognosis for complete remission.

Dental neoplasia

- epithelial.
- or odontogenic in origin:
  - cementomas, ameloblastomas, odontomas or other calcifying epithelial odontogenic lesions.
  - mesenchymal odontogenic tumours include myxomas and dentigerous cysts.
- dental tumours are invariably benign but may be locally invasive or expansive.
- some dental tumours can result in gross changes to dental apices and reserve crowns:
  - ameloblastomas (Fig. 2.89).
  - complex and compound odontomas (Fig. 2.90).
  - mandibular tumours of non-dental origin including:
    - osteomas, ossifying fibromas, and squamous cell carcinomas.

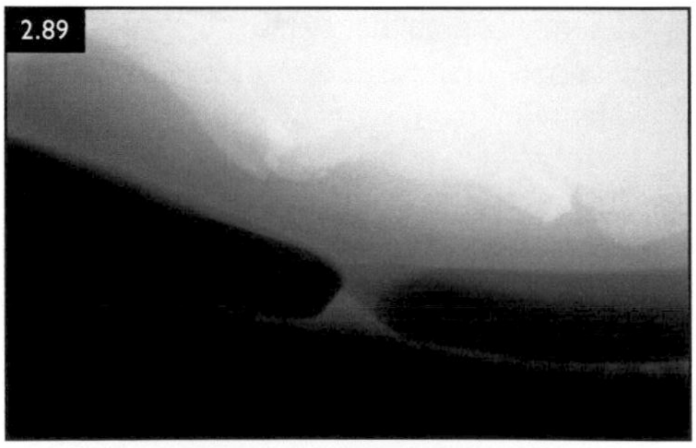

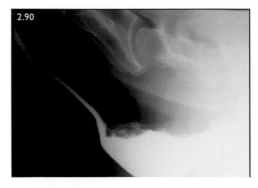

FIG. 2.89 An ameloblastoma in the cranial lower jaw about to undergo surgical resection (arrow).

FIG. 2.90 Radiograph of a compound odontoma within the paranasal sinuses (arrows) – a rare dentally derived tumour.

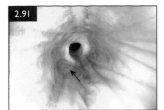

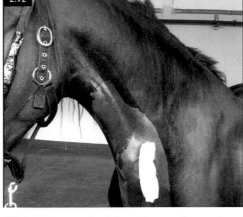

FIG. 2.92 Oroscopic picture of a small sarcoma at the caudal commissure under the oral mucosa.

FIG. 2.91 This adult horse has a large ossifying fibroma in the ventral mandible.

- may be accompanied by swelling of the affected alveolar bone, with increased or decreased radiopacity.
- dental tumours are variably mineralised, and usually well circumscribed.

Oral tumours of non-dental origin

- reports describing oral tumours of non-dental origin include:
  - mandibular ossifying fibromas (Fig. 2.91).

- osteomas and osteosarcomas.
- fibrosarcomas (Fig. 2.92).
- squamous cell carcinomas (Figs. 2.93, 2.94):
  - rare in the horse but typically produce destruction of the mandible or palate.
  - loss of mineral density and periodontal disease and loose teeth.
- spindle cell tumours.

Clinical presentation

- oral/dental tumours can present as asymmetric swellings of the maxilla and mandible:
  - may be associated with masticatory disorders.
- may be detected incidentally or in investigation of masticatory pain, hypersalivation, and halitosis.

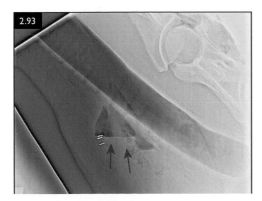

FIG. 2.93 Non-healing ulcers on the lip margins can signal squamous cell carcinoma.

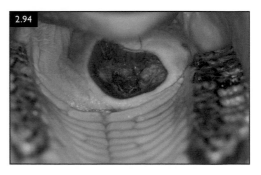

FIG. 2.94 Severe ulcerative necrosis of the soft palate with a squamous cell carcinoma.

- aggressive lesions may be associated with secondary dental disease.

Differential diagnosis

- dental pulpitis, fracture callus, foreign body granuloma, sialodeniasis, and fracture haematomas.

Diagnosis

- clinical appearance:
  - gross appearance of many lesions is similar.
  - non-neoplastic lesions such as exuberant granulation tissue and reactive inflammatory lesions can be mistaken for tumours.
  - histopathological examination is necessary for a specific diagnosis.
- oroscopic examination.
- diagnostic imaging:
  - radiography and CT:
    - CT offers the most extensive imaging in three dimensions.
    - vital in treatment planning, especially for dental and osseous tumours (Fig. 2.95).
    - MRI, where available, would be desirable for soft tissue lesions.

Management

- treatment options are often limited by:
  - advanced stage of the lesion.
  - anatomical location, which can preclude surgical access.
  - few treatment options available to the clinician.
- benign dental tumours are excisable, with a low recurrence rate:

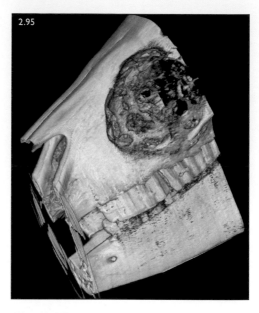

FIG. 2.95 3D surface reconstruction of a pony with a maxillary sarcoma.

- may also involve removal of teeth.
- non-dental tumours are usually poorly demarcated, at an advanced stage when diagnosed and adjacent to other vital structures.
- benign osteomas and fibro-osseous lesions can be treated by radical mandibulectomy:
  - welfare implications of radical surgery may deem euthanasia more appropriate.
- radiotherapy may have limited availability:
  - appropriate for easily accessible lesions no larger than a few cm^3.

DISEASES OF THE SALIVARY GLANDS

Introduction

- consist of paired parotid, sublingual and submaxillary glands:
  - parotid glands are the largest and produce the greatest volume of saliva.
- saliva contains electrolytes:
  - concentration of which is dependent on flow rate, which is variable.
  - up to 50 ml/min have been recorded in ponies.
- diseases are rare in horses, and most are acquired consequent to trauma.
- single case of congenital salivary tract atresia has been reported.

Trauma to salivary glands and ducts

Definition/overview
- parotid duct trauma is the most encountered salivary disorder.
- parotid salivary gland lobules drain via multiple small ductules, which converge and anastomose to form the parotid duct:
  - passes ventrally on the medial side of the mandible traversing its lateral border.
  - ascends rostral to the masseter muscle.
  - before entering the oral cavity via the parotid papilla at level of the 3rd cheek tooth.

Aetiology/pathophysiology
- trauma to the parotid duct occurs from:
  - kicks to the mandible and lacerations
  - surgical treatments including dental extraction and guttural pouch surgery.

Clinical presentation
- parotid duct damage occurs most commonly on the ventral aspect of the mandible where the duct passes from the medial to the lateral aspects.
- small wounds to the duct lead to saliva leakage with staining of the hair:
  - usually short-lived and resolve spontaneously (few days) as heals by granulation.

- large volumes of saliva continuously draining:
  - salivary fistula can develop.
  - skin heals, but the duct does not, a salivary mucocoele (Fig. 2.96).

Diagnosis
- clinical appearance and production of saliva in response to stimulation of food is normally diagnostic.
- retrograde contrast radiographs have been attempted.
- transcutaneous ultrasonography (Fig. 2.97).

Differential diagnosis
- sinus tracts due to foreign body penetration, dentigerous cysts, and tooth root infections.

Management
- wounds to the parotid gland and subsequent fistula usually heal by granulation.
  - when surgical debridement is indicated:
    - **care taken to avoid iatrogenic damage to branches of the salivary duct.**
- reduce salivary stimulation:
  - withholding of feed.
  - feeding via a nasogastric tube.

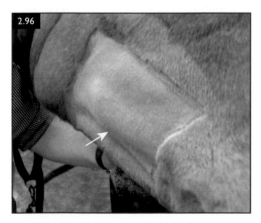

FIG. 2.96 This view of the right side of the face of a pony shows a marked swelling in the centre of the clipped area due to a salivary mucocoele under the skin (arrow).

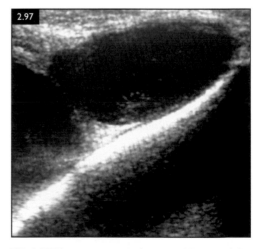

FIG. 2.97 Transcutaneous ultrasound image of the mucocoele shown in Fig. 2.76. Note the loculated hypoechoic well-described fluid swellings overlying the hyperechoic bone of the jaw.

- generally, meets with limited success.
- persistent salivary duct fistulae can be treated surgically:
  - ideally repair the damaged duct.
  - more simply the salivary duct proximal to the fistula can be ligated:
    - partial atrophy of the gland follows.
- sclerosis of the duct:
  - curetting and injecting with iodine solution.
  - 10% buffered formalin has also been used:
    - injected and kept in contact for 1–2 minutes.
  - side effects may include facial oedema.
- trauma to the sublingual glands can cause a sublingual salivary mucocoele:
  - located lateral to the frenulum.
  - easily be treated by marsupialisation into the oral cavity.

Salivary gland calculi (sialoliths)

Definition/overview

- precipitation of mineralised material within the salivary glands or ducts.

Aetiology/pathogenesis

- rare in horses and only clinically significant if lodged in the salivary papilla at the orifice of the parotid salivary duct.
- consist of calcium carbonate and sloughed cells.
- can reach several centimetres in size.

Clinical presentation

- distension of the duct proximal to the calculus may be detected by palpation or ultrasonographically.

Diagnosis

- calculi are often radiopaque and visible on plain radiographs.
- ultrasonography may reveal hyperechoic matter within the parenchyma of the salivary glands or within the ducts.
- CT, in the standing horse, gives a three-dimensional appraisal and enables more accurate and precise surgical planning (Fig. 2.98).

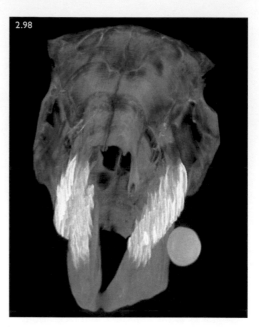

FIG. 2.98 3D bone algorithm reconstruction of a horse with a salivary calculus obstructing the parotid duct.

Differential diagnosis

- Parotiditis, parotid melanoma, retropharyngeal or submandibular lymphadenitis, guttural pouch enlargement.

Management

- calculus can be freed by incising the buccal mucosa via an oral approach in the sedated horse:
  - sialolith is expressed into the oral cavity and the duct heals by granulation.
- alternatively, via an external transcutaneous approach:
  - more technically difficult approach.
- permanent stenosis of the duct causes chronic distension and mucocoele formation.

Sialoadenitis (parotiditis)

Definition/overview

- inflammation of the salivary glands or ducts.

Aetiology/pathogenesis

- transient inflammation of the salivary gland can occur following trauma to the gland or after duct obstruction but is uncommon.
- may be observed in grazing horses in Europe and Australia, particularly in the early growing season, but it appears to be rare in the USA.

Clinical presentation

- glands are bilaterally swollen but non-painful a few days after grazing at pasture.
- does not affect mastication and is seasonally self-limiting.
- appears to be a response to changes in the content of grazed forage.
- may occur sporadically or as a herd outbreak.
- chronic cases of parotiditis can develop salivary gland abscessation due to infection with pyogenic organisms (Fig. 2.99):
  ○ extremely painful disease.
  ○ affected patients are dysphagic and painful to palpate.

Diagnosis

- history and clinical signs are often diagnostic.

- ultrasonography is useful to diagnose the distended ducts and affected glands.
- CT should be considered in chronic cases.

Management

- most cases resolve spontaneously when the horse is removed from the pasture, provided that the duct is unobstructed.
- chronic septic sialoadenitis can be treated using:
  ○ salivary lavage and attempts to encourage drainage via the parotid duct.
  ○ antimicrobial therapy based on culture and sensitivity.

Neoplasia

- affecting the salivary gland is rare:
  ○ adenocarcinomas, acinar cell tumours and mixed cell carcinomas reported.
- enlargement of the parotid gland associated with advanced melanoma is not uncommon in grey horses:
  ○ swelling may be sufficiently large to impinge into the pharynx and restrict airflow in extreme cases (Fig. 2.100).
  ○ dissection of the melanoma from the gland tissue is virtually impossible.
  ○ radiation therapy has been used to achieve remission in a few cases.

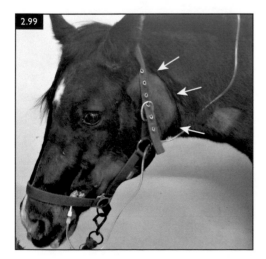

FIG. 2.99 This horse has gross distension of the parotid gland (arrows) due to an acutely painful bacterial infection.

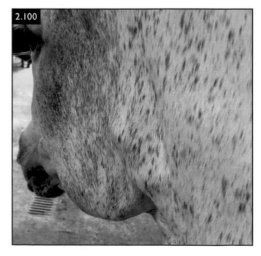

FIG. 2.100 Enlargement of the area immediately caudal to the left vertical mandible caused by a number of large parotid gland melanomas.

Ptyalism

- Ptyalism or excessive salivation may occur in response to:
  - oral pain including periodontal disease.
  - mucosal penetration by a foreign body.
  - ingestion of the fungus *Rhizoctonia legumincola*:
    - excess salivation is induced by the toxin slaframine (parasympathomimetic).
    - toxin may also induce lacrimation, anorexia, and diarrhoea.
- clinical signs may be associated secondarily with other diseases including:
  - rabies.
  - oesophageal obstruction and pharyngeal dysphagia.
  - stomatitis.
- investigation directed at identifying the primary cause and should include:
  - oral examination, pharyngeal endoscopy and passage of a nasogastric tube.

DISEASES OF THE OESOPHAGUS

Introduction

Anatomy of the equine oesophagus

- equine oesophagus consists of:
  - stratified squamous mucosa lining.
  - within a spiralling muscular tube:
    - striated and smooth muscle in the cranial two-thirds.
    - smooth muscle layers only in the caudal third.
  - no serosal layer and outer adventitial layer is suspended within the mediastinium.
  - occupies a position dorsal and slightly to the left of the trachea.
  - closely associated with:
    - carotid arteries within the carotid sheath.
    - cranial sympathetic trunk.
    - recurrent laryngeal nerves.

Clinical signs of oesophageal disease

- often presents as signs of swallowing difficulties.
- dysphagia, hypersalivation, and sweating are associated with oesophageal obstruction.
- dysphagia can have oral, pharyngeal, and oesophageal causes (Fig. 2.101):
  - due to inflammation, neurological dysfunction, pharyngeal or oesophageal trauma, or luminal obstruction.
- aspiration of food spilling from an obstructed oesophagus can result in:
  - coughing.
  - aspiration pneumonia.
- oesophageal perforation can lead to a painful mediastinal cellulitis.
- oesophageal reflux syndrome in foals can cause intermittent signs of oesophageal pain associated with food ingestion.

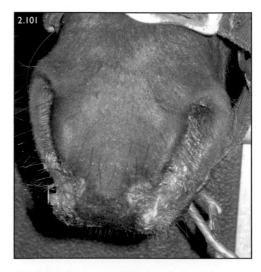

FIG. 2.101 Grass-stained bilateral nasal discharge associated with an oesophageal obstruction (choke).

Diagnosis of oesophageal diseases

Physical examination

- careful palpation of the neck from the larynx to the thoracic inlet for:
  - swelling, pain, oedema, cellulitis, crepitus or firm masses.
- general physical parameters such as:
  - circulatory function and hydration status.
  - haematological parameters and electrolytes.
  - neurological examination of the cranial nerves.
- cautious passage of a round-ended, well-lubricated nasogastric (NG) tube:
  - sedation may be necessary.
  - measuring scale marks helpful to assess distance of any obstruction from the nares.
  - NG tube usually seen descending the cervical oesophagus dorsal to the trachea on left side.
  - severe resistance to passage of NG tube indicates an oesophageal obstruction:
    - **attempts to force the tube through/past, the obstruction, contraindicated.**
    - may lead to oesophageal wall perforation.
- absence of swallowing reflex may indicate the presence of neurological dysfunction.
- thorough oral examination performed to check for any pharyngeal obstructions or causes of oral dysphagia.

Oesophagoscopy

- most effective way to examine the lumen of the oesophagus.
- safe and convenient to perform in the conscious sedated horse (Fig. 2.102).
- 2 metre endoscope is sufficient to reach the cardia in most horses:
  - 3 m gastroscope can also be used for gastroscopy.
- care taken when passing the endoscope into the pharynx:
  - avoid retroflexion of the endoscope into the oral cavity:
    - crushing of end of the endoscope.
  - avoided by use of:
    - Hausmann's gag.

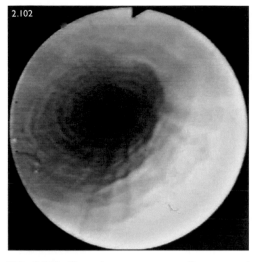

FIG. 2.102 Oesophagoscopy revealing normal oesophageal mucosa (distended).

- short wide-bore NG tube into the cranial oesophagus before introducing the endoscope.
- lubricated scope is passed all the way down the oesophagus:
  - inflate the lumen using the air pump to inspect the mucosa as far as the stomach.
  - usually, more easily viewed while withdrawing the endoscope distad to proximad.
  - constant irrigation necessary to remove any food or mucus and to identify small mucosal lesions or perforations.
- normal oesophagus is collapsed with longitudinal folds:
  - flatten when distended.
  - good distension avoids missing small focal/longitudinal oesophageal perforations.
- oesophagus obstructed with food:
  - cranial end of bolus and the type of feed can be identified.
  - visibility is poor in the presence of food and saliva in the lumen.
- mural or intrathoracic masses e.g. tumours or abscesses can occlude the lumen from externally, causing secondary obstruction (choke).

Radiography

- plain and contrast radiographs for a thorough investigation (Figs. 2.103, 2.104).
- oesophagus is soft tissue radiodensity:
  - not normally identified on plain films.
    - contrast against the air-filled trachea enables some distinction.
  - gas density shadow representing air in the lumen can be identified:
    - NG tube previously passed.
    - cranial oesophageal sphincter muscle disorder (4th branchial arch syndrome).
  - granular shadows caused by food stationary in lumen is an abnormal finding.
- contrast radiographs are indicated for:
  - swallowing defects.
  - irregularities or masses associated with the oesophageal lumen.
  - dynamic studies involving fluoroscopic imaging during swallowing are useful:
    - demonstrate duplication cysts or diverticula.
  - contrast radiographs and/or fluoroscopy helpful in diagnosis of:
    - external compression of the lumen by masses.
    - generalised cranial megaoesophagus, strictures, and vascular ring anomalies.
  - contrast achieved using gas, barium sulphate, or water-soluble iodinated solution:
    - barium sulphate mixed into paste with feed.
    - enables voluntary ingestion and swallowing to be imaged.
  - oesophageal wall perforation is suspected:
    - care must be taken with potentially irritant or toxic contrast media.
  - negative contrast is obtained by inflating the oesophagus via a cuffed NG tube placed in the cranial oesophagus:
    - useful for demonstrating foreign bodies, diverticula, and mural perforations.
  - normal peristalsis can create impression of irregular luminal folds and strictures on contrast films:
    - film taken immediately after injection of contrast media via a cuffed tube can avoid such artefacts.
  - evaluation of swallowing reflexes only attempted without sedation.

Transcutaneous ultrasonographic examination

- cervical area to identify:
  - mural thickening.
  - extraluminal masses.
  - luminal distension with fluid.
  - perioesophageal diverticula and oedema.
  - cellulitis and oedema caused by perforations leaking saliva and enzymes into surrounding tissues.

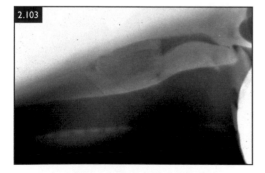

FIG. 2.103 Plain radiograph of the cranial neck in a horse presenting with choke. Note the regularly shaped foreign body in the cranial oesophagus, found subsequently to be a piece of wood.

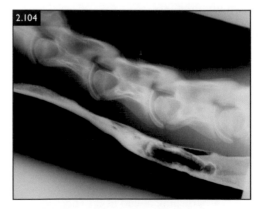

FIG. 2.104 Positive contrast oesophagram showing a partially obstructed lumen.

CONGENITAL AND DEVELOPMENTAL DISEASES OF THE EQUINE OESOPHAGUS

Congenital persistent right aortic arch

Definition/overview

- rare congenital anomaly where 4th right aortic arch develops into the functional aorta instead of the normal left vessel.

Aetiology/pathophysiology

- fibrous remnant of the ductus arteriosus occludes the oesophagus between the aortic arch and the left pulmonary artery.

Clinical presentation

- signs of oesophageal dysphagia and obstruction:
  - salivation.
  - cervical oesophageal distension.

Differential diagnosis

- Oesophageal obstruction, 4th branchial arch defects, and megaoesophagus.

Diagnosis

- based on clinical signs of oesophageal dysphagia.
- confirmed by plain and contrast radiographs:
  - dilatation of the oesophagus proximal to the ductus arteriosus.
- oesophagoscopy reveals a dilated proximal oesophagus with diffuse oesophagitis and an apparent stricture just cranial to the level of the heart.

Management

- successful surgical correction reported in one foal.
- euthanasia may be more practical.

Oesophageal duplication cysts and intramural duplication cysts

Definition/overview

- oesophageal cysts are congenitally replicated segments of the proximal oesophagus:
  - bifurcation of the embryonic oesophageal tube.
- intramural duplication cysts are evaginations within the wall of the oesophagus lined by stratified squamous epithelium:
  - separated and isolated from the main oesophagus.

Aetiology/pathophysiology

- lesions arise congenitally as elements of the embryonic alimentary endoderm become separated from the main alimentary tube.
- reported in young animals involving both the oesophagus and components of the oesophagus and trachea.
- lesions result in external compression on the oesophageal lumen causing obstruction.

Clinical presentation

- palpable, non-painful swelling may be present in the cervical oesophagus:
  - increases as the cysts enlarge.
  - usually not reducible.
- impingement of the true oesophageal lumen is possible:
  - may result in intermittent oesophageal dysphagia and signs of 'choke'.

Differential diagnosis

- oesophageal obstruction, thyroid masses, cervical abscessation, parotid salivary gland enlargement and oesophageal diverticula.

Diagnosis

- oesophagoscopy may reveal a lumen in the case of duplication cysts.

- contrast oesophagrams may show accumulation of contrast in the lumen of duplication cysts, which often communicates with the oesophageal lumen.
- transcutaneous ultrasonography is useful to identify encapsulated fluid-filled homoechoic structures:
  - ultrasound-guided aspiration may demonstrate squamous cells supporting a diagnosis of an oesophageal cyst.

Management

- successful treatment of the cysts by marsupialisation of the cyst.
- attempted removal of the cyst *in toto* may have complications.

Megaoesophagus

Definition/overview

- persistent dilatation of the oesophagus, resulting in:
  - failure of peristalsis and accumulation of ingesta in the oesophagus.

Aetiology/pathophysiology

- primary megaoesophagus is very rare in the horse:
  - consequence of motor dysfunction of the oesophageal musculature.
- congenital oesophageal dilatation syndrome also described:
  - involves neural and muscular components.

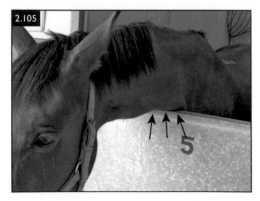

FIG. 2.105 Dilatation of the oesophagus on the left side of the neck in a horse with acquired megaoesophagus (arrows).

- secondary megaoesophagus can be associated with other conditions such as:
  - equine grass sickness.
  - botulism.
  - toxicity with lead, thallium or anticholinesterase.
  - following sedation with acepromazine and detomidine.
  - neurological dysfunction associated with acquired diseases such as:
    - ♦ equine protozoal meningitis (EPM).
    - ♦ equine herpesvirus-1 (EHV-1).
  - transient form after persistent oesophageal obstruction or indwelling NG tube placement.

Clinical presentation

- observation while grazing can reveal palpable dilatation of the oesophagus on the left-hand side of the neck, which may be reducible when the head is raised (Fig. 2.105):
  - more obvious when solid food is being ingested.
  - may not be obvious with liquid food.
- obstruction is incomplete and cases may compensate and maintain body condition.
- aspiration pneumonia is a possible secondary complication.

Differential diagnosis

- oesophageal obstruction and oesophageal diverticula.

Diagnosis

- plain and contrast radiographs:
  - obstruction at caudal oesophageal sphincter with damming of ingesta cranially.

Management

- dietary management will help avoid complete oesophageal obstruction and aspiration of food.
- transient secondary cases can gradually improve after conservative treatment.
- permanent megaoesophagus with persistent dysphagia carries a guarded prognosis.

Gastro-oesophageal reflux syndrome

Definition/overview

- gastric contents are refluxed into the caudal oesophagus.

Aetiology/pathophysiology

- reflux oesophagitis is the consequence of repeated episodes of gastric fluid regurgitation into the distal oesophagus.
- gastric acid results in chemical injury to the mucosa and eventually mucosal sloughing and ulceration.
- may occur in combination with:
  - gastric ulcer disease.
  - motility disorders including intestinal ileus.
  - distal oesophageal sphincter dysfunction.
- most common in weanlings and occasionally in adults.
- acquired oesophagitis can occur during:
  - indwelling NG tube placement, especially in foals.
  - frequent NG tube passage.
  - after oesophageal obstruction.

Clinical presentation

- clinical signs are non-specific and include:
  - signs similar to oesophageal obstruction.
  - discomfort when ingesting including:
    - ◆ gagging, bruxism, hypersalivation, and anorexia.
    - ◆ inflammation can cause oesophageal hypomotility:
      - – secondary obstruction with food if the horse continues to eat.

Differential diagnosis

- colic in foals, gastric ulceration, cardiac sphincter stenosis, and oesophageal obstruction.

Diagnosis

- thorough oesophagoscopy after clearing obstructions (Fig. 2.106):
  - patchy or linear ulceration is diagnostic for oesophagitis.
  - careful examination for any underlying cause including gastroscopy.

Management

- any primary cause such as oesophageal obstruction should be removed.
- treatment with H_2 receptor antagonists (e.g. ranitidine or cimetidine) or by using oral medication with omeprazole is beneficial:
  - reduce gastric acid production and chemical damage to the oesophageal mucosa.
  - alteration in feeding regimes to promote continuous gastric outflow may help reduce symptoms.
- NSAIDs may be indicated for their fibrinolytic activity:
  - help reduce likelihood of fibrous stricture formation at the distal oesophageal sphincter.
  - **careful use in neonates to avoid possibility of gastric ulceration.**
- gastric protectants such as sucralfate are of questionable benefit:
  - may give physical protection to the ulcerated mucosa.
- feeding of semi-liquidised food will help reduce likelihood of oesophageal obstruction at the distal oesophageal sphincter.
- stricture of the distal oesophageal sphincter because of fibrosis:
  - consequence of chronic reflux oesophagitis.
  - occasionally diagnosed in young and adult horses.

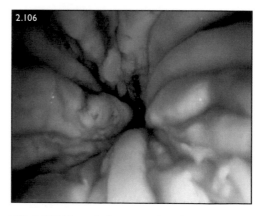

FIG. 2.106 Ulcerated mucosa in a foal with reflex oesophagitis.

ACQUIRED OESOPHAGEAL DISORDERS.

Oesophageal obstruction ('choke')

Definition/overview

- physical obstruction of the oesophagus with ingesta.

Aetiology/pathophysiology

- most common oesophageal disorder in the adult horse.
- inadequate soaking of proprietary or preserved foods is cited as the most frequent predisposing cause:
  - sugar beet pulp is the most implicated foodstuff in the UK.
- presence of motility disorders within the oesophagus may be a cause but is unproven.
- primary grass choke is rare and suggests an underlying problem.
- absorption of saliva by the food bolus results in it swelling.
- bolus may lodge in the oesophagus:
  - commonly at the thoracic inlet:
    - diameter is narrowest and oesophagus changes direction.
  - spasm of the oesophageal muscle distal to the bolus may occur:
    - prevents further passage by peristalsis.
- horses often continue to eat after oesophageal obstruction:
  - food accumulation can extend proximally almost to the larynx.
- oesophageal obstruction may be associated with autonomic dysfunction (equine grass sickness).

Clinical presentation

- signs of oesophageal obstruction include:
  - anxiety, with elevated pulse and respiratory rates and sweating of the neck.
  - inability to swallow despite ongoing saliva production can lead to:
    - dehydration and electrolyte disturbances including hypochloraemia.
  - nasogastric reflux of food and saliva can be observed from both nostrils.

Differential diagnosis

- oesophageal diverticula, congenital anomalies, cardiac sphincter incompetence, grass sickness, and botulism.

Diagnosis

- attempts to pass a NG tube will be met with resistance at the proximal end of the obstructing bolus.
- oesophagoscopy will reveal:
  - cranial extent of the bolus and saliva pooling.
  - can indicate the type of food (Fig. 2.107).
  - demonstrate luminal defects or a diverticulum.
  - view may be obscured by opaque liquid and suspended food.
- aspiration of food into the trachea will be observed endoscopically in many cases:
  - ensuing tracheitis will lead to coughing.

Management

- **oesophageal obstruction does not constitute an acute emergency:**
  - many horses tolerate obstruction for 24 hours or more without significant oesophageal mucosal damage.
- prompt investigation is warranted due to:

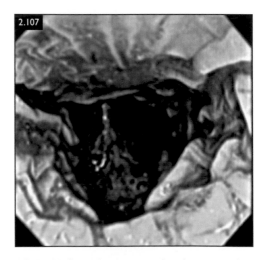

FIG. 2.107 Oesophagoscopy showing an atypical obstruction with grass.

- ○ distress to the horse and owner.
- ○ potential for electrolyte and fluid disturbances.
- ○ inhalation pneumonia and oesophageal ulceration.
- spontaneous clearing of the obstruction will occur in many cases if relaxation of the oesophageal muscle spasm can be achieved:
  - ○ smooth muscle relaxants e.g. N-butylscopolammonium bromide (Buscopan).
  - ○ phenothiazine tranquillisers including acepromazine.
  - ○ diazepam.
  - ○ alpha-2 agonists including xylazine, detomidine and romifidine:
    - ◆ additionally reduce anxiety and sedation:
      - – latter leads to lowering of the head.
      - – promotes orad drainage of any food and saliva from pharynx and trachea.
- limited access to small volumes of water can help with irrigation:
  - ○ **all food should be immediately withdrawn.**
- soften bolus by irrigation with warm water through a narrow NG irrigation tube:
  - ○ **care taken to avoid excessive force when advancing the tube.**
  - ○ avoids perforation of the delicate oesophageal mucosa.
  - ○ lower head with sedation to ensure that overflow exits the nostrils.
  - ○ infuse water slowly to allow drainage around the tube without excessive overflow into the trachea.
  - ○ bolus is softened and gradually removed with the egress water:
  - ○ allows cautious advancement of the tube.
  - ○ **patience is required when the bolus is extensive.**
  - ○ multilumen, cuffed oesophageal bougienage tubes are available to reduce the likelihood of aspiration during irrigation.
  - ○ process can be repeated at 2–4-hourly intervals, until the NG tube can be passed into the stomach.
  - ○ most cases will eventually clear.
  - ○ once cleared:

- ◆ oesophagus should be lavaged with saline to clear residual food.
- ◆ oesophagoscopy to inspect for mucosal ulceration or a primary cause.
- food restricted for the first 24–48 h and then introduced gradually with moistened food or grazing.
- functional oesophageal spasm may remain temporarily after clearance, especially where ulcers are present.
- treatment of any aspiration pneumonia is essential.

Oesophageal ulceration

Definition/overview
- full-thickness erosion of the oesophageal mucosa.

Aetiology/pathogenesis
- ulceration can occur secondary to impaction and may lead to re-impaction.
- circumferential ulceration is particularly hazardous:
  - ○ cicatrisation of the healing ulcer can lead to a permanent oesophageal stricture.
  - ○ repeated episodes of oesophageal obstruction at this site.
- ulceration in the distal oesophagus can be associated with gastro-oesophageal reflux.

Clinical presentation
- may present with hypersalivation.
- recurrent oesophageal obstruction.
- discomfort when swallowing food.
- chronic colic.

Differential diagnosis
- Squamous cell carcinoma of the oesophagus.

Diagnosis
- oesophagoscopy will reveal the red submucosa surrounded by the frayed edges of the eroded stratified squamous epithelium (Fig. 2.108).
- contrast oesophagrams may show some stricture at the site of a circumferential ulcer (Fig. 2.109).

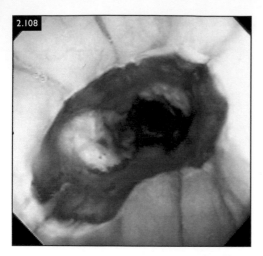

FIG. 2.108 Circumferential ulcer secondary to prolonged choke.

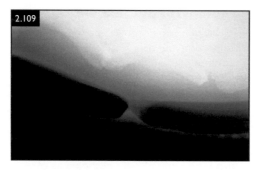

FIG. 2.109 Contrast oesophagram showing narrowing of the oesophageal lumen due to a circumferential oesophageal stricture.

Management

- NSAIDs such as phenylbutazone will delay fibrosis.
- before re-introducing a normal diet:
  - ○ repeated endoscopic monitoring of the healing lesion.
  - ○ feeding of moistened softened food.
- fibrosed strictures can involve all layers or just the muscular and adventitial layers:
  - ○ full-thickness strictures:
    - ♦ form after deep, circumferential ulcers.
    - ♦ observed endoscopically and demonstrated on contrast oesophagrams.
    - ♦ treatment by various types of surgery.
  - ○ partial-thickness strictures:
    - ♦ do not involve the mucosa.
    - ♦ successfully treated by oesophagomyotomy.
    - ♦ oesophageal bougienage dilation has met with very limited success.
- prognosis for persistent circumferential strictures is poor:
  - ○ many cases suffer repeated episodes of choke.

Oesophageal diverticula

Definition/overview

- pathological evaginations of the oesophageal mucosa resulting from a defect in the muscularis.

Aetiology/pathogenesis

- usually acquired lesions and two types have been described.
- **Traction diverticula:**
  - ○ result of traction from the fibrosis and adhesion of perioesophageal scar tissue following a partial- or full-thickness wound.
  - ○ following the second-intention healing of a ventral oesophagotomy.
- **Pulsion diverticula:**
  - ○ form when a defect of the oesophageal muscularis occurs.
  - ○ intact oesophageal mucosa prolapses through the defect without perforation, and subsequently increases in size as the diverticulum becomes impacted with food.

Clinical presentation

- diverticula should be suspected when:
  - ○ horse presents with chronic intermittent choke, particularly when out at grass.
  - ○ swelling of the cervical neck over the oesophagus:
    - ♦ does not prevent passage of a NG tube.
    - ♦ be careful when passing the tube to avoid the end passing into the diverticulum and perforating the mucosa.

Diagnosis

- oesophagoscopy will often reveal flattening of the lumen, and food accumulating in the diverticulum.
- diverticulum type is demonstrated with contrast oesophagrams:
  - ventral defect on the oesophageal lumen in the case of traction diverticula.
  - pathognomonic 'hour-glass' image in pulsion diverticula (Fig. 2.110).

Management

- traction diverticula rarely cause obstruction and most cases do not require intervention.
- pulsion diverticula can be treated by surgery but recurrence is the main complication.
- careful feeding of soft food for 4–6 weeks is advised in all cases.

Foreign body penetrations and oesophageal fistula

Definition/overview

- foreign bodies may cause focal perforation of the oesophageal mucosa.
- consequences include:
  - cellulitis, abscessation, and oesophageal dysfunction.
- uncommon in horses because they are relatively fastidious feeders.

Aetiology/pathogenesis

- perforation of the oesophageal mucosa by sharp ingested foreign bodies leads to:
  - egress of saliva into the interstitium.
  - development of an initial cellulitis, which eventually suppurates:
    - ◆ perioesophageal cellulitis or an abscess may cause pain on swallowing and oesophageal dysfunction.
    - ◆ abscess may burst into the oesophageal lumen or subcutaneously to form an oesophageal fistula.
  - results in pain, peristaltic dysfunction and food impaction proximal to the site.

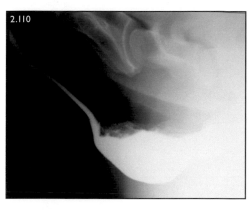

FIG. 2.110 Contrast oesophagram showing a pulsion diverticulum.

  - some cases develop a mediastinitis and endotoxic shock.

Clinical presentation

- dysphagia.
- oesophageal obstruction (choke).
- painful swellings of the neck.
- hypersalivation.
- pyrexia and acute endotoxic shock.

Differential diagnosis

- primary choke.
- injection abscesses.
- diverticula.
- mediastinitis from other sources.

Diagnosis

- oesophagoscopy may reveal the mucosal defect when the oesophageal lumen is fully dilated with air, although these can prove to be elusive (Fig. 2.111).
- contrast oesophagrams may be helpful although false-negative images are possible.
- inoculation of the mediastinum with bacteria and saliva provokes:
  - acute inflammatory sepsis with pain, swelling, and rapid shock (Fig. 2.112).
  - lesions are challenging to identify once such inflammation is present.

Management

- some foreign bodies can be retrieved from the oesophagus endoscopically:

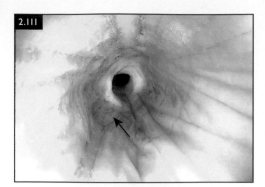

FIG. 2.111 Oesophagoscopy of a perforated oesophagus indicating the difficulty identifying the perforation (arrow).

- contrast radiography may be necessary to demonstrate their location.
- endoscopic retrieval using basket forceps, or a snare is the least traumatic method.
- some cases, advancement into the stomach is possible where extraction proves impossible.
- sharp barbed twigs or thorns can be extremely traumatic to the lumen during retrieval:
  - lubrication or ensheathing in a NG tube may help reduce this.
- surgical exploration under general anaesthesia may be necessary to remove the foreign body and allow effective drainage of any surrounding septic exudates.
- perioesophageal infections should be cultured to optimise antibiotic administration.

Oesophageal rupture

Definition/overview
- traumatic disruption of the oesophageal mucosa and other layers.

Aetiology/pathogenesis
- follow prolonged obstruction, overaggressive NG tube use or ingestion of foreign bodies.
- drainage of saliva results in rapid cervical swelling due to cellulitis.
- swallowed air can disperse to form subcutaneous emphysema:

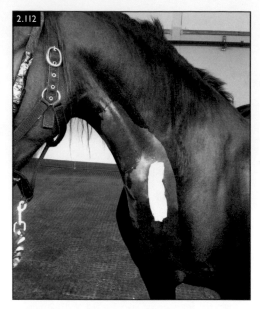

FIG. 2.112 Exudation from the oesophagus can cause a painful dissecting cellulitis.

  - demonstrated on radiographs (Fig. 2.113).
- development of cervical cellulitis to an extensive mediastinitis carries a guarded prognosis.

Clinical presentation
- cervical swelling, dysphagia, and dyspnoea are typically present.
- signs of systemic toxaemia may be apparent.

Diagnosis
- oesophagoscopy and contrast radiographs are critical.
- transthoracic ultrasound can demonstrate perioesophageal abscesses.

Management
- small, acute defects may be treated by surgical repair.
- all chronic or heavily contaminated defects are treated by:
  - surgical drainage of the affected area.
  - oesophagostomy caudal to the rupture, to allow continued feeding.
  - damaged area is then left to heal by secondary intention.

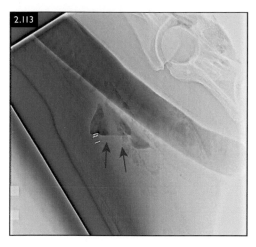

FIG. 2.113 Contrast oesophagram of a horse with gas shadows in the perioesophageal tissue (arrows) subsequent to an iatrogenic oesophageal rupture.

Oesophageal neoplasia

- rare in the horse.
- oesophageal extension of gastric mucosa squamous cell carcinoma is the most common.
- prognosis for such lesions is very guarded and for resection is dubious.

The Lower Gastrointestinal Tract

Physical examination

- evaluation of the GI tract should include:
  - animal's history:
    - signalment and occupation of the horse.
    - diet and feeding practices.
    - recent management changes.
    - deworming and dental care schedule.
    - temperament and vices.
    - availability and quality of water.
    - medication received.
    - duration and occurrence of the problem.
  - evaluation of horse and its surroundings:
    - water source, housing condition, and pasture.
    - attention given to assessing:
      - physical appearance of the horse and body condition.
      - abdominal contour and skin trauma.
- thorough physical examination should be performed including:
  - evaluation of other body systems such as:
    - cardiovascular, respiratory, neurological, musculoskeletal, and reproductive.
    - GI problems can be mistaken for other body system abnormalities and vice versa.
  - examine the mouth:
    - full dental examination:
      - abnormalities may be associated with anorexia or abnormal eating patterns.
    - presence of feed material in the oral cavity should be noted.
  - neurological examination where there are concerns about the horse's ability to eat properly:
    - observation of eating can be useful.

- palpate the neck for the presence of masses, crepitus, or pain:
  - oesophagus normally runs down the left side but examine both sides.
  - passage of a NG tube is helpful in:
    - oesophageal abnormalities.
    - during a colic examination.
- gut motility may be assessed by calculating gut transit time:
  - passage of mineral oil in faeces following administration via a NG tube should be observed after 8–12 hours.
- consistency, colour, and volume of faeces should be noted:
  - presence of sand, gravel, or large food particles.

Gastrointestinal tract auscultation and percussion

- auscultation is an important part of GI tract examination.
- results taken in the context of the entire clinical presentation and not overinterpreted.
- multiple locations should be evaluated:
  - dorsal and ventral quadrants should be auscultated over both abdominal walls.
- frequency and character of borborygmi should be noted:
  - be patient as borborygmi are often intermittent, particularly those associated with caecal contraction.
  - decreased or absent sounds are indicative of decreased intestinal motility.
  - increased sounds suggest hypermotility.
  - fluid sounds may be present in colic or impending colitis cases.
  - simultaneous auscultation and percussion should be performed to detect 'pings', which indicate underlying gaseous distension.

DOI: 10.1201/9781003427711-3

Palpation per rectum

- evaluation of the intestinal tract per rectum is a useful diagnostic tool:
  - **should be performed, if possible, on all horses with colic.**
  - only approximately 40% of the abdomen palpable in an average horse.

- iatrogenic rectal tears can occur:
  - ♦ proper restraint (including chemical restraint) and technique can greatly reduce the risk.
  - ♦ horse should be handled by an experienced person.
  - ♦ sedated if required.
  - ♦ ample lubrication should be used.
  - ♦ patience is important and excessive force should never be used:
    - – forcing an arm forward in a straining horse may lead to a rectal tear.
  - ♦ reduce straining:
    - – rectal infusion of lidocaine (60 ml of 2% lidocaine per 450 kg horse).
    - – and/or administration of N-butylscopolammonium bromide (Buscopan®), 0.1–0.3 mg/kg i/v.

  - good knowledge of the normal anatomy and understanding of displacement and change that can occur in different pathologies is required.

Normal findings

Left abdomen
- pelvic flexure located cranially and ventrally to brim of the pelvis:
  - knee-shaped, and bands felt if content within it.
- thin, sharp, caudal edge of the spleen present against the abdominal wall.
- nephrosplenic ligament and posterior pole of the left kidney palpable dorsomedially to spleen.
- cranial mesenteric artery can sometimes be felt caudally and medially to the left kidney, running forward along the aorta.

Right abdomen
- caecum (particularly its ventral taenial band) felt running forward and down.

Mid-abdomen
- small colon characterised by the presence of faecal balls, sacculations, and an antimesenteric taenial band.
- bladder found just cranial to the pelvic rim.
- small intestine is usually not palpable.
- in males evaluate the inguinal rings for any abnormal content such as omentum or small intestinal loops.
- in mares, the uterus and ovaries should be palpated.

Potential abnormal findings

Stomach
- not palpable.
- with excessive distension, the spleen can be displaced caudally.

Small intestine
- distension characterised by presence of one or more loops of >5 cm diameter, smooth-surfaced viscera:
  - not always palpable immediately, depending on location of the loops.
- palpation of the wall of the intestine performed to evaluate the degree of oedema.

Caecum
- distinct contents within the caecum or a tight ventral taenial band running in a vertical plane:
  - indicative of caecal tympany or impaction.
- with gas distension, the apex of the caecum may be directed dorsally and the ventral taenial band may be in an oblique or transverse position.
- some large colon displacements, the caecum may not be found in its normal location.

Large intestine
- large colon impactions are usually located in the left ventral colon and, less commonly, in the right dorsal colon.
- feed impaction usually feels like firm bread dough:
  - easily indented by digital pressure with the impressions remaining.
  - free taenial bands of the colon are palpable and run longitudinally.

- sacculations are not palpable because of the distension.
  - impaction of the right dorsal colon:
    - mass felt in the right quadrant in small horses.
- gas or fluid distension:
  - colon can be indented, but the impression does not remain.
  - gas-distended pelvic flexure is often displaced on the right side or cranially.
- oedema of the colonic wall usually indicative of large colon torsion.
- tympany and/or impaction of left colon with band running dorsally toward the nephrosplenic space:
  - consistent with left dorsal displacement of the large colon.

Small colon
- Small colon impaction on palpation:
  - doughy, sausage-like structure about 10 cm in diameter and usually longer than 30 cm.
- other abnormalities that may be palpable *per rectum* include intraluminal foreign bodies, enteroliths, or intussusception.

Rectum
- absence of faeces, or the presence of mucus-covered faeces:
  - indicates decrease in GI transit, often secondary to an obstructive disease.
- blood present locally or on rectal sleeve:
  - palpate rectum carefully for the presence of a rectal tear.

Others
- peritoneal wall should be felt for roughening or a gritty feeling:
  - indication of peritonitis following bowel rupture.

Diagnostic tests

Haematology and biochemistry

- haematology of variable usefulness in the investigation of gastrointestinal disease.
- minimum blood work should include full haematological and biochemical analysis plus fibrinogen and serum amyloid A.
  - acute, one-off episode of colic:
    - usually unremarkable or non-specific changes.
    - not commonly indicated.
  - blood work is indicated in:
    - acute colic presentation is atypical.
    - chronic or recurrent colic.

- chronic undifferentiated gastrointestinal disease.
- decrease in serum proteins useful indicator of chronic gastrointestinal disease.

Nasogastric (NG) intubation

- NG intubation is an essential component of colic examination in all horses:
  - identification and relief of accumulated fluid or gas in the stomach.
  - identification of oesophageal obstruction.
  - provides an administration route for water, electrolyte solutions, mineral oil, or other substances.
- creation of a siphon, by priming the tube with water, is required to confirm the presence of gastric reflux:
  - often no spontaneous reflux, even with severe gastric distension.
- passage of the tube:
  - appropriately sized tube.
  - adequate manual or chemical restraint to prevent injury to horse or humans.
  - essential to confirm present in oesophagus before anything is administered.

Radiography

- abdominal radiography has limited applications in adult horses:
  - mainly used to identify sand accumulation or enteroliths.
- more useful in foals and small horses (Figs. 3.1, 3.2):
  - gaseous distension of the stomach, small intestine, and large intestine.
  - intestinal obstructions.
  - presence of free gas in the abdomen.
- combination of lateral and ventrodorsal radiographs is most useful.
- contrast radiography can be used for the diagnosis of meconium impactions and assess intestinal patency and gastric emptying.

Ultrasonography

- useful in the diagnosis of GI disease:
- limitations:
  - inexperience of the ultrasonographer.
  - only adequate penetration of 25–30 cm into the abdomen:

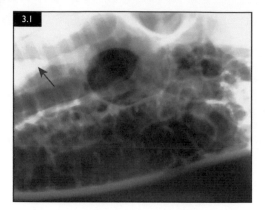

FIG. 3.1 Survey abdominal radiograph in a foal with meconium impaction. Note the radiodense meconium in the cranial abdomen (arrow).

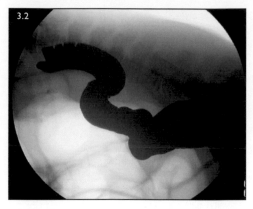

FIG. 3.2 Barium enema in a foal with meconium impaction. The contrast dye stops at the level of the impaction.

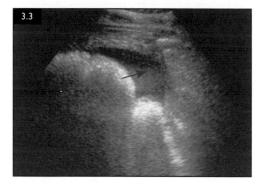

FIG. 3.3 A pocket of peritoneal fluid (arrowed) is evident ultrasonographically in a horse with acute colic.

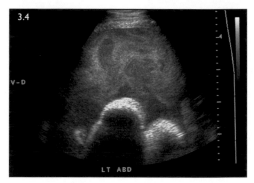

FIG. 3.4 Ultrasonographic appearance of haemoperitoneum in a horse with blunt abdominal trauma.

- ◆ combination of transabdominal and transrectal approaches.
- ◆ significant percentage of the abdomen can be examined.
- ○ intestinal gas can result in interference.
- examination approached in an organised manner to ensure that all relevant areas of the abdomen are examined:
  - ○ adult horses, 2.5–3.5 MHz probes are typically used.
  - ○ foals, 5.0–7.5 MHz probes.
  - ○ alcohol or methylated spirits applied to the haircoat in horses without excessive coat:
    - ◆ image quality not adequate, then the haircoat should be clipped.
- useful for identification of:
  - ○ peritoneal effusion (Fig. 3.3) and haemoperitoneum (Fig. 3.4).
  - ○ distended small intestine.
  - ○ thickened intestinal walls.
  - ○ adhesions, masses, and intussusceptions.
  - ○ left dorsal displacement of the large colon.
  - ○ splenic abnormalities.
  - ○ qualitative diagnosis of sand accumulation:
    - ◆ radiography more accurate in quantifying the sand accumulation.

Abdominocentesis

- utilised to assist in determining whether colic surgery, or euthanasia, is indicated.
- useful in evaluation of fever of unknown origin, or peritoneal effusion.
- controversy exists as to its use in:
  - ○ chronic weight loss.
  - ○ chronic diarrhoea.
  - ○ chronic inflammatory bowel disease.

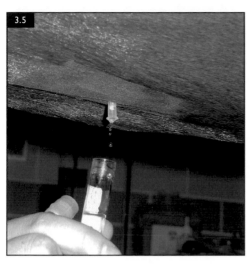

FIG. 3.5 Free-flowing abdominal fluid during abdominocentesis.

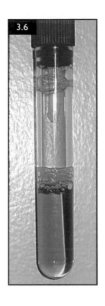

FIG. 3.6 Serosanguineous abdominal fluid from a horse with a strangulating small intestinal lesion.

- preferred site is approximately 10 cm caudal to the xiphoid and 5–10 cm to the right of midline:
  - area clipped and surgically prepared.
  - 18-gauge, 1.5-inch needle is adequate for most horses.
  - larger needle may be required for very fat animals and those with ventral oedema.
  - change in resistance or 'pop' may be felt when the peritoneum is entered, or fluid may flow spontaneously (Fig. 3.5).
  - small volume (1–2 ml) of air can be aseptically injected into the needle to dislodge any tissue that may be blocking flow.
  - no fluid is obtained, a second needle can be inserted 3–6 cm from the first.
  - alternatively, a teat cannula can be used:
    - insertion site skin infiltrated with 2% lidocaine.
    - stab incision made through the skin and superficial tissue.
    - pass canula into peritoneal cavity with controlled force.
- abdominocentesis does not always yield fluid and this is not an abnormal or unexpected finding.
- visual examination of the fluid, plus determination of total protein or specific gravity (SG) is adequate in most cases:
  - normal peritoneal fluid is clear to slightly yellow in colour:

- dark yellow or orange and turbid with peritonitis or compromised intestinal viscera (Fig. 3.6).
- bloody or red-tinged fluid can be iatrogenic with bleeding discolouring a normal sample.
  - total protein level should be <25 g/l (2.5 g/dl).
  - high PCV is suggestive of splenic puncture:
    - determination of total protein content of the supernatant is not reliable in such cases.
- intestinal contents may be evident as dark, flocculent, foul-smelling fluid:
  - enterocentesis is possible, particularly when a needle is used.
  - rapid initiation of broad-spectrum antimicrobials via a single intravenous dose is indicated:
    - further therapy not typically required.
    - patient should be monitored closely for signs of peritonitis.
- fluid suggestive of rupture of an intestinal viscus:
  - repeat sampling at one or more distant sites.
  - ultrasonography useful to distinguish rupture:
    - large volume of free fluid seen in such cases.
- cytological examination of peritoneal fluid useful in certain circumstances:

o differentiation of enterocentesis versus intestinal rupture:
  ♦ intracellular bacteria and degenerate neutrophils present if intestinal rupture.
o total nucleated cell count should be <5 × 10^9/l.
o bacterial culture should be performed if septic peritonitis or chronic inflammation is suspected:
  ♦ Gram stain may be useful in guiding initial antimicrobial therapy.

Carbohydrate absorption tests

- used to assess small intestinal absorption:
  o chronic weight loss or hypoproteinaemia.
  o suspected inflammatory bowel disease.
- monosaccharides (i.e. D-xylose, glucose) are normally readily absorbed in the small intestine:
  o oral administration of the carbohydrate is followed by analysis of serial blood samples for the specific carbohydrate.
  o unlike glucose, xylose is not metabolised, so blood levels more closely represent intestinal absorption.
  o xylose is more expensive, and glucose is more readily available.
- both tests performed following an 18–24-hour fast:
  o beyond 24 hours may potentially impact the test results.
- baseline blood sample is collected.
- xylose or glucose (0.5–1.0 g/kg as a 10–20% solution in water) administered via a NG tube:
  o avoid sedation as affects gastric emptying.
- blood samples collected every 30 minutes for 3 hours, or until an adequate increase in blood carbohydrate level is observed:
  o blood glucose levels should increase by at least 85%.
  o blood xylose levels should reach 1.33–1.68 mmol/l (20–25 mg/dl):
    ♦ peak glucose or xylose typically occurs within 60–90 minutes.
- flattened absorption curve suggests impaired small intestinal absorption:
  o delayed gastric emptying can cause similar results.

- decrease of blood glucose levels of <15%:
  o considered complete malabsorption and may be a poor prognostic indicator.
- **care should be taken in interpreting results:**
  o attenuated absorption curves have been reported in normal horses.
  o consider tests in the context of the animal's clinical state and other findings.
  o 'normal' test results do not necessarily indicate normal small intestine:
    ♦ segmental disease may not be identified.

Rectal mucosal biopsies

- useful adjunctive diagnostic tool in the evaluation of chronic gastrointestinal disease.
- limitations should be recognised, and they are rarely diagnostic in isolation.
- performed as part of a thorough diagnostic work-up of chronic gastrointestinal disease.
- samples readily collected using uterine biopsy forceps.
- sedate horse and remove all faecal matter.
- 20–50 ml of 2% lidocaine is infused into the rectum.
- insert the biopsy forceps into the rectum shielded by a gloved hand:
  o sampling at approximately 15–20 cm of depth and at 10 and 2 o'clock positions.
  o small tag of mucosa is pulled ventrally, and the biopsy forceps are applied.
  o remaining mucosa is then separated, and the forceps removed.
  o procedure is repeated 3–4 times.
  o biopsy is well tolerated when performed correctly and no specific aftercare (i.e. antimicrobials) is required.
- histopathological evaluation of biopsies should be performed by a pathologist experienced with mucosal pathology in the horse.

Use of analgesics in colic

- goal is to:
  o relieve pain to facilitate examination.
  o benefit animal welfare.

- ○ prevent self-induced trauma.
- ○ lessen pain-induced ileus.
- ○ allow for safe transportation to a referral facility.
- 'standard' regimen for analgesia is not available and analgesic administration should be tailored towards each case (Table 3.1).
- overly aggressive analgesic therapy should be avoided so deterioration of the disease is not masked:
  - ○ particularly when early surgical intervention may be required.
  - ○ where surgical intervention is not an option then more aggressive analgesic therapy should be pursued in the interests of animal welfare.
- flunixin meglumine is most used at a dose of 1.1 mg/kg i/v.
- other NSAIDs such as phenylbutazone, ketoprofen, meloxicam, and dipyrone have lesser analgesic properties but can also be used.
- N-butylscopolammonium bromide (Buscopan®) is an antispasmodic and anticholinergic that may relieve intestinal spasm and is useful in spasmodic colic.
- alpha-2 adrenergic agonists have a potent analgesic effect:
  - ○ adverse effects on GI motility.

- ○ reserved for situations where:
  - ♦ poor response to NSAIDs.
  - ♦ NSAIDs are contraindicated.
  - ♦ rapid onset of analgesia and sedation is required.
- ○ xylazine, alone or in combination with butorphanol, can be very useful:
  - ♦ short-term (15–30 minutes alone, 30–120 minutes with butorphanol) analgesia, and sedation.
- ○ detomidine is more potent, but it should be used judiciously:
  - ♦ deleterious effects on intestinal motility and blood pressure.
- constant-rate infusion of butorphanol, ketamine, or lidocaine may be useful:
  - ○ severely painful horses, particularly postoperative cases.
  - ○ where surgical intervention is not an option.
- morphine is not commonly used:
  - ○ potential for hyperexcitability and ileus.
  - ○ useful in some non-responsive cases.
- acepromazine has no analgesic effects and causes peripheral vasodilation:
  - ○ **contraindicated in dehydrated or hypotensive horses.**
  - ○ should be avoided.

TABLE 3.1 Analgesic drugs used for the treatment of colic

DRUG	DOSE	ROUTE	COMMENT
Flunixin	1.1 mg/kg q8–12h	i/v	Good analgesic effect
Dipyrone	5–22 mg/kg	i/v	Less potent than flunixin
Ketoprofen	2.2 mg/kg	i/v	
Meloxicam	0.6 mg/kg	i/v	COX-1 sparing, may have reduced adverse effects
Phenylbutazone	2.2–4.4 mg/kg	i/v	Not generally recommended for colic. No advantage over other NSAIDs
Buscopan®	0.3 mg/kg	i/v	Antispasmodic, only for spasmodic colic
Xylazine	0.25–0.5 mg/kg	i/v or i/m	Short-term sedation/analgesia
Detomidine	10–20 µg/kg	i/v or i/m	Potent analgesic, more likely to cause hypotension and ileus
Butorphanol	0.02–0.1 mg/kg	i/v or i/m	Use with α-2 agonist
	13 µg/kg/hour	i/v	CRI
Lidocaine	1.3 mg/kg loading dose over 15 minutes, then 0.05 mg/kg/min	i/v	Neurotoxicity may occur rarely

GENERAL DISORDERS OF THE LOWER GASTROINTESTINAL TRACT

Ileus

Definition/overview

- impairment of aboral transit of ingesta due to abnormal or absent intestinal motility:
  - secondary to an obstructive intestinal disease (obstructive ileus).
  - can be paralytic (adynamic).

Aetiology/pathophysiology

- any intestinal insult can induce a dynamic ileus:
  - local insults include:
    - intestinal distension or impaction.
    - enteritis/colitis.
    - abdominal surgery, or peritonitis.
  - electrolyte imbalances (esp. hypokalaemia, hypomagnesaemia or hypocalcaemia).
  - certain drugs (alpha-2 agonists or opioid analgesics).
  - endotoxaemia.
  - pain.
  - general anaesthesia.
  - vascular or obstructive intestinal injuries will cause an obstructive ileus:
    - torsion, entrapment, and strangulation.
- extrinsic and local enteric nervous systems control GI motility:
  - extrinsic nervous system:
    - motility stimulated by parasympathetic activity (acetylcholine).
    - sympathetic stimulation (norepinephrine) has an inhibitory effect.
    - imbalance between these two components results in ileus.

Clinical presentation

- ileus is often secondary and clinical findings of the primary disease may predominate.
- adynamic ileus associated with depression, mild to severe abdominal pain, anorexia, and decreased faecal output:
  - borborygmi are usually absent or reduced.
  - heart and respiratory rate are often elevated.
  - signs associated with hypovolaemia due to intestinal sequestration of fluids.
  - fluid accumulation in the stomach due to lack of progressive motility can result in severe pain, or gastric rupture.
- obstructive ileus, the clinical signs are usually more severe and endotoxaemia can be present.

Differential diagnosis

- adynamic ileus should be differentiated from obstructive disease that requires surgical intervention.

Diagnosis

- distended small intestinal loops often palpable per rectum.
- ileus involving the large intestine, caecal or large intestinal distension can be palpated.
- **passage of a nasogastric tube is a vital diagnostic and therapeutic procedure:**
  - record the volume of reflux.
- blood samples:
  - PCV often increased.
  - total protein levels may be increased/ decreased depending on degree of intestinal protein loss and haemoconcentration.
  - leucopenia present if ileus associated with an acute inflammatory response.
  - sequestration of fluid in the intestines may result in:
    - hypokalaemia, hypocalcaemia, hypochloraemia, and hyponatraemia.
- peritoneal fluid is usually normal in non-surgical cases.
- abdominal ultrasonographic examination important to characterise:
  - intestinal size, wall thickness, and motility.

TABLE 3.2 Prokinetic drugs that have been used for the treatment of ileus

DRUG	ACTION	DOSE
Cisapride	Acts on entire GI tract. Oral administration may not be effective if significant gastric reflux is ongoing. Rectal administration is not effective. Should not be used in horses treated with certain drugs such as erythromycin	0.1–0.6 mg/kg p/o q8h
Erythromycin lactobionate	Improves small- and large-intestinal motility	1 mg/kg in 1 litre saline given i/v for 1 hour q6h
Metoclopramide	Improves gastric and proximal small intestinal motility	0.1 mg/kg/hour CRI
Lidocaine	May act by reducing the release of catecholamines systemically, suppressing the reflex inhibition of gut motility, stimulating smooth muscles directly, or by decreasing the inflammation locally	1.3 mg/kg i/v bolus over 15 minutes, followed by 0.05 mg/kg/minute in saline CRI
Bethanecol	Stimulates cholinergic (muscarinic) receptors, resulting in increased peristaltic activity in the stomach and intestinal tract	(1) 2.5 mg s/c 2 and 5 hours postoperatively (2) 0.025–0.1 mg/kg s/c q6–8h (3) 0.3–0.4 mg/kg p/o q6–8h
Neostigmine	Competes with acetylcholine for acetylcholinesterase, resulting in accumulation of acetylcholine and increased intestinal muscle tone	0.004–0.022 mg/kg i/v

Management

- supportive therapy is critical and should include:
  - intravenous fluid therapy:
    - rates calculated on initial fluid deficit, maintenance requirements, and ongoing losses.
    - urine output and urine SG are effective way of measuring ongoing hydration.
  - withhold feed and water.
  - frequent gastric decompression:
    - NG tube passed or indwelling.
  - electrolyte imbalances should be corrected as negatively affect motility:
    - hypokalaemia, hypomagnesaemia, and hypocalcaemia.
- analgesia is often required.
- drugs with inhibitory effects on intestinal motility should be avoided if possible.
- multiple prokinetic drugs have been used (Table 3.2):
  - none have proven completely satisfactory.
  - undesirable side effects or an inconsistent response.
- large colon stasis cases:
  - enhanced motility via the gastrocolic reflex may result when laxatives are administered by NG tube and recommendations include:
    - mineral oil (10 ml/kg).
    - sodium sulphate (0.15–0.5 g/kg).
    - magnesium sulphate (0.5–1.0 g/kg).
    - all in 4 litres of warm water.
    - or dioctyl sodium succinate (DSS) (10–30 mg/kg of a 10% solution).
  - more recently, frequent (q1–2h) administration of 10–20 ml/kg balanced electrolyte solution via nasogastric tube has been shown to be superior to traditional laxative therapy.
- ileus persists or an underlying obstructive cause is suspected:
  - exploratory laparotomy to decompress the intestine or correct a primary problem.

Prognosis

- cases of obstructive ileus, the prognosis will depend on the underlying cause.
- cases of adynamic ileus, the prognosis is good to fair.

Intestinal stricture

Definition/overview

- reduction of the intestinal lumen that typically occurs following local trauma.

Aetiology/pathophysiology

- formation of a stricture related to an enterotomy or intestinal resection:
  - usually at the surgical site.
- site of resolved entrapment, non-perforating duodenal ulceration, and possibly from duodenitis/proximal jejunitis.
- proximal duodenal stricture caused by severe gastroduodenal ulceration is classically found in foals more than 2 months of age.
- stricture at the ileocaecal valve may result from tapeworm injury.
- strictures usually result from local ulceration or inflammation:
  - subsequent formation of fibrous tissue.
  - eventually remodel and contract.
  - potentially resulting in decreased lumen diameter.

Clinical presentation

- varies with the region affected:
  - **Duodenal stricture:**
    - ◆ poor growth, depression, anorexia, fever, bruxism, reduced gastric emptying, severe equine gastric ulcer syndrome (EGUS), and intermittent colic may be observed.
  - **Ileal stricture:**
    - ◆ ranges from chronic mild intermittent colic to, less commonly, severe peracute colic similar to obstructive lesions.
  - **Stricture of the pelvic flexure or small colon:**
    - ◆ characterised by intermittent colic, recurrent impactions, or intestinal tympany.

Differential diagnosis

- depends on the degree of intestinal obstruction and the location of the stricture.

Diagnosis

- **Duodenal stricture:**
  - laboratory findings can include:
    - ◆ dehydration and azotaemia.
    - ◆ hypochloraemia and hyponatraemia.
  - contrast radiography (barium series) demonstrates delayed gastric emptying:
    - ◆ barium remains pooled in the stomach for >90 minutes.
  - nasogastric reflux may be present, but small intestine distension is not palpable.
  - endoscopic examination of the gastric and duodenal mucosa may be useful:
    - ◆ identify a stricture, the underlying cause.
    - ◆ secondary problems such as EGUS.
- **Ileal stricture:**
  - chronic adaptive small intestinal distension may occur:
    - ◆ may be palpable per rectum.
    - ◆ identified ultrasonographically.
  - total obstruction, severe intestinal distension with decreased intestinal motility.
- **Stricture of the pelvic flexure or small colon:**
  - impaction at the pelvic flexure or the small colon often palpable per rectum.
  - gaseous distension of the large intestine +/– small intestine may be present if the obstruction is severe.
  - narrowing of the lumen may be felt in some cases.
- regardless of the location, exploratory surgery is often required to definitively identify the stricture.

Management

- **Duodenal stricture:**
  - surgery is required.
- **Ileal stricture:**
  - surgery is required.
- **Stricture at the level of the pelvic flexure or small colon:**
  - surgery is required.

Prognosis

- fair to poor for duodenal stricture, good to fair for other locations.

Cantharidin toxicosis (blister beetle toxicosis)

Definition/overview

- Cantharidin is a highly irritating toxin.
- GI, urogenital, and cardiac damage is possible following ingestion.

Aetiology/pathophysiology

- found in a variety of blister beetles, particularly those of the *Epicauta* species:
  - found over much of the USA, particularly in the southwestern part.
- horses are usually exposed via ingestion of alfalfa hay containing dead beetles trapped in the hay during harvesting:
  - simultaneous cutting and crimping of the forage may increase the chance of blister beetle contamination.
  - usually not evenly distributed between or within bales of hay from the same cutting.
  - concentration of cantharidin in beetles can be variable.
  - ingestion of 4–6 g of dried blister beetle may be fatal.
- Cantharidin is very irritating to mucous membranes and skin:
  - causes acantholysis and vesicle formation.
  - sloughing of GI mucosa may occur following ingestion, particularly in proximal regions.
  - intestinal mucosal damage may result in:
    - ♦ fluid and protein loss.
    - ♦ alteration of electrolyte homeostasis.
    - ♦ absorption of bacterial toxins normally excluded by the mucosal barrier.
    - ♦ dehydration, hypovolaemic shock, toxaemia, and abdominal pain may develop rapidly.
- renal tubular necrosis and ulceration of the renal pelvis, ureters, and bladder mucosa is common.
- cardiac toxicity is less common but may occur:
  - characterised by ventricular myocardial necrosis and pericardial effusion.
- hypocalcaemia develops for unknown reasons.

Clinical presentation

- signs may be apparent hours to days following cantharidin ingestion.
- severity of clinical signs is dose dependent.
  - GI, urinary, cardiac, and systemic signs may be apparent:
    - ♦ abdominal pain, anorexia, depression, sweating, and frequent drinking or soaking the muzzle in water are most common.
  - oral mucous membranes are hyperaemic, with a prolonged CRT:
    - ♦ oral ulceration is uncommonly observed.
    - ♦ profuse salivation is sometimes present.
  - body temperature, heart rate, and respiratory rate are usually elevated.
  - if myocardial damage is present, heart rhythm may be abnormal.
  - pollakiuria and stranguria may be observed:
    - ♦ grossly evident haematuria may be present later in the disease.
  - synchronous diaphragmatic flutter, muscle fasciculation, and weakness may be present due to hypocalcaemia.
  - horses sometimes have a stiff gait suggestive of acute myositis.
  - sudden death occurs in some cases.

Differential diagnosis

- other causes of GI, urinary, and systemic disease must be considered.

Diagnosis

- clinical and laboratory findings are non-specific.
- history of eating alfalfa hay or other alfalfa products supports the suspicion in endemic regions.
- identification of blister beetles in hay is highly suggestive:
  - failure to identify blister beetles does not rule out the disease.
- blood samples:

- PCV is usually elevated.
- total protein is usually normal or elevated initially:
  - hypoproteinaemia may develop over time.
- neutrophilia may be present.
- hypocalcaemia, hyperglycaemia, and hypomagnesaemia.
- serum urea and creatinine levels may be elevated:
  - urinalysis performed to differentiate prerenal from renal disease.
  - hyposthenuria may be present for unknown reasons in some cases.
- microscopic haematuria evident early in the disease:
  - gross haematuria occurs later.
- elevation in creatine kinase (CK) may be present in severely affected animals:
  - may indicate a poorer prognosis.
- oesophageal and gastric inflammation or ulceration may be evident endoscopically.
- Cantharidin can be identified in urine or intestinal contents in first few days of disease:
  - availability of testing may be limited.
  - urine (minimum 500 ml) or gastric contents (minimum 200 g) submitted.

Management

- no antidote.
- early and aggressive treatment is required.
- supportive therapy is essential:
  - intravenous fluid therapy (balanced electrolyte solution) should be commenced:
    - supplementation with calcium borogluconate may be required:
      - ideally based on repeated evaluation of serum calcium levels.
      - magnesium supplementation is less commonly required.
  - analgesics may be required.
- hay source should be changed to prevent further intoxication.
- removal of recently ingested cantharidin attempted via NG administration of:
  - mineral oil (4–6 litres) or activated charcoal (1–3 g/kg).
- diuretics (furosemide, 1 mg/kg i/v or i/m q6h) recommended to increase cantharidin excretion:

- only when horse has been rehydrated.
- Sucralfate (20 mg/kg p/o q6–8h) useful if gastritis or EGUS has developed.
- broad-spectrum antimicrobials frequently recommended based on concerns of bacterial translocation from affected intestine:
  - little evidence to support this concern.
  - nephrotoxic antimicrobials such as aminoglycosides should be avoided.
- treatment of other potentially exposed horses with mineral oil or activated charcoal may be indicated.

Prognosis

- depends on amount of toxin ingested and severity of disease at the time of treatment.
- poor overall.
- persistent tachycardia, tachypnoea, and elevated CK levels are poor prognostic indicators.

Spasmodic colic

Definition/overview

- probably the most common type of colic in adult horses.

Aetiology/pathophysiology

- specific aetiology is unclear.
- association between *Anoplocephala perfoliata* (tapeworm) infestation and spasmodic colic has been reported.
- changes in diet and a history of recent anthelmintic administration are important risk factors.
- individual horses may be predisposed to recurrent spasmodic colic for unknown reasons.
- abnormal contractions, or spasms, of the intestine may result in the development of abdominal pain through stimulation of stretch receptors.
- intestinal spasms are transient and do not result in intestinal obstruction.

Clinical presentation

- usually display signs of mild to moderate abdominal pain, including:
  - anorexia, rolling, flank-watching, kicking at the abdomen, pawing,

recumbency, and straining to urinate or defaecate.
  - pain is usually intermittent:
    - ♦ severe pain is uncommon but can be observed transiently.
  - heart rate normal or elevated consistent with degree of pain (rarely exceeds 60 bpm).
- borborygmi are usually increased.
- faeces may be normal or soft.

Differential diagnosis

- variety of causes of colic should be considered:
  - particularly tympanic colic and large colon impaction.

Diagnosis

- physical examination findings are suggestive but not diagnostic:
  - usually, no abnormalities palpable per rectum.
  - gastric reflux is not present.
  - borborygmi are increased.
  - intestinal hypermotility may be evident ultrasonographically.
  - peritoneal fluid and haematology are unremarkable.
  - presumptive diagnosis often made on clinical presentation and response to therapy.

Management

- may require no treatment:
  - analgesics are commonly administered, and their use is logical.
  - analgesic/spasmolytic drug combination may be useful (Table 3.1).
- fluid therapy is rarely necessary:
  - may help restore normal intestinal motility and ensure adequate hydration.
  - 10–20 ml/kg of water or balanced electrolyte solution via NG tube considered.
- feeding should be restricted until signs of colic and effects of analgesics have abated.

Prognosis

- excellent for full recovery.
- most affected horses respond to a single treatment.

- progressive pain or poor response to analgesics:
  - reconsider diagnosis.
- recurrence warrants an attempt made to identify an underlying cause.

Ileocolonic aganglionosis (Overo lethal white syndrome)

Definition/overview

- inherited (homozygous recessive), congenital disorder of white-patterned horses characterised by myenteric aganglionosis and fatal functional intestinal obstruction.

Aetiology/pathophysiology

- results when a foal inherits two copies of the lethal white gene:
  - breeding of two horses that are heterozygous for this gene results in this condition in approximately 25% of foals.
  - most horses carrying the gene display the Overo colour pattern:
    - ♦ most common in American Paint horses, but also found in other breeds, particularly Quarter horses, Pintos, and Saddlebreds.
- autosomal recessive condition, and therefore the abnormal gene must be acquired from both parents.
- abnormal gene codes for endothelin receptor B:
  - unclear how the alteration in endothelin B receptor produces the disease.
  - complete absence of myenteric ganglia from the terminal ileum to small colon.

Clinical presentation

- foals may be entirely white or have small areas of pigmentation, mainly on the forelock and tail (Fig. 3.7).
- irises are white.
- foals are normal at birth but develop signs of colic within the first 4–24 hours of life:
  - abdominal pain and distension are progressive as intestinal distension develops.
  - small volume of faeces occasionally passed following enema administration.

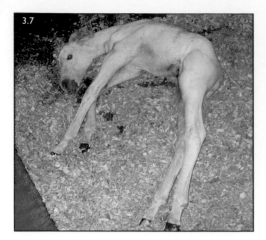

FIG. 3.7 Foal with ileocolonic aganglionosis displaying signs of colic.

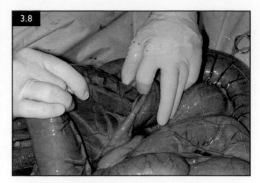

FIG. 3.8 Jejunojejunal intussusception. The intussusceptum (left side of the picture) is clearly observed to invaginate into the lumen of the intussuscipiens (right side of the picture).

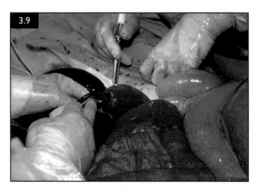

FIG. 3.9 Note the haemorrhagic strangulation lesion on the intussusceptum (left side of the picture).

Differential diagnosis

- other causes of colic and abdominal distension should be considered, including:
  - intestinal accident, meconium impaction and intestinal atresia.
  - severe enteritis with impending diarrhoea.
  - uroperitoneum.

Diagnosis

- progressive abdominal distension and lack of defaecation in a white foal of an Overo–Overo mating within the first 48 hours of life is highly suggestive.
- abdominal radiographs or ultrasound only demonstrate intestinal distension.
- confirmation of the diagnosis at necropsy:
  - demonstration of lack of myenteric ganglia in the small colon.
  - demonstration that the foal is homozygous for the gene mutation.

Management

- no treatment options are available.
- breeding stock should be tested for the genetic mutation:
  - heterozygote should not be bred to another heterozygote.

Prognosis

- fatal condition and foals should be euthanased.

Intussusception

Definition/overview

- condition where the intestine telescopes into itself (Figs. 3.8, 3.9):
  - consists of an intussusceptum, the leading edge of the orad intestine telescoping into the outer distad segment, the intussuscipiens.
- frequency of intussusception varies geographically and anatomically:
  - more common in younger horses (<3 years).
  - may be more common in Standardbreds, Thoroughbreds, and ponies.
  - most common locations include jejunoileal, ileocaecal, caecocaecal, and caecocolic sites.

o other sites such as the ascending and descending colon have also been reported.

Aetiology/pathophysiology

- aetiology hypothesised as a physical consequence of motility waves in a certain structure meeting a structure of different mechanical and functional properties.
- may occur at sites of anatomical differences, such as at the jejunoileal junction or at the ileocaecal valve.
- intestine may become predisposed to intussusception by alteration of the mechanical function or by the presence of intestinal parasites:
  o tapeworm *Anoplocephala perfoliata* often associated with intussusception.
  o larval cyathostomes have been implicated.
- other potential risk factors include motility-modifying drugs, enteritis, and surgical modification to the intestine.
- consequence of an intussusception is that the intestinal lumen is reduced and the blood supply to the intussusceptum may be compromised:
  o damage to the latter can cause oedema and necrosis of the intussusceptum.

Clinical presentation

- two discrete clinical presentations have been reported:
  o acute colic and chronic low-grade colic.
  o length of the intussusception partially explains the different clinical presentation:
    ◆ short intussusceptions cause partial intestinal obstruction and low-grade chronic colic.
    ◆ longer intussusceptions result in marked luminal obstruction and more acute, severe signs of discomfort.
- poor physical condition with varying degrees of intermittent or continual abdominal pain is characteristic of the chronic presentation:
  o affected horses are frequently anorexic and depressed.
- acute presentation, signs of acute colic are present with severe pain, and elevated heart rate:
  o signs of toxaemia present if significant intestinal compromise.

Differential diagnosis

- causes of chronic ill-thrift including:
  o heavy parasite burdens, intestinal neoplasia, and inflammatory intestinal infiltrates.
- acute colic difficult to differentiate from other causes of small intestinal entrapment/obstruction.

Diagnosis

- clinical findings are frequently consistent with luminal obstruction of varying degrees:
  o palpation of distended small intestine per rectum.
  o nasogastric reflux.
  o abnormalities on abdominocentesis are inconsistent.
  o palpation of an ileocaecal intussusception (right dorsal quadrant) consistent finding in some studies.
- abdominal ultrasonographic 'target' or 'bullseye' lesion consisting of concentric rings of intestine may be seen (Fig. 3.10).
- definitive diagnosis on exploratory laparotomy.

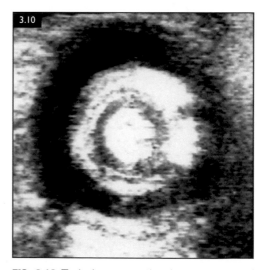

FIG. 3.10 Typical cross-sectional appearance of the ultrasonographic image of a small intestine intussusception. In this image the intussusception wall appears as concentric rings.

Management
- surgical correction is required.

Prognosis
- reducible intussusceptions are fair and depends on:
  - portion of intestine involved.
  - chronicity.
  - amount of damaged tissue.
  - surgical procedure required to correct the lesion.
- irreducible intussusceptions, the prognosis is poorer:
  - surgical techniques for correction are more technically demanding.
  - postoperative complications are common.

Foreign bodies

Definition/overview
- ingestion of items that are not normal components of the diet.
- may result in obstruction of and/or damage to the intestinal tract.

Aetiology/pathophysiology
- may occur due to accidental ingestion of foreign material contained in feed.
- intentional ingestion of abnormal items (pica).
- irregular shape and indigestibility of foreign bodies may cause them to lodge anywhere in the GI tract.
- slower intestinal transit leads to accumulation of ingesta within/around foreign bodies:
  - adherent ingesta begins to solidify, increasing the size of the mass (enterolith).
  - stops breakdown and increases chances of the mass lodging in the intestine.
- gas/fluid distension of the bowel proximal to the obstruction:
  - may lead to gastric distension and reflux.
  - more likely in the small intestine (large bowel obstruction occasionally).
- bowel adjacent to a lodged foreign body may have ischaemia and pressure necrosis:
  - increases likelihood of intestinal rupture at the site of the obstruction.

- less commonly, rupture proximal to obstruction due to marked bowel distension.
- penetrating foreign bodies may lead to abscess or sinus formation:
  - may result in adhesion formation.
  - leakage has the potential to cause severe peritonitis.

Clinical presentation
- ingestion of foreign bodies may occur in horses of any age, but younger horses are more commonly affected due to their adventurous nature.
- clinical signs are usually non-specific and may manifest over several weeks.
- vary according to the location of the foreign body and severity of intestinal obstruction.
- most common clinical signs are:
  - colic of variable frequency and severity
  - anorexia, lethargy, and weight loss.
  - abdominal distension.
  - passage of faeces may continue depending on location/completeness of obstruction.
  - acute peritonitis without any preceding signs secondary to intestinal perforation.

Differential diagnosis
- other causes of non-strangulating obstruction:
  - phytobezoars and food impaction.

Diagnosis
- rectal palpation may reveal distended bowel, but not usually the foreign body.
- gastroscopy is effective at diagnosing gastric foreign bodies.
- nasogastric reflux indicates a proximal obstruction but is not specific to foreign bodies.
- ultrasonographic examination may show bowel distension but not usually the obstruction.
- radiography is useful for the diagnosis of enteroliths if suitable equipment is available.
- definitive diagnosis usually made during an exploratory laparotomy.

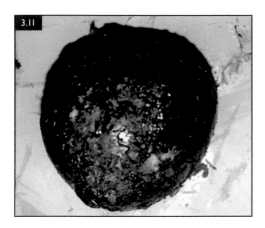

FIG. 3.11 Large solitary (round) enterolith.

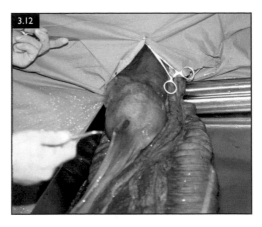

FIG. 3.12 Intraoperative view of the right dorsal colon, where two stay sutures have been applied before performing an enterotomy to exteriorise a large round enterolith.

Management

- some cases managed medically by hydrating the bowel using frequent, large volume enteral fluids.
- unresponsive cases require an exploratory laparotomy and enterotomy:
  - identify and remove foreign body and associated damaged bowel (Figs. 3.11, 3.12).
- behavioural reasons for foreign body ingestion addressed to minimise likelihood of recurrence.

Prognosis

- for full recovery is good if the obstruction is resolved medically.
- for surgical cases is dependent on extent of bowel damage and accessibility of the obstruction:
  - guarded if large amount of bowel damage or vascular supply compromised.
  - grave for leakage of ingesta and peritonitis.

Lymphocytic/ plasmacytic enteritis

Definition/overview

- form of inflammatory bowel disease.
- no age, sex or breed predilection.

Aetiology/pathophysiology

- aetiology is unknown, and the pathophysiology is unclear.

- infiltration of intestinal wall with lymphocytes and plasmacytes into the lamina propria.
- lesions tend to occur diffusely throughout the gastrointestinal tract:
  - fibrotic changes are occasionally observed but not granulomatous changes.

Clinical presentation

- most common presenting complaints are weight loss, diarrhoea and recurrent colic.
- behavioural changes and persistent leucopenia may also occur.

Differential diagnosis

- other causes of protein and weight loss should be considered, including:
  - protein-losing nephropathy.
  - eosinophilic enterocolitis.
  - intestinal lymphosarcoma.
- other differentials for non-specific chronic gastrointestinal disease, such as:
  - EGUS and sand enteropathy.

Diagnosis

- blood samples:
  - hypoproteinaemia, consisting mainly of hypoalbuminaemia, is common.
  - anaemia is common.
  - WBC count usually normal but may be decreased.

- urinalysis and abdominocentesis are usually normal.
- abdominal ultrasound examination is usually unremarkable.
- carbohydrate absorption testing should be performed:
  - decreased absorption is usually present, except in early disease or focal lesions.
  - rectal mucosal biopsy can be diagnostic if the disease involves the rectum.

Management

- treatment can be rewarding:
  - initial therapy consists of prednisolone 1 mg/kg p/o q 24h for 21 days:
    - ♦ initial positive response to treatment is a good prognostic indicator.
    - ♦ failure to respond leads to a poorer prognosis.
  - further treatment consists of systemic dexamethasone.

Prognosis

- variable.
- important prognostic indicators are magnitude of hypoproteinaemia and response to treatment.

Granulomatous enteritis

Definition/overview

- form of inflammatory bowel disease.
- most reported in Standardbred horses and a familial predisposition has been postulated.
- young horses (1–5 years old) are most affected.

Aetiology/pathophysiology

- aetiology is unknown, and the pathophysiology is unclear.
- characterised by intestinal wall infiltration with macrophages and epithelioid cells.
- villus atrophy subsequently develops, resulting in malabsorption and maldigestion.
- impaired dietary protein absorption and small intestinal mucosal ulceration may contribute to hypoproteinemia.

- more common and severe in the small intestine, particularly the ileum.
- large colon less frequently affected.

Clinical presentation

- most common presenting complaints are weight loss and anorexia.
- peripheral oedema may develop, depending on the degree of protein loss.
- diarrhoea and colic are less commonly observed.
- small intestinal fluid loss can be masked by absorptive capacity of normal large colon.
- attitude normal initially, but depression and weakness may develop over time.

Differential diagnosis

- other causes of protein loss and weight loss should be considered, including:
  - protein-losing nephropathy.
  - lymphocytic–plasmacytic enteritis.
  - eosinophilic enterocolitis.
  - intestinal lymphosarcoma.

Diagnosis

- hypoproteinaemia, consisting mainly of hypoalbuminaemia, is common.
- anaemia is common resulting from chronic disease or immune-mediated haemolytic anaemia (IMHA).
- WBC count usually normal.
- urinalysis and abdominocentesis are usually normal, although aseptic peritonitis may be present in some cases.
- abdominal ultrasound examination is usually unremarkable.
- carbohydrate absorption testing should be performed:
  - decreased absorption is usually present, except in early disease or focal lesions.
- rectal mucosal biopsy can be diagnostic if disease also involves the rectum.
- surgical biopsy of the ileum has the highest diagnostic value.
- many cases are only diagnosed definitively at necropsy.

Management

- treatment is often unrewarding:
  - poor response to treatment.

- severity of disease when diagnosed or suspected.
- long-term dexamethasone has been reported to be successful in a few cases:
  - 40 mg/adult horse i/m q96h for 4 weeks.
  - then 35 mg/adult horse i/m q96h for 4 weeks, with continued tapering of dose.
- parenteral nutrition may be required initially in severely affected animals.
- surgical resection of the affected area is unlikely to be practical as a large portion of the intestinal tract is usually involved.

Prognosis

- poor.
- most horses are euthanased because of poor response to medical treatment and deterioration of condition.

Eosinophilic enterocolitis/ multisystemic eosinophilic epitheliotropic disease

Definition/overview

- Eosinophilic enterocolitis (EE) is an uncommon form of inflammatory bowel disease.
- Multisystemic eosinophilic epitheliotropic disease (MEED) involves the intestinal tract and other organs.

Aetiology/pathophysiology

- aetiology is unknown.
- no breed or familial predispositions have been reported for EE.
- most cases of MEED have been in young (<4 years of age) Standardbred horses.
- EE is characterised by eosinophilic infiltration of all layers of the intestine and fibrosis.
- MEED is characterised by infiltration of the mucosa and submucosa of the intestine with eosinophils, lymphocytes, and macrophages, as well as invasion of other organs:
  - liver and pancreatic disease is common.
  - Basophilic enterocolitis is thought to be a variant of MEED.

Clinical presentation

- most reported presentation of EE is abdominal pain:
  - weight loss is uncommon, and diarrhoea is rare.
- weight loss is invariably present, and diarrhoea is common in horses with MEED:
  - approximately two-thirds of horses with MEED have skin lesions:
    - exudative dermatitis of the face, limbs, and ventral abdomen.
    - ulcerative coronitis and loss of chestnuts may also occur.
  - lingual and buccal ulceration may be present.

Differential diagnosis

- variety of differential diagnoses must be considered, depending on clinical presentation:
  - colic, weight loss, hypoproteinemia, and skin lesions.

Diagnosis

- EE:
  - haematological abnormalities are uncommon.
  - carbohydrate absorption tests are typically normal.
  - diagnosis based on surgical biopsy and histological examination:
    - circumferential fibrous bands may be present in the intestinal wall, resulting in intestinal distension.
- MEED:
  - hypoproteinaemia, mainly from hypoalbuminaemia, is common.
  - WBC numbers are usually normal but may be a marked eosinophilia.
  - biochemistry results depend on the involvement of other organ systems.
  - rectal mucosal biopsy can be diagnostic in many cases:
    - identification of eosinophilic granulomas associated with vasculitis and fibrinoid necrosis of intramural vessels.

Management

- long-term prognosis is guarded.

- oral corticosteroids (prednisolone, 1 mg/kg p/o q12h for 28 days, followed by gradual tapering) may be effective in EE.
- intestinal obstruction by fibrous circumferential bands may cause recurrent colic:
  - some horses can be managed by feeding small meals of a pelleted complete ration.
  - resection of the affected area(s) may be required in others.
- treatment of MEED is usually unrewarding.
- administration of larvicidal anthelminthics has been suggested for both EE and MEED:
  - nematode larvae have been postulated in the pathogenesis of the diseases.

Prognosis

- EE is reasonable:
  - horses that respond to corticosteroid therapy often have no recurrence of disease.
  - presence of fibrous circumferential bands worsens the prognosis, but surgical intervention may be successful.
- MEED is very poor.

Chronic and recurrent colic

Definition/overview

- frustrating problems that are often difficult to diagnose and manage.
- chronic colic has been defined as colic persisting for 3 days or longer:
  - definition encompasses cases of acute colic that are poorly responsive to initial therapy.
- recurrent colic is defined as multiple, distinct episodes of colic.

Aetiology/pathophysiology

- causes of chronic and recurrent colic are varied and often difficult to identify.
- extensions of acute colic episodes:
  - large colon impaction, caecal impaction, peritonitis, or enteritis.
- other causes include:
  - colonic displacement, diaphragmatic hernia, ileal obstruction, pyloric stenosis.

- inflammatory bowel disease.
- peritonitis, pleuritis, verminous arteritis.
- lymphosarcoma and other GI neoplasms.
- intestinal adhesions, abdominal abscess, enteroliths, intussusceptions.
- EGUS.
- grass sickness.
- sand impaction.
- right dorsal colitis (NSAID toxicity).
- urinary tract and liver disease.
- reproductive tract abnormalities.
- varied pathophysiology depending on the inciting cause.

Clinical presentation

- intermittent or continuous colic of 3 days' duration or longer.
- pain may range from mild and intermittent to severe and continuous.
- weight loss and poor body condition evident in some cases, especially recurrent colic.

Differential diagnosis

- many other GI and extraintestinal disorders.

Diagnosis

- thorough history is essential (Table 3.3).
- complete physical examination:
  - identify intestinal and extraintestinal abnormalities:
  - palpate linea alba for a scar from a previous laparotomy if history is unknown.
  - not unusual to find no significant abnormalities.
- thorough diagnostic testing plan is usually required (Table 3.4):
  - necessary to rule out differentials.
  - provisional diagnosis can be reached in most cases.

Management

- varies with the inciting cause and specific treatments are described elsewhere.
- management of idiopathic cases is frustrating.
- absence of specific clinical signs:
  - treatment for a presumed impaction with fasting and large volume, frequent

TABLE 3.3 Important historical information in the investigation of recurrent colic

- Age
- Duration of ownership
- Appetite
- Ability to maintain good body condition
- Faecal consistency
- **Reproductive status**: pregnant, recently bred, recently foaled
- **Pain**: duration, recurrent/continuous, frequency, intensity, response to analgesics, patterns of onset (e.g. associated with feeding)
- **Deworming history**: deworming programme, recent deworming
- **Diet**: type, quality, amount, frequency of feeding, recent changes
- **Management changes**: exercise, turnout, change in routine, co-mingling with new horses, place in hierarchy with co-mingled horses
- Dental prophylaxis
- **Previous medical problems**: colic, abdominal surgery, extraintestinal infection (i.e. *S. equi*), NSAID therapy
- **Water**: access, quality, change in source, intake

TABLE 3.4 Diagnostic options for chronic colic

COMMON INITIAL TESTING

- Haematology: complete blood cell count, serum biochemical profile, plasma fibrinogen and serum amyloid A assay
- Palpation per rectum
- Gastroscopy
- Abdominal ultrasonography
- Abdominocentesis
- Abdominal radiography

FURTHER TESTING

- Carbohydrate absorption test
- Rectal mucosal biopsy
- Thoracic radiography
- Thoracic ultrasonography
- Reproductive tract examination
- Cystoscopy
- Liver biopsy
- Urinalysis
- Exploratory laparoscopy
- Exploratory laparotomy with multiple intestinal biopsies

enteral fluids for 2–3 days may be rewarding.
- variety of other treatments can be attempted including:
  - diet change:
    - ready access to good-quality hay or pasture with minimal grain or pelleted ration.
    - some cases respond to elimination of hay from the diet and switching to complete pelleted feeds.
    - nutritional analysis and consultation may be useful.
  - change in location.
  - deworming with moxidectin (0.4 mg/kg p/o) is often attempted.
  - antiulcer treatment.

Prognosis

- highly variable and depends on the inciting cause, ranges from:
  - very good (i.e. EGUS).
  - very poor (i.e. GI neoplasia, grass sickness, and intestinal adhesions).
- overall, frustrating condition in many cases as an aetiology is often not identified.

Grass sickness (equine dysautonomia, mal seco)

Definition/overview

- equine grass sickness (EGS) is a geographically important debilitating and frequently fatal cause of GI disease.
- most widely reported in the UK:
  - also present in several mainland European countries.
  - termed 'mal seco' in South America.
  - anecdotal reports of EGS in North America and Australia.

Aetiology/pathophysiology

- polyneuropathy affecting both the central and peripheral nervous systems.
- EGS is a seasonal disease, with case occurrence peaking in April to June in the northern hemisphere.
- virtually all affected horses are grazing animals, often in good condition.
- risk of disease highest in horses aged 2–7 years.
- previous identification of cases on the farm and recent changes in pasture use are risk factors.

- clusters of cases are not uncommon.
- suggested that changes in feed, pasture, weather conditions, and parasite burden may affect the GI microflora and allow for *C. botulinum* growth and toxin production.
- pathophysiology is still unclear:
  - widespread neuroanatomical distribution of degenerative neuronal lesions.
  - autonomic and enteric nervous systems most consistently and severely affected.
  - severity of disease and gross pathological findings are largely determined by the extent of enteric neuronal loss.
  - potential role of either *Clostridium. botulinum* neurotoxins or ingested pasture-derived mycotoxins:
    - increasing evidence of the role of *Clostridium botulinum* type C.

Clinical presentation

- acute, subacute, and chronic forms are recognised:
  - **Acute:**
    - predominately depression, anorexia, and mild to moderate colic.
    - initially in good body condition.
    - borborygmi decreased/absent and progressive abdominal distension.
    - muscle tremors are common and may be severe:
      - particularly over the shoulders, triceps, flank, and quadriceps.
    - patchy sweating is common in all forms of the disease (Fig. 3.13).
    - tachycardia may be severe and higher than expected considering the apparent degree of abdominal pain.
    - body temperature normal to slightly elevated.
    - pytalism is common, as is dehydration, which may be severe.
    - nasogastric reflux may be present:
      - stomach rupture, with ensuing peritonitis, may occur if gastric decompression is not performed.
    - dysphagia may not be recognised because of the anorexia that accompanies severe disease.
    - bilateral ptosis is invariably present in all forms of the disease (Fig. 3.14).
  - **Subacute:**
    - similar to acute form, although of lesser severity.
    - tachycardia is usually present.
    - signs of distress or severe abdominal pain are uncommon.
    - nasogastric reflux is uncommon.
    - dry faeces are commonly present.
  - **Chronic:**
    - insidious onset.
    - weight loss, depression, a 'tucked-up' or 'wasp-like' abdomen, weakness, and dysphagia.
    - mastication is typically slow and laboured.

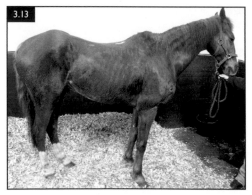

FIG. 3.13 Horse with subacute grass sickness showing marked patchy sweating, muscle fasciculations, and a mild tucked-up abdomen.

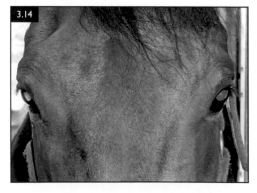

FIG. 3.14 Horse with acute grass sickness showing bilateral upper eyelid ptosis.

- ◆ oesophageal spasm may be noted after swallowing.
- ◆ intermittent diarrhoea, bilateral nasal discharge, paraphimosis in entire males, and chronic rhinitis sicca may be noted.

Differential diagnosis

- variety of other causes of acute colic, chronic colic, chronic weight loss, and dysphagia.
- most important differentiation is from causes of colic requiring surgical intervention.

Diagnosis

- palpation per rectum to identify other causes of colic:
  - ○ dry, mucus-covered faeces are common.
  - ○ distended loops of small intestine (also on transabdominal ultrasonography).
  - ○ large colon and caecal impactions in the chronic cases (Fig. 3.15):
    - ◆ reflects large intestinal ileus and desiccation of the fibrous ingesta.
- voluminous foul-smelling gastric reflux may be present with the acute form:
  - ○ reflects generalised gastrointestinal ileus.
- clinical signs, signalment, identification of risk factors (recent change in grazing or previous disease on premises) and exclusion of other differential diagnoses is suggestive of EGS.
- temporary reversal of ptosis following:
  - ○ topical application of 0.5% phenylephrine ophthalmic solution to conjunctival sac.
  - ○ confirms neurogenic smooth muscle paralysis as the cause of ptosis.
- barium swallow studies or oesophagoscopy may confirm:
  - ○ retrograde flow of gastric fluid and abnormal oesophageal motility.
- ileal biopsy:
  - ○ histological identification of neuronal loss and chromatolysis within myenteric and submucosa nerve plexuses provides a 100% definitive diagnosis.
- post-mortem confirmation of the diagnosis is more common:

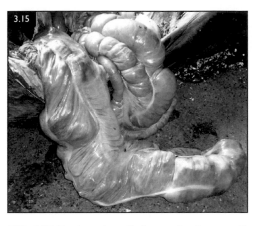

FIG. 3.15 Post-mortem findings of a horse with chronic grass sickness showing marked chronic impaction of the entire large colon and caecum with a very dried out, clamped-down appearance of the gut wall, typical in these cases.

  - ○ characteristic neural degeneration.
- *C. botulinum* type C more commonly identified in the intestinal contents of horses with EGS:
  - ○ found in some normal horses (intestinal culture is not useful).

Management

- treatment of acute and subacute forms is not indicated:
  - ○ **affected horses invariably die.**
- some horses with chronic EGS can recover:
  - ○ selection of appropriate cases to treat is difficult.
  - ○ ideally should still be able to swallow to some degree.
  - ○ have some remaining appetite.
  - ○ absence of continuous moderate to severe abdominal pain.
  - ○ owners must be prepared for considerable commitment in time, nursing care and finances.
  - ○ treatment predominantly requires:
    - ◆ intensive nursing care.
    - ◆ profound inappetence is the major obstacle to survival and adequate level of voluntary feed intake is key:
      - – highly palatable, high-energy and high-protein feed.

- – different components and consistencies to suit individual needs.
    - – two-hourly small feeds are initially useful.
  - ♦ regular hand walking and short periods turned out to grass may be helpful.
  - ♦ judicious use of non-steroidal anti-inflammatory drugs is often beneficial:
    - – probably controls low-grade abdominal pain and systemic inflammation.
  - ♦ broad-spectrum antimicrobial drugs in cases with aspiration pneumonia.
  - ♦ long-term treatment (months) is required, and cases should always be stabled.
- affected horses and herd mates should be removed from the affected pasture, if possible.
- reduction in grazing time, particularly of young horses, and supplementation of feeding have been used, but the effect of these measures is unclear.
- vaccination with *C. botulinum* type C toxoid may be a preventive option in the future and this possibility is being evaluated.

Prognosis

- mildly affected horses with the chronic form may recover fully given adequate supportive care:
  - ○ significant expenditure of time and money is required:
    - ♦ approximately 50% of chronic cases survive with intensive nursing care.
    - ♦ over 1 year may be required for return to full competitive work.
  - ○ horses that recover may return to normal function:
    - ♦ peak performance may be affected.
    - ♦ residual problems with eating dry fibrous food may persist.
    - ♦ mild, recurrent colic may persist in some cases.
- **acute and subacute cases are invariably fatal and prompt euthanasia is indicated.**

Intestinal adhesions

Definition/overview

- problems associated with abdominal adhesions include recurrent abdominal pain with or without intestinal obstruction.

Aetiology/pathophysiology

- usually form following abdominal surgery:
  - ○ particularly small intestinal surgery or repeat coeliotomy.
  - ○ peritonitis or prolonged ileus may also induce their formation.
  - ○ foals under 30 days old are reported to be more susceptible to postoperative adhesion formation:
    - ♦ dependent on the degree of underlying systemic illness
- abdominal adhesions form at a peritoneal injury site due to an imbalance between fibrin deposition and fibrinolysis:
  - ○ inflammation and ischaemia increase fibrin deposition and decrease fibrinolysis.
  - ○ adhesions begin to form within 48 hours of an injury as a fibrin cover appears on the injured serosal bed.
  - ○ well formed by 5–7 days.
  - ○ after 7 days not reversible:
    - ♦ collagen content increases to a level that cannot inherently be broken down.
  - ○ permanent fibrous adhesions are usually formed by 7–14 days.
- extensive well-defined adhesions are often covered by mesothelium and contain blood vessels and connective tissue fibres, including elastin.

Clinical presentation

- most common clinical sign is recurrent colic.
- acute non-strangulating or strangulating intestinal obstruction can occur.
- poor body condition and inability to consume a high-roughage diet also associated with mild restrictive adhesions.
- clinical signs associated with postoperative abdominal adhesions are usually observed 1–4 weeks after surgery.

Differential diagnosis

- any clinical condition leading to acute non-strangulating or strangulating intestinal obstruction, recurrent colic, and poor body condition.

Diagnosis

- abdominal adhesions are diagnosed most frequently during exploratory laparotomy (Figs. 3.16, 3.17).
- rarely, palpated per rectum as a tight band running from one viscus to either the body wall or another viscus.
- ultrasonography may be helpful with diagnosis.
- history of previous coeliotomy and appropriate clinical signs.
- palpate ventral midline for evidence of previous surgery, particularly when health history is unknown.

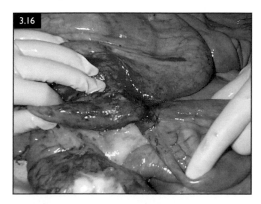

FIG. 3.16 Example of fibrinous adhesions that cover injured serosal surfaces.

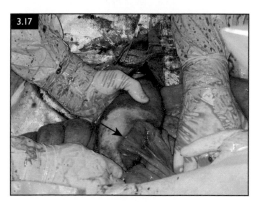

FIG. 3.17 Example of a focal mesentery-to-intestine adhesion. Note the ischaemic (pale) area on the intestinal surface that most likely induced the formation of this adhesion (arrow).

Management

- signs of colic are mild: medical treatment can be attempted and includes:
  - use of enteral fluids, analgesics, and modified diets.
  - low-residue feeds, such as completely pelleted feeds or alfalfa cubes:
    - ◆ may pass through small intestine more easily and reduce risk of obstruction.
    - ◆ after several weeks on modified feeding regimen may be possible to re-institute a normal diet if the fibrous adhesions have remodelled and become less obstructive.
    - ◆ some cases, pelleted feed may be required for the duration of a horse's life.
- surgical treatment for bowel obstruction associated with adhesions includes resection and anastomosis or bypass of the affected bowel, with or without adhesiolysis.
- laparoscopic adhesiolysis has been used successfully in a small number of equine cases.

Prevention

- intraoperative methods for preventing postoperative adhesion formation have been evaluated and now form part of standard laparotomy procedure:
  - unfortunately, no definitive method has been developed.

Prognosis

- adhesions causing clinical signs have a reported prognosis of between 0 and 20% for long-term survival.

Gastrointestinal neoplasia

Definition/overview

- relatively rare in horses.
- lymphosarcoma is the most common condition (Figs. 3.18, 3.19).
- gastric SCC is the second most common (Fig. 3.20).
- other, rarely encountered neoplasias include:
  - gastric leiomyosarcoma, leiomyoma, and adenocarcinoma.

- o intestinal leiomyosarcoma, leiomyoma, adenocarcinoma, myxosarcoma.
- o disseminated leiomyomatosis, omental fibrosarcoma, and mesothelioma.

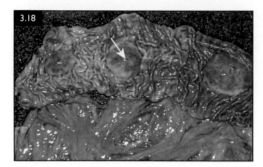

FIG. 3.18 Mucosal surface of the small intestine in a horse with intestinal lymphosarcoma. Note the markedly enlarged Peyer's patches (arrow).

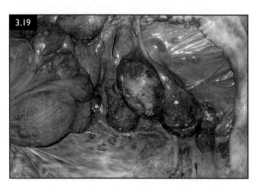

FIG. 3.19 Multiple large mesenteric lymph nodes are evident in this horse with intestinal lymphosarcoma.

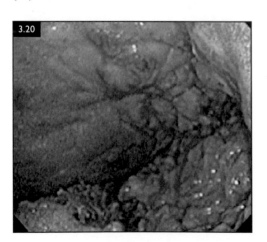

FIG. 3.20 Gastric squamous cell carcinoma in a 19-year-old horse that presented for weight loss.

Aetiology/pathophysiology

- aetiology is unknown.
- pathophysiology is variable and clinical signs develop subsequent to:
  - o intestinal obstruction.
  - o maldigestion/malabsorption.
  - o blood loss.
  - o peritoneal effusion.
  - o chronic inflammatory response.

Clinical presentation

- varies with tumour type and location.
- weight loss and recurrent colic are the most common abnormalities:
  - o appetite may be decreased, normal, or increased.
- weakness, acute colic, depression, or abdominal distension may also be present.

Differential diagnosis

- variety of causes of weight loss and chronic colic must be considered.

Diagnosis

- specific diagnosis of GI neoplasia may be difficult.
- anaemia may be present because of chronic disease, bone marrow infiltration, or blood loss.
- WBC count and morphology are usually normal.
- hypoproteinaemia is common because of maldigestion, protein loss, or chronic inflammation.
- elevations in certain enzymes may reflect involvement of other organ systems.
- hypercalcaemia is less common in horses than in other species, but it does occur.
- firm masses or abnormal intestine may be palpable per rectum.
- oesophageal, gastric, and proximal duodenal tumours may be visualised and biopsied endoscopically.
- abdominocentesis may yield neoplastic cells, particularly with mesotheliomas.
- rectal mucosal biopsy may be useful with diffuse or distal disease:
  - o can be used to differentiate intestinal neoplasia and inflammatory bowel disease.
- carbohydrate absorption tests assess small intestinal absorption but cannot specifically diagnose neoplasia.

- transabdominal ultrasonography may reveal abnormal segments of bowel.
- exploratory laparotomy or laparoscopy and biopsy is preferred.
- definitive diagnosis is often only made at necropsy.

Management

- treatment of GI neoplasia is usually unrewarding.
- focal, benign lesions may be removed surgically.
- resection may also be successful with some other tumours provided adequate margins are resected.
- prior to surgery ensure that metastasis has not occurred:
  - ○ radiographs of thorax.
  - ○ ultrasonographic examination of the liver.

- ○ potentially, bone marrow biopsy.
- often, palliative therapy is attempted:
  - ○ parenteral dexamethasone used with variable success in certain neoplasms.
  - ○ variety of antineoplastic drugs have been tried on limited numbers of horses, with inconclusive results.
  - ○ nutritional support is often required in conjunction with medical treatment.

Prognosis

- guarded to grave for virtually all GI neoplasms:
  - ○ usually not detected until a relatively advanced stage.
- rarely is complete surgical excision a possibility.
- occasionally, small GI tumours may be detected during coeliotomy for other reasons.

DISORDERS OF THE STOMACH

Gastric squamous cell carcinoma

Definition/overview

- SCC is the most common neoplasm of the equine stomach.

Aetiology/pathophysiology

- aetiology is unknown.
- affected horses are usually ≥ 6 years of age.
- SCC originates from the squamous epithelium of the stomach or distal oesophagus:
  - ○ metastasis reported in 50–75% of cases, particularly into the thoracic cavity.
  - ○ spread may be via direct invasion of adjacent tissues or through blood or lymphatic vessels.

Clinical presentation

- signs of SCC are non-specific and include:
  - ○ weight loss, anorexia, chronic colic, pyrexia, halitosis, weakness, and lethargy.
  - ○ oesophageal or cardia involvement:

    - ♦ dysphagia, chronic choke, or ptyalism may be present.
- other clinical signs depending on whether the tumour has metastasised.

Differential diagnosis

- other causes of chronic colic, weight loss, and non-specific disease.
- SCC is usually diagnosed during thorough evaluation of weight loss or chronic colic.

Diagnosis

- non-specific haematological changes may be present including:
  - ○ anaemia, leucocytosis, hyperfibrinogenaemia, and hypoalbuminaemia.
- peritoneal fluid is variable:
  - ○ normal to turbid with an increased total protein and nucleated cell count:
  - ○ neoplastic cells are uncommonly identified.
- gastroscopy is important and allows direct visualisation of the tumour:
  - ○ multiple biopsies taken to confirm the diagnosis.
- stomach can be visualised ultrasonographically:

- ○ ultrasound-guided biopsy can be performed if gastroscopic biopsy not possible.
- ○ examination of the liver, spleen, and pleura.
- thoracic radiography may demonstrate metastatic masses.

Management

- no viable treatment options.

Prognosis

- grave.

Gastric parasitism: *Habronema* spp. and *Draschia* sp.

Definition/overview

- gastric parasitism caused by *Habronema* and *Draschia* occurs sporadically worldwide.
- varying clinical significance:
  - ○ gastric habronemiasis of lesser significance than cutaneous habronemiasis.
  - ○ *Draschia* infection is more likely to produce clinical gastric disease.

Aetiology/pathophysiology

- parasitic nematodes *Habronema muscae, H. microstoma,* and *Draschia megastoma.*
- eggs are passed in the faeces of infected animals.
- L1 larvae are ingested by muscid fly larvae which mature.
- adult fly feeds around the mouth of a horse:
  - ○ infective L3 parasitic larvae migrate from the mouthparts to the skin of the horse.
  - ○ swallowed or, less commonly, the fly is swallowed whole.
- adult worms develop in glandular portion of the stomach over approximately 2 months:
  - ○ may induce mild haemorrhagic gastritis.
  - ○ nodules of adult worms and necrotic debris develop with *Draschia* infection.

Clinical presentation

- infection is usually inapparent.
- rarely, nodule formation may affect gastric outflow via physical obstruction of the pylorus.

Differential diagnosis

- EGUS, gastritis, gastric SCC, and other gastric tumours considered in severe cases.

Diagnosis

- lack of clinical signs means that diagnosis of gastric *Habronema* and *Draschia* infection is often made incidentally during gastroscopy:
  - ○ mild gastritis (*Habronema*).
  - ○ presence of nodules (*Draschia*) – endoscopic biopsy of nodules can be diagnostic.

Management

- ivermectin (0.2 mg/kg p/o) or moxidectin (0.4 mg/kg p/o) are effective.
- measures to control flies would be beneficial.

Prognosis

- excellent unless gastric outflow is obstructed:
  - ○ unclear with obstruction, and response to treatment must be observed.

Gastric parasitism: *Gasterophilus* spp. and *Trichostrongylus axei*

Definition/overview

- gastric infection by *Gasterophilus* spp. (bots) or *T. axei* is very common and typically of little significance.

Aetiology/pathophysiology

- multiple bot species may be encountered:
  - ○ *G. nasalis, G. hemorrhoidalis,* and *G. intestinalis* are most common and are found worldwide.
  - ○ *G. pecorum* may be involved in Europe, Africa, and Asia.
  - ○ *T. axei* may also cause gastric parasitism.

- adult *Gasterophilus* flies usually attach eggs to the hairs of the legs, shoulders, lips, or intermandibular space during the late summer and fall:
  - eggs are 1–2 mm in length and creamy-white to orange.
  - eggs around the mouth hatch spontaneously.
  - eggs at other sites may hatch in response to warmth provided by licking.
- *G. pecorum* eggs are deposited in pasture and ingested during grazing.
- larvae enter the mouth, penetrate the tongue or buccal mucosa, and reside in these tissues for several weeks before entering the stomach via the pharynx and oesophagus.
- *G. nasalis* larvae tend to attach to the pylorus and duodenum.
- *G. intestinalis* to the non-glandular mucosa around the cardia.
- *G. haemorrhoidalis* to the duodenum and rectum.
- L3 larvae are then passed in faeces and pupate in the soil.
- only one generation per year in temperate areas.
- infective L3 of *T. axei* are ingested on pasture and tunnel into the gastric wall:
  - gastritis may result.
  - small erosions produced by a high density of parasites in a small area.

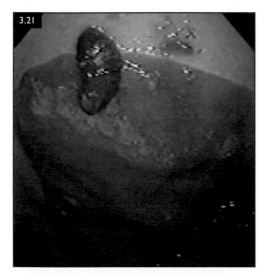

FIG. 3.21 *Gasterophilus intestinalis* (bot) larva is present in the stomach of a normal horse.

Clinical presentation

- infection is usually inapparent.
- adult bot flies may be of greater significance because of annoyance while they are flying around horses and depositing their eggs.

Diagnosis

- Bot infection can be inferred by the finding of eggs deposited on the horse.
- L3 larvae may be identified in faeces.
- *G. intestinalis* larvae often identified incidentally during gastroscopy (Fig. 3.21).
- *T. axei* infection, gastritis may be evident endoscopically:
  - larvae are small (<7.0 mm) and may be difficult to identify.
  - *T. axei* eggs may be identified in faecal flotation.

Management

- ivermectin (0.2 mg/kg p/o) and moxidectin (0.4 mg/kg p/o) are effective against bots.
- infestation is rarely associated with disease.
- annual boticidal therapy is recommended:
  - temperate areas, administered in midwinter post any exposure to bot eggs.
- physical removal of eggs deposited on the skin but may not be particularly useful.
- *T. axei* is susceptible to most anthelmintics.

Prognosis

- excellent.

Equine gastric ulcer syndrome (EGUS)

Definition/overview

- common problem, affecting a wide range of horse types and usages.
- equine stomach comprised of two distinct areas:
  - glandular.
  - non-glandular (squamous).
- equine squamous gastric disease (ESGD) refers to disease of the squamous mucosa.

- equine glandular gastric disease (EGGD) refers to disease of the glandular mucosa.
- risk factors, prevalence, and response to treatment of ESGD and EGGD are different.
- glandular mucosa is protected primarily by mucus and bicarbonate secretion and prostaglandin-mediated mucosal blood flow.
- non-glandular mucosa has fewer protective mechanisms and is more prone to damage by hydrochloric acid and pepsin.
- ESGD is most common in high performance horses, particularly close to the margo plicatus, which is the most acidic non-glandular area.
- EGGD is most common in sport horses with Warmbloods predisposed.

Aetiology/pathophysiology

- EGUS is a multifactorial condition that results when the protective mechanisms of the gastric mucosa are overwhelmed.
- recognised risk factors for ESGD include:
  - high carbohydrate diets.
  - infrequent feeding.
  - decreased roughage in the diet.
  - intense exercise.
  - relatively linear relationship between increasing intensity of exercise and grain feeding, and increased risk of ESGD.
- causes of EGGD are not known but it is believed that 'stress' may play a central role:
  - breed disposition and management factors related to behavioural stress such as multiple handlers and riders.
  - exercising >4 and >5 days per week has been shown to increase the risk of EGGD in racehorses and show horses, respectively:
    - ♦ suggests rest days may be important in reducing EGGD risk.
- widely believed NSAID administration is associated with ulceration of the glandular mucosa in adults and both the glandular and non-glandular mucosa in foals:
  - no epidemiological evidence to support this when NSAIDs are used at correct doses.

- high-dose NSAID therapy is associated with the development of EGGD lesions.
- extended duration therapy may be associated with increased risk of EGGD.
- no evidence that *Helicobacter pylori* plays a role in EGUS.
- relatively linear relationship between exercise and ESGD is not seen in EGGD:
  - EGGD affects a wide range of horses not typically considered at high risk of ESGD.

Clinical presentation

- adult horses:
  - decreased appetite (particularly for concentrates).
  - decreased performance.
  - weight loss.
  - changes in behaviour or rideability.
- foals:
  - intermittent, low-grade colic.
  - poor haircoat and lethargy.
  - anorexia, bruxism, salivation, and diarrhoea.
- some horses have severe lesions without any clinical signs.
- gastric rupture secondary to ulceration is very rare in adults and uncommon in foals:
  - can occur without preceding signs.
- clinical examination is often unremarkable in both adults and foals:
  - possible exception of decreased body condition.

Differential diagnosis

- variety of causes of mild colic, partial anorexia, or ill-thrift.
- EGUS can occur concurrently with other diseases.

Diagnosis

- clinical signs may be suggestive but are not diagnostic:
  - haematology is typically unremarkable:
    - ♦ anaemia and hypoproteinaemia are uncommon even with severe ulceration.
  - faecal occult blood testing is unreliable.
  - sucrose permeability testing is not useful in adult horses.
- gastroscopy provides a definitive diagnosis:
  - full examination of the stomach is essential.
  - absence of ESGD lesions cannot be used to predict the presence, or absence, of EGGD lesions.
  - grading system can be used to evaluate ESGD (Table 3.5 and Figs. 3.22–3.26).
  - descriptive terminology is preferred for EGGD.

- ○ identification of severe EGUS in a foal should prompt an evaluation of gastric emptying:
  - ♦ gastric outflow problems can produce severe ulceration.
- ○ positive response to therapy is supportive of a diagnosis of EGUS:
  - ♦ does not differentiate ESGD from EGGD:
    - − when diagnosis is based on response to treatment, gastroscopy should be performed prior to discontinuation of therapy.

TABLE 3.5 Grading System for ESGD

GRADE	DESCRIPTION
0	Intact mucosa with a completely normal appearance and there is no appearance of hyperkeratosis
1	Mucosa is intact but there are areas of hyperkeratosis
2	Small (<2 cm) single ulcer or smaller multifocal ulcers
3	Large (>2 cm) single ulcer or large multifocal ulcers
4	Extensive ulceration that may involve coalescence of multiple ulcers. Bleeding may be evident

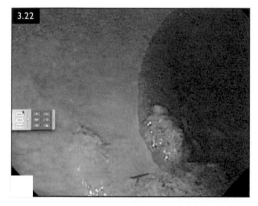

FIG. 3.22 stomach (Grade 0). The area of glandular mucosa is to the right of the image and the non-glandular area is to the left.

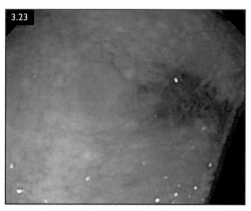

FIG. 3.23 Grade 2 ESGD characterised by a single superficial ulcer.

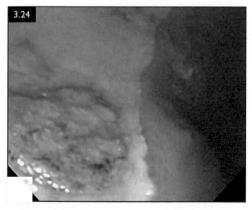

FIG. 3.24 Grade 3 ESGD. A large ulcer that is deeper than the ulcer in Fig. 3.23 is evident, as are smaller ulcers in the distance.

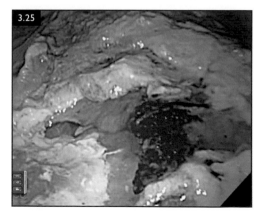

FIG. 3.25 Grade 4 ESGD. Note the bleeding ulcer.

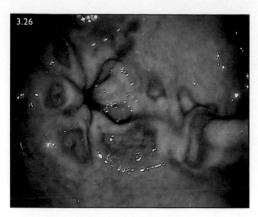

FIG. 3.26 A severe EGGD lesion involving the pyloric antrum.

Management

- combination of drug therapy and management changes is important.
- variety of drugs are available for the treatment of EGUS (Table 3.6):
  - Omeprazole is the best evaluated drug.
  - H_2 antagonists may be useful:
    - may be effective at relieving clinical signs rather than promoting full healing.
  - antacids have not been shown to be beneficial:
    - may temporarily ameliorate clinical signs in early treatment with H_2 antagonists or proton pump inhibitors.

- treatment duration depends on lesion type and disease severity:
  - typically, at least 21–28 days should be given.
- gastroscopy should be repeated prior to cessation of treatment.
- animals with severe or recurrent EGUS not taken out of training may benefit from preventive therapy following treatment.
- management changes are critical:
  - hay- or pasture-based diet with roughage available at all times.
  - turnout is preferred.
  - concentrates should be decreased or withheld.
  - moderate to severe cases, performance should cease during the treatment period.
  - possible stressors should be addressed.

Prognosis

- excellent if appropriate treatment is provided.
- recurrence is likely if long-term management changes are not made.
- perforation of EGUS carries a grave prognosis.
- routine antiulcer prophylaxis of sick or hospitalised horses is controversial:
  - sick horses, particularly foals, may not respond adequately to antiulcer therapy.
  - raising gastric pH may be a risk factor for the development of infectious colitis.

TABLE 3.6 Options for the treatment of gastric ulceration

DRUG	CLASS	DOSE	ROUTE	INTERVAL	COMMENT
Ranitidine	H_2 antagonist	6.6 mg/kg	p/o	q6–8h	Oral administration is preferable. Inconsistent efficacy as a therapeutic
		1.0–1.5 mg/kg	i/v	q8h	
Omeprazole	Proton pump antagonist	2–4 mg/kg	p/o	q24h	Best evaluated treatment
		1–2 mg/kg 4 mg/kg	p/o i/m	q24h q7d	Preventive therapy Novel long-acting formulation
Sucralfate		20–40 mg/kg	p/o	q6–8h	Adjunctive therapy for EGGD. Not recommended as a sole treatment
Misoprostol	PGE analogue	5 µg/kg	p/o	q12h	Potentially useful alternative for EGGD

Gastric dilation

Definition/overview

- distension of the stomach by gas or fluid can cause signs of colic and potentially result in gastric rupture.

Aetiology/pathophysiology

- dilation may be primary or secondary:
  - primary dilation due to excessive:
    - gas production following ingestion of highly fermentable feed material.
    - consumption of water following exercise.
  - secondary dilation due to:
    - obstructive small intestinal lesion.
    - excessive intestinal secretion.
    - disrupted intestinal motility.
    - stomach distends with ingested fluid, gas, and small intestinal fluid reflux.
- gastric dilation occurs if aboral movement of gas does not equal production.
- distended stomach tightly closes the cardia, and fluid and gas cannot move from the stomach into the oesophagus.
- signs of colic may develop as dilation increases.

Clinical presentation

- non-specific signs of colic are most common:
  - severe pain (markedly elevated heart rate [>100 bpm]) with increased distension.
  - tachypnoea due to compression of thoracic cavity by a large, distended stomach.
  - other clinical abnormalities relating to the underlying disease process in secondary gastric dilation.

Differential diagnosis

- other causes of colic should be investigated:
  - especially small intestinal disorders that may result in gastric distension.

Diagnosis

- gastric dilation is identified/relieved by nasogastric tube passage (part of colic exam).
  - uncomplicated cases:
    - should result in near complete resolution of clinical signs.
    - presence of pain or tachycardia should prompt further evaluation of other differentials.
- no abnormalities are typically detectable per rectum unless:
  - gastric dilation is secondary to a small intestinal lesion.
  - marked gastric dilation displaces the spleen caudally.
- gastric distension may be evident ultrasonographically:
  - also evaluate abdomen for small intestinal lesions.

Management

- decompression of the stomach and resolution of the primary cause.
- large volumes of gas or fluid reflux obtained:
  - leave nasogastric tube in place or intubation repeated hourly.
  - remove the tube once gas and fluid reflux are minimal.
- surfactants such as DSS are not effective.
- surgical intervention required if an obstructive small intestinal lesion is present.
- primary gastric dilation is suspected, diet and management should be evaluated.

Prognosis

- depends on the cause:
  - primary gastric dilation is excellent.
  - secondary dilation depends on the severity of the inciting lesion:
    - spontaneous reflux is a poor prognostic indicator:
      - potential for complications such as aspiration pneumonia.

Gastric impaction

Definition/overview

- uncommon cause of colic.

Aetiology/pathophysiology

- accumulation of excessive amounts of ingesta in the stomach may result in gastric impaction.

- impacted ingesta become dessicated, firm, and resistant to rehydration.
- gastric distension may result in signs of abdominal pain.
- many cases are idiopathic.
- dental disorders, EGUS, poor-quality diet, abnormal GI motility (e.g. grass sickness) and gastric outflow obstruction may be associated with gastric impaction.
- gastric impactions can occur concurrently with large colon impactions.

Clinical presentation

- non-specific signs of colic ranging from mild to severe:
  o heart rate is elevated consistent with the degree of pain.
- signs of toxaemia or cardiovascular compromise not evident.

Differential diagnosis

- variety of other causes of acute colic must be considered.
- primary gastric impaction must be differentiated from secondary causes:
  o abnormalities of gastric motility or gastric outflow such as pyloric stenosis and grass sickness.

Diagnosis

- medical diagnosis of gastric impaction is difficult:
  o difficulty passing a stomach tube through the cardia may suggest that gastric distension is present.
  o palpation per rectum is usually unremarkable.
  o abdominocentesis is normal unless gastric rupture has occurred.
- gastroscopy is very useful:
  o difficult to differentiate an impaction from a full stomach.
  o feed withheld for 18–24 hours and a large volume of feed material is present, then an impaction is likely.

Management

- no food until the impaction has resolved; but free access to water should be provided.
- nasogastric tube left in place or passed frequently.

- o 10–20 ml/kg balanced electrolyte solution via tube every 2–4 hours.
  o **not too much pressure when infusing water lessens chances of gastric rupture:**
    ♦ gravity flow is preferred over hand pumps.
    ♦ horse appears to be in pain, infusion should be stopped.
- use of carbonated beverages has been recommended:
  o little benefit aside from cases of persimmon seed impaction.
- bethanecol (0.02 mg/kg s/c q6–8h) has been recommended:
  o theoretical increased risk of gastric rupture.
  o appears to offer little benefit over frequent infusion of fluids alone.
- gastroscopy used to evaluate response to treatment and confirm impaction has passed.
- risk factors should be identified and addressed.

Prognosis

- frustrating because of the time required for some impactions to resolve.
- good prognosis for recovery unless serious primary problem (grass sickness or pyloric obstruction) is present.
- long-term prognosis is poor with recurrence, although some animals can be managed on low-bulk diets.

Pyloric stenosis

Definition/overview

- rare condition that results in delayed gastric outflow.

Aetiology/pathophysiology

- congenital lesion.
- occurs secondary to severe gastric and duodenal ulceration:
  o particularly in foals, weanlings, and yearlings.
- inhibited gastric outflow leads to accumulation of food material and gastric acid.

Clinical presentation

- intermittent colic, lethargy, and chronic weight loss are the most common clinical signs.
- salivation, bruxism, and anorexia may also occur.

Differential diagnosis

- EGUS and duodenal ulceration are the main differential diagnoses.
- all other causes of weight loss and chronic colic should be considered.

Diagnosis

- haematological changes, if present, are non-specific.
- palpation per rectum and abdominocentesis are usually normal.
- nasogastric reflux depending on the severity of gastric outflow disruption.
- EGUS will be evident endoscopically:
  - not possible to determine whether it is primary or secondary.
  - attempt to enter the duodenum.
- ultrasonographic examination of the abdomen can be used to assess:
  - gastric distension, duodenal thickness, and duodenal motility.
- other methods to evaluate gastric emptying include:
  - nuclear scintigraphy, oral glucose absorption testing, and acetaminophen absorption testing.
- barium radiography can be used to evaluate gastric emptying, particularly in foals.
- definitive diagnosis is made at surgery.

Management

- medical treatment should be attempted initially in case gastric outflow is being affected by inflammation, not stenosis:
  - proton pump inhibitors should be administered as for EGUS.
  - systemic administration is preferred to oral administration.
  - inhibitors are acid labile and delayed gastric emptying may reduce oral bioavailability.
  - general supportive care, including intravenous fluid therapy, may be required.
  - dietary change instituted initially, depending on the severity of clinical signs:
    - frequent feeding of small meals of grass, slurries, or a pelleted ration.
    - oral feeding not tolerated:
      - parenteral nutrition considered, particularly in foals.
  - bethanecol (0.025–0.10 mg/kg s/c q6–8h or 0.3–0.4 mg/kg p/o q6–8h) or metoclopramide (0.05–0.25 mg/kg s/c q6–8h or 0.6 mg/kg p/o q4h):
    - used to increase rate of gastric emptying.
    - both drugs can be associated with adverse clinical signs.
  - medical treatment, particularly nutritional support, may be most useful for improving the horse's condition prior to surgery.
  - surgical intervention required if improvement is not evident within 5 days:
    - success via gastrojejunostomy or gastroduodenostomy has been reported.

Prognosis

- lack of prompt response to treatment, medical therapy is unlikely to be effective.
- successful surgical treatment has been reported.
- overall, the prognosis is guarded to poor.

Gastric rupture

Definition/overview

- fatal condition usually secondary to distension of the stomach with gas, ingesta, or fluid.

Aetiology/pathophysiology

- variety of situations can result in gastric distension and subsequently gastric rupture:
  - primary distension:
    - excessive gas production, grain engorgement, and excessive water consumption after exercise.
  - secondary distension:
    - obstructive small intestinal lesions, proximal duodenitis/jejunitis, and ileus.

- less commonly, gastric impaction or infarction of the stomach:
  - ◆ perforation of gastric ulcers is uncommon.
  - no apparent age, breed, or gender predisposition.
- stomach of an average adult horse capacity of 15–25 litres under maximal distension:
  - rupture due to excessive distension and/or ischaemic necrosis of the gastric wall.
- majority of tears occur along the greater curvature.
- upon perforation, severe septic peritonitis will rapidly develop.

Clinical presentation

- stomach ruptures:
  - short period where the horse appears to improve clinically.
  - pain associated with gastric distension is relieved.
  - septic peritonitis develops and there is a rapid deterioration.
- progressive signs of:
  - depression and colic.
  - toxaemia, dehydration, cardiovascular compromise, sweating, and shaking.
  - heart rate increases (>100 bpm).
  - mucous membranes may be dark red, purple, or blue.
  - CRT may be markedly prolonged.
  - borborygmi will be decreased or absent.

Differential diagnosis

- septic peritonitis of other causes.

- severe enterocolitis, septicaemia, and pleuritis.

Diagnosis

- **presence of gastric reflux does not rule out gastric rupture.**
- haematology may be normal initially:
  - neutropenia with a left shift and degenerative change will develop.
  - total plasma protein levels decrease as peritonitis progresses and PCV increases.
- excessive flocculent peritoneal fluid will be evident ultrasonographically +/– fibrin.
- **abdominocentesis should be performed:**
  - fluid may have gross appearance of ingesta.
  - variable increase in WBC count and degenerative changes in neutrophils.
  - peritoneal fluid may be normal in some cases:
    - ◆ rupture has occurred very recently.
    - ◆ gastric contents sequestered initially by omentum.
  - definitive diagnosis at surgery or necropsy.

Management

- severe septic peritonitis develops rapidly after rupture.
- limited reports of successful surgical repair of some types of tears.
- there are no viable treatment options with gross contamination of the abdomen.

Prognosis

- gastric rupture with abdominal contamination is invariably fatal.

DISORDERS OF THE SMALL INTESTINE

Duodenal ulceration

Definition/overview

- less common than EGUS
- more difficult to diagnose and can be more serious.
- EGUS is usually present concurrently.
- most common in horses less than 2 years of age:
  - foals only a few days old may be affected.

- perforating ulcers are more common in the first 2 months of life.

Aetiology/pathophysiology

- aetiology is not well understood.
- duodenal ulceration develops when protective mechanisms are overwhelmed:
  - most important mechanism is presence of bicarbonate-rich secretions.
  - factors affecting these mechanisms have not been clearly identified.

- segmental ulceration is most common:
  - often in area at entrance of the bile duct.
  - inflammation associated with ulceration can result in duodenal stricture:
    - may subsequently affect gastric emptying.
- perforation of duodenal ulcers can occur, often with few prodromal signs.

Clinical presentation

- clinical signs are the same as those from severe EGUS (often present concurrently).
- **foals:**
  - bruxism, excessive salivation, rolling on back, and anorexia.
  - diarrhoea may be present.
  - pyrexia and/or depressed.
- **older horses:**
  - mild to moderate colic signs.
  - decreased appetite (particularly for grain), weight loss, and ill-thrift.
  - duodenal stricture:
    - poor growth, bruxism, and excessive salivation.
    - depression, intermittent colic, and fever.

Differential diagnosis

- EGUS is the main differential.
- variety of other causes of intermittent colic and diarrhoea.

Diagnosis

- duodenoscopy (Fig. 3.27):
  - performed in all animals with consistent clinical signs.
  - those with severe EGUS or evidence of decreased gastric outflow.
- contrast radiography (barium series) used to identify delayed gastric emptying (>2 hours) and duodenal strictures.

Management

- suppression of gastric acidity achieved by a variety of drugs (Table 3.6):
  - omeprazole most effective available drug:
    - systemic administration should be considered.
    - variable absorption of oral formulations:

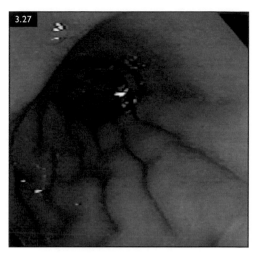

FIG. 3.27 Endoscopic view of a normal duodenum.

- especially where delayed gastric emptying present.
  - concurrent treatment with sucralfate is indicated.
  - duration of treatment is unclear (minimum of 1 month usually indicated).
- proper gastric emptying is important for decreasing secondary EGUS and for delivering administered drugs to the small intestine:
  - gastric emptying delayed:
    - bethanecol (0.025–0.10 mg/kg s/c q6–8h or 0.3–0.4 mg/kg p/o q6–8h).
    - metoclopramide (0.05– 0.25 mg/kg s/c q6–8h or 0.6 mg/kg p/o q4h).

Prognosis

- variable, depending on the degree of duodenal damage (Fig. 3.28).
- duodenal stricture carries a guarded prognosis.
- peritonitis from a perforating duodenal ulcer carries a grave prognosis.

Lawsonia intracellularis infection (proliferative enteropathy)

Definition/overview

- important disease in foals that is occasionally seen in older horses.

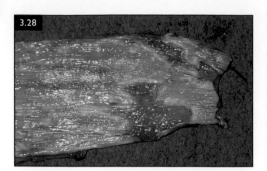

FIG. 3.28 Multifocal erosions of the duodenal mucosa.

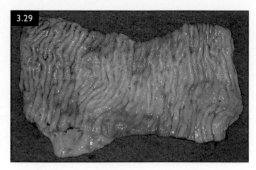

FIG. 3.29 Mucosal surface of the ileum of a 6-month-old foal with *Lawsonia intracellularis* infection. Note the thickened, corrugated mucosa.

Aetiology/pathophysiology

- *Lawsonia intracellularis* is an obligate intracellular organism that can cause proliferative enteropathy in a number of species, particularly pigs.
- infection via the faecal–oral route:
  - source of infection is typically not identified.
  - post-ingestion, organism invades enterocytes, particularly in jejunum and ileum.
  - affected cells proliferate, causing hyperplasia (Fig. 3.29).
- pathophysiology is not completely understood.
- large intestine is not affected:
  - faecal consistency may be normal even with severe small intestinal disease.

Clinical presentation

- foals 3–7 months of age most affected.
- development of disease is often slow and insidious:
  - clinical abnormalities often not noted until disease is quite advanced.
- most common presenting complaints:
  - weight loss, depression, oedema, diarrhoea, and ill-thrift.
  - colic, but is not typical.
- foals usually:
  - poor body condition.
  - ventral and limb oedema.
  - pot-bellied appearance.
  - poor haircoat.
- severe weakness may be present in advanced cases.
- often, multiple foals on a farm will be affected.

Differential diagnoses

- depends on clinical presentation:
  - intestinal parasitism, malnutrition, maldigestion, severe EGUS and duodenal ulceration
  - clostridial diarrhoea, salmonellosis, NSAID toxicosis, and protein-losing enteropathy.
  - protein-losing nephropathy, hepatic disease, and plant or chemical intoxication.

Diagnosis

- severe hypoproteinaemia (<40 g/l [4g/dl]):
  - marked hypoalbuminaemia (<15 g/l [1.5 g/dl], occasionally <10 g/l [1.0 g/dl]).
  - degree of hypoproteinaemia usually more severe than expected with severity and duration of the diarrhoea (if present).
- leucocytosis, with a neutrophilia, may be present.
- mild to moderate hyponatraemia, hypokalaemia, hypochloraemia, and hypocalcaemia, particularly in diarrhoeic foals.
- transabdominal ultrasonography:
  - thickened loops of small intestine with classic 'target' appearance:
    - not always present.
- presumptive diagnosis based on clinical presentation, severe hypoproteinaemia, and exclusion of other causes of disease.
- specific testing should be performed:
  - testing for *L. intracellularis* involves serological testing or PCR testing of faeces.

- more beneficial for population monitoring than individual diagnosis.
- coinfection with other enteropathogens can occur:
  - such as *Salmonella* spp. and *C. difficile.*
  - testing for multiple pathogens should be performed.
- post-mortem examination:
  - much of the small intestine, mainly the jejunum and ileum.
  - usually thickened and corrugated.
  - *L. intracellularis* detected histologically using silver stains.
- confirmation of diagnosis on intestinal tissues via immunohistochemistry or PCR.

Management

- antimicrobial therapy is indicated:
  - must be able to penetrate intracellularly.
  - oxytetracycline (6.6 mg/kg i/v q12 h) and doxycycline (10 mg/kg p/o q12 h).
  - erythromycin estolate 25 mg/kg p/o q6–8 h or erythromycin phosphate 37.5 mg/kg p/o q12 h), with or without rifampin (10 mg/kg p/o q24 h), and chloramphenicol (50 mg/kg p/o q6 h) have been used with anecdotal success.
  - required duration of therapy is unclear:
    - foals often treated for a minimum of 21–28 days.
    - treatment until resolution of clinical signs, normal ultrasonography, and normal serum total protein and albumin.
- fluid therapy may be required in diarrhoeic foals:
  - **use sparingly because of the hypoproteinemia.**
  - oncotic support with plasma or synthetic colloids often required:
    - not to return total protein levels to normal.
    - alleviate any negative consequences of hypoproteinaemia.
- parenteral nutrition may be required in severely affected foals.
- **one affected foal on a farm:**
  - all other foals should be considered at risk.
  - pay close attention to the body condition of at-risk foals.

- regular assessment of total protein and albumin levels may allow early identification and treatment.

Prognosis

- reasonable for affected foals with appropriate treatment.
- worse in foals with severe weight loss and hypoproteinaemia.
- foals that are weak and recumbent carry a poor prognosis:
  - even with aggressive support, including parenteral nutrition.
- rapid clinical response to therapy has been observed but gross small intestinal changes and hypoproteinaemia require weeks to months to resolve.

Rotavirus enteritis

Definition/overview

- common cause of diarrhoea in foals less than 3–6 months of age:
  - foals as young as 1–2 days of age can be affected.
- most identified cause of diarrhoea in young foals in some areas.
- outbreaks can occur.

Aetiology/pathophysiology

- variety of different equine rotavirus serotypes identified:
  - prevalent in the horse population.
  - most horses are likely to be exposed early in life.
- foals are infected via the faecal–oral route.
- following ingestion, rotavirus invades villous epithelial cells in the small intestine:
  - fluid absorption is decreased, and secretion can be increased.
  - lactase-producing cells at the tips of the villi may be damaged.
  - secondary lactose intolerance may be an important aspect of this disease.
- foals can shed rotavirus and be a source of infection:
  - before clinical signs develop, while diarrhoeic, and for variable lengths of time after resolution of disease.
  - some foals can shed rotavirus for up to 8 months.

- adult horses do not develop clinical disease but may be a source of infection.
- rotavirus can persist in the environment for long periods of time (up to 9 months):
  - once on a farm, can be difficult to eradicate.

Clinical presentation

- most affected foals are diarrhoeic, mildly depressed, partially anorexic, and pyrexic.
- other signs may precede diarrhoea by 24 hours.
- depression and anorexia may worsen as dehydration develops.
- young foals are usually more severely affected.
- older foals may only develop very mild disease.
- typical clinical course is 3–5 days:
  - diarrhoea may persist for longer periods in some cases.
  - signs of toxaemia and sepsis should not be present.

Differential diagnosis

- Foal heat diarrhoea, salmonellosis, clostridial enteritis, and parasitic diarrhoea.

Diagnosis

- identification of rotavirus in faeces via:
  - PCR, ELISA, a latex agglutination test, or electron microscopy.
  - interpretation complicated by potential for virus shedding by subclinical carriers.
- prudent to test for *Salmonella*, *Clostridium difficile* and *C. perfringens* to identify coinfection.
- **testing is important**:
  - identification of disease for which specific treatments are indicated.
  - determining appropriate infection control practices.

Management

- specific management depends on the severity of disease and the age of the foal:
  - very young foals are more likely to require intensive treatment.
  - fluid therapy is most important aspect of treatment:

- intravenous fluid therapy (balanced electrolyte solution) often required in dehydrated foals.
  - nutritional support may be required, particularly in young foals.
  - diagnosis and management of lactose intolerance should be considered.
- Rotavirus is not invasive and does not typically cause significant mucosal damage:
  - low risk of bacterial translocation and antimicrobial therapy not usually indicated.
  - considered in young, severely compromised foals and any suspected case of septicaemia.
- isolate infected foals and their dams.
- good general farm management for prevention of rotavirus diarrhoea including:
  - implementation of isolation and quarantine protocols.
  - proper disinfection.
  - rotavirus can persist in the environment for several months.

Prognosis

- very good to excellent if adequate supportive care can be provided.
- complications are uncommon.

Duodenitis/proximal jejunitis

Definition/overview

- also termed anterior enteritis or proximal enteritis, duodenitis/proximal jejunitis (DPJ).
- inflammatory condition resulting in fluid distension of the small intestine, gastric reflux, toxaemia, colic, and depression.
- reported more commonly in the USA and sporadically elsewhere in the world:
  - anecdotally greater prevalence in southern USA.
- most cases occur in the summer months for unclear reasons.
- vast majority of cases are in horses more than 2 years old.

Aetiology/pathophysiology

- aetiology is unknown but an infectious cause is highly suspected:

- o   recent evidence has implicated *Clostridium difficile*.
- lesions tend to be restricted to the duodenum and proximal jejunum.
- inflammation of areas of small intestine results in increased net movement of fluid into the lumen.
- intestinal motility may not be coordinated and progressive:
  - o   small intestinal distension develops.
  - o   ileus may occur due to distension, electrolyte disturbances, toxaemia, or pain.
  - o   eventually, gastric distension may occur:
    - ♦   typically causes more severe signs of colic.
    - ♦   gastric rupture if the stomach is not decompressed.

Clinical presentation

- acute onset of colic most common presentation:
  - o   occasionally, depression and fever noted before colic signs.
  - o   colic largely attributable to gastric distension.
  - o   large volumes of gastric reflux may be produced.
  - o   variable appearance of gastric reflux:
    - ♦   reddish colour and foetid odour suggest enteritis, but these are not consistent.
  - o   post-stomach decompression, horses often appear more depressed than painful:
    - ♦   compared to a strangulating small intestinal lesion.
  - o   tachycardia is common and can be marked (80–120 bpm).
- varying degrees of dehydration, fever, and toxaemia may be present.
- laminitis is a common complication, occurring in up to 30% of cases.

Differential diagnosis

- early on, strangulating and non-strangulating obstructive small intestinal lesions.
- less commonly, primary ileus can produce the same clinical signs.
- diagnostic challenge is determining whether a surgical or medical lesion is present.

Diagnosis

- multiple loops of distended small intestine are usually palpable per rectum.
- ultrasonographic examination of the abdomen:
  - o   typically displays multiple loops of distended small intestine.
  - o   loops are generally more motile than strangulating lesions (not always).
- abdominocentesis useful in some cases but results are variable:
  - o   high total protein (>30 g/l [3 g/dl]) with normal cell count (<5 × 10⁹ cells/l).
  - o   changes are typically not as severe as with strangulating lesions.
- surgical exploration is the only definitive diagnostic test and should be considered when there is a reasonable suspicion of a strangulating lesion:
  - o   pre-surgery differentiation is critical but is not always possible.
  - o   DPJ is suggested by:
    - ♦   fever and depression following gastric decompression.
    - ♦   hypermotility of intestinal loops on ultrasonographic examination.
    - ♦   increased abdominal fluid total protein with a normal cell count.

Management

- initial goals are stabilisation of the patient and deciding whether surgical exploration is required.
- gastric decompression is critical and should be performed early.
- leave a nasogastric tube in place or pass one frequently:
  - o   large volumes of reflux can be produced.
  - o   > 5 litres of reflux, decompress stomach hourly.
  - o   as amount decreases, the frequency of decompression can be decreased.
- intravenous fluid therapy is indicated because of dehydration, toxaemia, and an inability to provide oral water:
  - o   > 100 litres/day may be required in some cases.
  - o   electrolyte abnormalities can be associated with poor intestinal motility:

- ◆ monitor serum or plasma electrolyte levels if possible.
- ◆ supplement balanced electrolyte solutions with potassium chloride or calcium borogluconate.
- ◆ total potassium supplementation should not exceed 1.0 mEq/kg/ hour.
- hypoproteinaemia may develop, and oncotic support may be required:
  - ○ plasma beneficial if signs of endotoxaemia are present.
  - ○ synthetic colloids used if plasma is not available.
- unclear whether antimicrobials are required, either for treatment of a primary infection or prevention of bacterial translocation:
  - ○ penicillin is often used because clostridial organisms may be involved.
  - ○ broad-spectrum coverage is not unreasonable:
    - ◆ care taken with aminoglycosides because of the potential for nephrotoxicity.
  - ○ metronidazole (25–50 mg/kg per rectum q8–12h) has been used because of the suspected involvement of C. *difficile*, but its efficacy is unclear.
- flunixin meglumine (1.1 mg/kg i/v q12h) is useful for controlling pain, attenuating pain-induced ileus, and for purported 'anti-endotoxin' effects.
- other antiendotoxin therapies such as administration of polymyxin B (6000 IU/kg i/v q12h) should be considered in toxaemic horses.
- prokinetic therapy has not been shown to be effective.
- exploratory laparotomy is commonly performed to prevent a surgical lesion being overlooked.
- cases closely monitored for complications such as laminitis or catheter site thrombophlebitis.
- food and water should be withheld until refluxing has ceased.
- parenteral nutrition may be required in horses that continue to reflux for several days.
- oral medications should be avoided because of unpredictable absorption.

Prognosis

- reasonable if aggressive supportive care can be provided:
  - ○ reported survival rates range from 25 to 94%.
- response to treatment is highly variable:
  - ○ some horses may cease refluxing within 24 hours.
  - ○ others may continue to reflux for more than 1 week.
  - ○ horses that stop refluxing within 72 hours have a good prognosis.
- typical course of disease is 3–7 days.
- complications such as laminitis are not uncommon.
- euthanasia maybe required for economic reasons if prolonged treatment is required.

Lactose intolerance

Definition/overview

- occasionally identified in foals.

Aetiology/pathophysiology

- occurs following damage to the small intestinal villi:
  - ○ often secondary to infectious causes of enterocolitis.
  - ○ initial cause may not be identified in all cases.
  - ○ primary lactose intolerance has not been reported in foals.
- lactase is normally present in enterocytes on the tips of villi in the small intestine:
  - ○ enzyme responsible for converting lactose into glucose and galactose.
- secondary lactose intolerance occurs when lactase-producing cells have been damaged:
  - ○ usually associated with infectious enteritis in foals.

Clinical presentation

- main presenting signs are persistent diarrhoea and intermittent colic.
- other clinical abnormalities are uncommon.
- foals are typically bright and alert.
- experienced previous episode of suspected infectious enteritis:
  - ○ intolerance may be present transiently with enteritis of any aetiology, but

not readily apparent because of the primary disease.

Differential diagnosis

- clostridial enteritis, salmonellosis, rotaviral enteritis, idiopathic colitis, and other causes of diarrhoea, maldigestion, and malabsorption.

Diagnosis

- other causes of diarrhoea (*Salmonella, C. difficile, C. perfringens*, rotavirus) should be ruled out or treated:
  - lactose intolerance may be concurrent.
- response to supplementation with oral lactase is suggestive but not diagnostic.
- oral lactose tolerance test is most widely used for diagnosis (Table 3.7).

Management

- standard approach is supplementation with oral lactase (1500–3000 IU p/o q4–12h).
- weaning considered in older foals, particularly if oral supplementation is problematic.
- supportive treatment or treatment of the primary cause should be provided if necessary.

Prognosis

- excellent if adequate supportive care is provided.
- lactase production should be restored in a few days to weeks, depending on the severity of the primary insult.

Ascarid infection

Definition/overview

- common in horses, particularly those:
  - housed on crowded pastures with frequent mixing of horses.
  - inadequate parasite control programmes.
- Ascarid impaction is an uncommon but life-threatening problem:
  - typically occurs after deworming weanlings with large parasite burdens.

Aetiology/pathophysiology

- infection following ingestion of infective *Parascaris equorum* larvae that develop

TABLE 3.7 Protocol for lactose tolerance testing in foals

1 Fast the foal for approximately 4 hours
2 Obtain a baseline blood glucose level. Stallside testing with a glucometer can be performed. Red blood cells will consume glucose *in vitro*. If samples must be stored or shipped for >1 hour before testing, plasma or serum should be separated or tubes containing sodium fluoride should be used
3 Administer 1 g/kg lactose, as a 20% solution in water, via bottle or nasogastric tube
4. Determine blood glucose levels every 30 minutes for 3 hours
5 Increase in blood glucose of <2 mmol/l indicates maldigestion or malabsorption. The peak value is usually obtained at 60–90 minutes
6 Glucose absorption test should be performed on all foals with an abnormal lactose tolerance test to differentiate maldigestion from malabsorption
7 Glucose absorption test is performed as described for the lactose tolerance test, substituting lactose with 1 g/kg glucose. An increase in blood glucose of at least 75% should occur

within 10 days on pasture from faeces of infected horses.

- following ingestion, larvae migrate through the wall of the small intestine, pass through the liver via the portal vein, and eventually reach the pulmonary circulation.
- larvae moult in the lung, ascend the trachea, and are swallowed.
- final moulting and maturation occur in the small intestine.

Clinical presentation

- ascarids can be present in the small intestine without any obvious clinical signs.
- clinical infestation is usually non-specific and characterised by:
  - pot-bellied appearance and varying degrees of decreased growth rate.
  - poor haircoat and lethargy.
  - concurrent low-grade respiratory disease is not uncommon.
- ascarid impaction is a serious condition characterised by:

o acute, often severe, colic.
o consider in all colic cases presenting shortly after deworming of foals.
o intestinal rupture may occur, with associated peritonitis.

Differential diagnosis

- variety of other causes of ill-thrift such as:
  o malnutrition, poor management, other intestinal parasites, and chronic infection.
- other causes of colic may produce similar clinical signs to those of ascarid impaction.

Diagnosis

- faecal flotation test should be performed:
  o ascarid eggs are readily identified after the 10–12 weeks prepatent period.
- foals with ascarid impaction have signs of small intestinal obstruction:
  o gastric reflux.
  o ultrasonographic identification of distended small intestine.
  o occasionally, ascarids are identified in:
    ♦ gastric reflux, on gastroscopy or via ultrasound (Fig. 3.30).

Management

- routine deworming started in foals at 6–8 weeks of age.

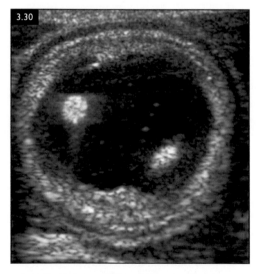

FIG. 3.30 Cross-sectional ultrasound image of a foal with ascarid impaction. Note the two cross-sectional images of ascarids within the intestinal lumen.

- repeated every 8 weeks for the first 6–12 months.
- broodmares dewormed regularly, including in third trimester, to decrease environmental contamination.
- resistance to various anthelmintics is widespread in ascarids:
  o knowledge of regional patterns is essential for adequate control.
  o faecal egg reduction tests should be regularly performed.
- large ascarid burden suspected:
  o deworm initially with slower-acting anthelmintics (e.g. fenbendazole), rather than avermectins, to reduce the chance of ascarid impaction.
- deworming programmes for yearlings and adult horses should be designed for the individual farm based on:
  o farm type, horse numbers, and horse movement.
  o pasture crowding, and ability to properly manage pastures.
- ascarid eggs can remain viable on pasture for years, so prevention of pasture contamination is important:
  o proper pasture management is essential:
    ♦ avoidance of overstocking.
    ♦ removal of faeces.
    ♦ pasture rotation.
    ♦ routine deworming of all animals with access to the pasture.
  o faecal egg count reduction tests useful for evaluating effectiveness of deworming programme.
- emergency surgery is required in foals with ascarid impaction and signs of intestinal obstruction (Fig. 3.31).

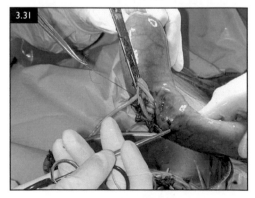

FIG. 3.31 Enterotomy to remove ascarids in a foal with an ascarid impaction.

Strangulating lipoma

Definition/overview

- common cause of small intestinal strangulation in older horses.

Aetiology/pathophysiology

- lipomas are fatty masses that can develop in the mesentery of older horses:
  - probably most common in fat, older horses and ponies.
  - inconsequential unless they enlarge and develop a pedicle.
  - may wrap around a section of small intestine, resulting in strangulation (Fig. 3.32).
  - vasculature compromise leads to affected intestine rapidly losing viability (Fig. 3.33).

Clinical presentation

- acute, severe colic is the most common presentation:
  - very painful with marked tachycardia (up to 120 bpm).
- immediate nasogastric intubation may relieve some pain via easing gastric distension.
- tachycardia and signs of colic usually continue to be severe.
- signs of toxaemia (hyperaemic mucous membranes, prolonged CRT) and cardiovascular compromise are often present.
- borborygmi often absent.
- response to analgesics may be poor.

Differential diagnosis

- other causes of small intestinal distension, including small intestinal volvulus, epiploic foramen entrapment, proximal enteritis, ileal impaction, and intussusception.

Diagnosis

- nasogastric reflux usually present.
- multiple loops of distended small intestine typically palpable per rectum:
  - detected ultrasonographically (Fig. 3.34):
    - round, distended, non-motile small intestine suggests intestinal compromise.
- peritoneal fluid changes occur as intestine becomes compromised:

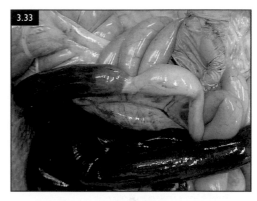

FIG. 3.33 After removal of the lipoma depicted in Fig. 3.32, a marked line of demarcation is evident at the site of strangulation.

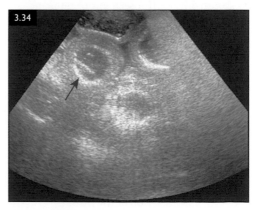

FIG. 3.34 Small intestinal distension in a horse with strangulating lipoma. Note the extremely thickened intestinal wall (arrow).

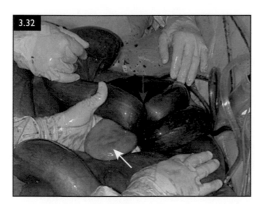

FIG. 3.32 Pedunculated lipoma (white arrow) causing strangulation of the small intestine (red arrow).

- o initially protein levels and WBC numbers increase.
- o followed shortly by changes in colour and turbidity (Fig. 3.6).

Management

- nasogastric tube passed to relieve gastric reflux:
  - o tube left in place if reflux is present.
- nothing given per os or via nasogastric tube.
- prompt surgical intervention is required.
- stabilisation is required prior to surgery:
  - o intravenous fluid therapy, gastric decompression, and analgesia administration.

Prognosis

- guarded to fair.
- length of affected intestine and the degree of compromise are important factors.
- intestinal resection is usually required.
- complications are not uncommon including:
  - o adhesions, anastomosis site abscessation, dehiscence, or intestinal stricture.
  - o postoperative prolonged ileus and laminitis are common.

Small intestinal volvulus

Definition/overview

- rotation of more than 180° around the long axis of the mesentery of the small intestine.
- can involve only a segment of intestine (Fig. 3.35) or the entire small intestine if the rotation is at the base of the mesentery.
- most often occurs in horses less than 3 years of age.

Aetiology/pathophysiology

- volvulus can be primary or secondary to another lesion such as:
  - o anastomosis site, entrapped bowel or a mesodiverticular band.
  - o these lesions probably act as a fixed axis for rotation of the bowel.
  - o volvulus in mesenteric portion of the small intestine from jejunum to distal ileum.

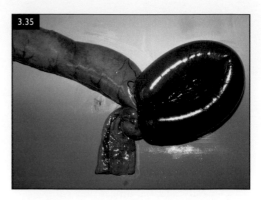

FIG. 3.35 Post-mortem specimen of a small intestine volvulus. Note the typical appearance of small intestine haemorrhagic strangulation. (Photo courtesy S Laverty)

- after the intestine rotates around an axis:
  - o peristalsis of the intestine orad to the lesion causes further mesenteric twisting.
  - o brings both orad and aborad intestine into the volvulus.
- post-volvulus increased intestinal movement is noted initially, followed by a decrease and eventually absence of motility (ileus).
- venous and luminal occlusion results in:
  - o fluid accumulation in the affected segment of small intestine.
  - o increased intraluminal pressure.
  - o secretion of more fluid by the intestinal wall worsens the condition.
- arterial blood usually continues to enter the affected segment leading to further oedema.
- intestine orad to the volvulus becomes distended leading to gastric distension.
- sequestration of fluid in the small intestine may produce dehydration.
- intestinal necrosis creates leakage of protein, RBCs, and bacteria:
  - o resulting in peritonitis and endotoxic shock.

Clinical presentation

- acute onset of often violent colic:
  - o pain may decrease in some cases concurrent with intestinal necrosis.
- moderate abdominal distension can be evident.

- marked elevation in heart rate and concurrent respiratory rate increase.
- body temperature is usually normal but may decrease in advanced stages of disease.
- spontaneous nasogastric reflux is uncommon.

Differential diagnosis

- other causes of small intestinal strangulation including:
  - pedunculated lipoma, intussusception, epiploic entrapment, and herniation.

Diagnosis

- small intestinal distension is usually palpable per rectum:
  - thickening of the intestinal wall may be appreciated in some cases.
- nasogastric tube passage often yields spontaneous or provoked reflux fluid:
  - gastric decompression may not result in any improvement in clinical signs.
- abdominocentesis usually yields a serosanguineous fluid with increased nucleated cell count and total protein level.
- ultrasonographic examination:
  - distension of small intestinal loops (>5 cm).
  - absence of motility.
  - increase in intestinal wall thickness may be present.

Management

- surgical intervention is required.
- cardiovascular compromise is common, and stabilisation is required prior to GA induction.

Prognosis

- generally poor to fair due to:
  - large amount of small intestine that can be involved:
    - >60% of small intestine involved, euthanasia is usually recommended because of the potential for maldigestion and malabsorption.
  - frequency of complications associated with small intestinal resection:
    - intestinal adhesions, abscessation of the anastomosis site, and functional obstruction of the anastomosis.

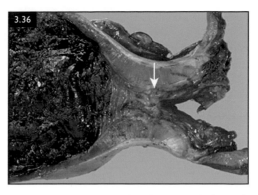

FIG. 3.36 A case of severe ileal hypertrophy (arrow).

Muscular hypertrophy of the ileum

Definition/overview

- hypertrophy with accompanying reduction of the intestinal lumen, can result in obstruction (Fig. 3.36).

Aetiology/pathophysiology

- muscular hypertrophy may be primary or secondary:
  - secondary cases usually associated with stenosis of the ileum or ileocaecal valve.
  - causes of the stenosis include:
    - ileocaecal intussusception, strongyle larvae migration, or mucosal/mural lesions.
  - muscular hypertrophy occurs as a compensatory mechanism.
- idiopathic hypertrophy of the ileum may also occur in primary cases:
  - aetiology believed to be an autonomic nervous system imbalance and dysfunction at the ileocaecal valve.
  - may be an increased risk with a heavy tapeworm burden.
- both circular and longitudinal muscular layers of the ileum are affected.
- abnormalities can extend to the distal jejunum or several segments of the small intestine.
- hypertrophied muscle narrows the lumen, causing a partial obstruction.
- obstruction can result in local impaction and distension of the small intestine orad to the lesion.

Clinical presentation

- clinical signs depend on the degree of obstruction:
  - intermittent colic (especially after eating), anorexia, and chronic weight loss.
  - 1–6 months duration.
  - partial obstruction may result in mild/moderate intermittent signs of colic.
  - total obstruction leads to more severe signs.
  - nasogastric reflux depending on severity and duration of the luminal obstruction.

Differential diagnosis

- variety of other obstructive or strangulating lesions of the small intestine.
- intestinal lymphosarcoma may also result in thickened small intestine.

Diagnosis

- distended loops of small intestine may be palpable per rectum:
  - loops with thickened wall may be palpable in the upper right abdominal quadrant.
- these findings may be observed on ultrasound examination:
  - objective assessment of wall thickness:
    - intestinal wall up to 25 mm thick in severe cases.
  - small intestinal distension orad to lesion if obstructive.
- nasogastric reflux present if a complete obstruction has developed.
- abdominocentesis usually yields normal fluid.
- haematology is unremarkable.

Management

- severity/frequency of clinical signs are used to determine whether surgery is required.
- mild cases, where surgery is not an option, may be treated conservatively:
  - laxative diet.
  - deworming programme evaluated, with particular attention paid to tapeworms.
  - all other cases should be presented for an exploratory laparotomy.

Prognosis

- lesion localised and does not involve the remainder of small intestine:
  - fair to good.
- surgical anastomosis (with or without resection) is performed:
  - local dehiscence of anastomosis site, stricture, and adhesions can occur.

Ileal impaction

Definition/overview

- obstruction of the ileum from accumulation of ingesta orad to the ileocaecal opening.
- most common as a primary condition, but also occurs secondary to ileal pathology.

Aetiology/pathophysiology

- more often seen in Europe and southeastern USA:
  - USA possibly related to feeding coastal Bermuda hay (often dry and fibrous):
    - more common between June and November.
  - Europe may be secondary to local infestation with tapeworms or mesenteric vascular thrombotic disease:
    - oedema and ulceration created by tapeworm attachment around the ileocaecal orifice.
    - disturbs motility and lumen diameter.

Clinical presentation

- impaction causes simple mechanical obstruction:
  - clinical signs are usually mild early in the condition.
- progression of ileal distension increases signs of pain:
  - usually not as severe as those seen with surgical lesions.
  - usually subside in 6–10 hours.
- abdominal pain then returns as gastric and orad small intestinal distension increases.
- gastric reflux is possible if the condition is chronic.

- borborygmi are usually decreased.
- heart rate is variably elevated.
- dehydration with secondary circulatory compromise arises following sequestration of fluid in the intestine and reduced oral intake.

Differential diagnosis

- main differential diagnoses are adynamic ileus and DPJ.
- more advanced cases, obstructive small intestinal conditions.

Diagnosis

- small intestinal distension usually palpable per rectum.
- approximately 25% of cases, impaction is palpable in the midline medial to the caecum.
- gastric reflux may be present, depending on the chronicity.
- abdominocentesis:
  ○ usually yields normal fluid.
  ○ if intestinal compromise develops from chronic and/or severe intestinal distension:
    ◆ protein level usually increases.
    ◆ long-standing impaction may result in local necrosis and peritonitis.

Management

- supportive medical therapy may be successful in early cases:
  ○ intravenous fluid therapy and analgesics.
- intermittent gastric decompression may be required:
  ○ nasogastric tube should be left in place or passed regularly.
- surgical intervention with an exploratory laparotomy is common:
  ○ diagnosis can be difficult.
  ○ impaction may be secondary to another lesion.

Prognosis

- fair to good:
  ○ better than most other small intestinal disorders.
  ○ shorter the duration before surgical intervention, the better the prognosis.
- postoperative ileus is common.

Meckel's diverticulum

Definition/overview

- embryonic remnant of the vitelline duct.
- results in formation of a blind sac that communicates with the lumen of the small intestine.

Aetiology/pathophysiology

- diverticulum can become impacted with ingesta, resulting in chronic colic.
- severe impaction can lead to necrosis followed by peritonitis.
- inflammation of the diverticulum may produce adhesions to other loops of intestine.
- diverticulum may wrap around other loops of small intestine causing strangulation.
- persistent vitelloumbilical bands may act as an axis for small intestinal volvulus.

Clinical presentation

- clinical signs are most common in adult horses:
- non-specific, if luminal obstruction is not present:
  ○ may be intermittent and chronic.
  ○ signs of abdominal discomfort with possible periods of inappetence.
- severe signs if a strangulation or volvulus.
- diverticulum also identified as incidental finding on exploratory laparotomy or necropsy.

Differential diagnosis

- vast array of causes of chronic or acute colic.

Diagnosis

- palpation per rectum:
  ○ small intestinal distension if total luminal obstruction is present.
  ○ sometimes palpable impacted diverticulum (blind sac with firm contents).
- transabdominal ultrasonography may reveal distended small intestine aborally to the diverticulum.
- peritoneal fluid WBC count and total protein may be elevated with a necrotic diverticulum.
- haematology is non-specific and variable.

3

Management

- exploratory laparotomy is indicated with severe signs of small intestinal obstruction, peritonitis, or chronic signs of colic.

Prognosis

- good if rupture and resulting peritonitis are not present or if resection is not needed.
- fair in the presence of strangulation or volvulus.

Mesodiverticular band

Definition/overview

- congenital abnormality forming a band extending from one side of the mesentery to the antimesenteric surface of the small intestine.
- persistence of the paired vitelline vessels as they extend from the aorta to the umbilicus.

Aetiology/pathophysiology

- triangular space is created:
  - mesodiverticular band forms one edge of a triangular hiatus.
  - adjacent mesentery and jejunum form the others.
  - forms a sac where herniation can occur.
- incarceration of the small intestine:
  - loop, most commonly the jejunum, passes into the depths of the hernial sac.
  - becomes trapped within it (Fig. 3.37).
- distension of the entrapped intestine creates pressure on the mesentery:
  - results in a mesenteric rent.
  - strangulation of a segment of jejunum in the rent (Fig. 3.38) may provide a fulcrum around which the surrounding intestine may form a volvulus.

Clinical presentation

- clinical signs are consistent with small intestine strangulation and include:
  - mild to severe signs of colic and moderate to severe elevations in heart rate.
  - eventual gastric reflux.

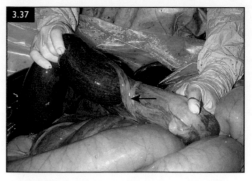

FIG. 3.37 A mesodiverticular band that was associated with a small intestine volvulus (arrow). This picture was taken after correction of the volvulus. Note the haemorrhagic strangulation lesion on the small intestine (left side of the picture).

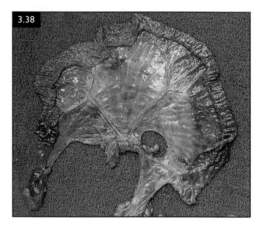

FIG. 3.38 Post-mortem specimen of a mesenteric rent located close to the root of the jejunal mesentery.

- incidental finding on exploratory laparotomy or necropsy.
- no age or sex predilection.

Differential diagnosis

- any other obstructive lesion of the small intestine, such as:
  - volvulus, strangulated lipoma, or mesenteric rent.

Diagnosis

- distended loops of small intestine are typically palpable per rectum.
- nasogastric reflux may be present, depending on the duration of obstruction.

- transabdominal ultrasonography may demonstrate distended small intestinal loops, potentially with intramural oedema.
- abdominocentesis when necrosis has occurred:
  - serosanguineous fluid.
  - increased nucleated cell count and total protein.

Management

- surgical correction is required.

Prognosis

- fair when resection is needed.
- worse if small intestinal volvulus is present concurrently.

Epiploic foramen entrapment (EFE)

Definition/overview

- epiploic foramen is a virtual space on the visceral surface of the liver (Fig. 3.39):
  - small intestine can become incarcerated within it.
- uncommon condition.
- Thoroughbreds and crosses, and male animals appear to be predisposed.

Aetiology/pathophysiology

- foramen lies on the visceral surface of the liver near the portal fissure:
  - narrow opening (approximately 4–10 cm diameter).

- cranially is the hepatoduodenal ligament.
- caudally junction between the pancreas and mesoduodenum.
- structures bordering the epiploic foramen are:
  - caudate process of the liver.
  - caudal vena cava dorsally.
  - right lobe of the pancreas, and the portal vein ventrally.
- hypothesised:
  - caudate process of the liver atrophies with age.
  - potential opening of the epiploic foramen becomes wider.
  - facilitates entrapment of small intestine.
- link between aerophagia and entrapment also reported.
- many cases occur in the winter months in the UK, when animals are stabled.
- distal jejunum and ileum most involved (long mesentery).
- entrapment from right to left or left to right:
  - right to left:
    - ♦ small intestine passes from peritoneal cavity through foramen and into omental bursa (left side) (Fig. 3.40).
  - left to right is more common:
    - ♦ intestine enters from visceral side of liver to lie between right liver lobe and the dorsal body wall.

Clinical presentation

- clinical signs are inconsistent, which may hamper diagnosis.

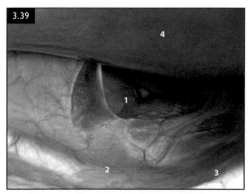

FIG. 3.39 Laparoscopic view of the opening of the epiploic foramen (1), the pancreas (2), the duodenum (3), and the liver (4).

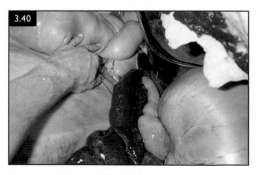

FIG. 3.40 Post-mortem view of a right-to-left epiploic foramen entrapment. Note the typical appearance of small intestine haemorrhagic strangulation.

- acute violent onset of colic, which subsides and is followed by depression.
- other cases may show no signs of abdominal pain and/or gastric reflux.
- despite presence of necrotic bowel, some horses have normal vital parameters:
  - infarcted bowel in an enclosed area may slow down absorption of endotoxin.
- severe hypovolaemic shock or sudden collapse if the portal vein or vena cava ruptures.

Differential diagnosis

- any other small intestinal obstructive disease such as:
  - strangulated lipoma, volvulus, intussusception, and mesenteric entrapment.

Diagnosis

- may be difficult.
- small intestine is incarcerated very cranially in the abdomen:
  - distention may not be palpable per rectum.
- nasogastric reflux may not be present until late in the disease:
  - typical involvement of distal portions of the small intestine.
- increase in peritoneal fluid lactate and protein levels in most cases:
  - fluid WBC count may also be increased (not consistent).
  - free blood in the abdomen if rupture of a main vessel.
- abdominal ultrasonography:
  - special attention for right middle body wall region.
  - suspect EFE if non-motile and oedematous small intestinal loops in this region.
- definitive diagnosis at surgery.

Management

- surgery is required:
  - usually, the intestine is nonviable and requires resection.
- rupture of the vena cava or portal vein is possible while trying to reduce the entrapment:
  - fatal complication.

Prognosis

- guarded to fair depending on whether resection is necessary or not.
- long-term outcomes vary from around 35 to 70%:
  - often poorer than other small intestinal surgical conditions.
  - ileus is a common complication postoperatively.

Inguinal rupture

Definition/overview

- result from herniation of intestine through the inguinal canal followed by rupture of:
  - peritoneum.
  - less commonly, vaginal tunic.
  - leads to intestinal loops in subcutaneous tissues of scrotal region.
  - often referred to as a direct inguinal hernia.

Aetiology/pathophysiology

- most common in foals after parturition:
  - secondary to traumatic rupture of vaginal tunic or peritoneum.
  - probably caused by compression during parturition.
- intestine passes through a rent in the parietal tunic and scrotal fascia.
- adult horses caused by trauma of a fall or a jump:
  - associated with a considerable length of intestinal herniation.

Clinical presentation

- foals usually presented for depression or mild colic signs:
  - pendulous swelling from inguinal region to cranial aspect of the prepuce.
- colic signs more severe with strangulation.
- friction between the swelling and the inner thigh may result in:
  - cold, oedematous, or necrotic skin locally.
- loops of bowel usually palpable subcutaneously:
  - evidence of peristalsis underneath the skin in some cases.
- usually difficult or impossible to reduce compared with a non-ruptured inguinal hernia.

- rupture in the adult occurs in both sexes and produces similar signs.

Differential diagnosis

- non-ruptured inguinal hernia, scrotal haematoma, seroma, or hydrocoele.

Diagnosis

- physical examination and haematology usually normal unless intestinal strangulation or concomitant disease.
- palpation of intestine outside the inguinal region and presence of swelling and abrasions are diagnostic.
- ultrasonography may reveal:
  - small intestine loops surrounded by subcutaneous fluid.
  - absence of vaginal tunic enclosing the intestine.
  - intestinal wall thickened and motility decreased if strangulation present.

Management

- surgery is advised to avoid strangulation, local adhesions of the small intestine, or total rupture:
- both testicles are removed at the same time in males.

Prognosis

- good if there is absence of strangulation or full-thickness trauma at the level of the skin.
- complications are limited to seroma formation, local infection and postoperative ileus.

Scrotal hernia

Definition/overview

- inguinal hernia results from passage of abdominal contents into the inguinal canal:
  - through external inguinal ring and into scrotum (scrotal hernia).

Aetiology/pathophysiology

- direct or indirect:
  - indirect hernia, herniated intestine located inside vaginal tunic beside the testis.
  - direct hernia, intestine herniates through rent in peritoneum and lies subcutaneously.
- indirect hernias are more common.
- condition may be congenital or acquired:
  - congenital is present at birth and considered an inherited defect:
    - secondary to an abnormal vaginal ring.
  - acquired hernias in adults are usually unilateral:
    - may occur secondary to conditions that increase the intra-abdominal pressure such as breeding or trauma.
    - can develop post-castration for up to a few days.

Clinical presentation
Congenital hernia in the foal

- usually observed in first few days of life.
- Standardbred and draught breeds are predisposed.
- may be unilateral or bilateral.
- often observed after straining to pass meconium.
- palpation of the scrotum:
  - fluid-filled intestinal loops can be detected.
  - borborygmi may be audible locally.
  - most of the hernia is easily reducible:
    - re-herniation occurs immediately when pressure is removed.
- foal may present with signs of colic if strangulation occurs (rare).

Acquired hernia in the adult

- most are unilateral (Fig. 3.41).
- variably reducible and more commonly acute intestinal strangulation (Fig. 3.42).
- scrotum and inguinal region may be swollen and cold to the touch.
- thickening at the neck of the testicle is usually present.
- usually presented for colic because of incarcerated small intestine:
  - mild to severe signs of abdominal pain with decreased/absent intestinal motility.
  - nasogastric reflux depending on duration of the obstruction.

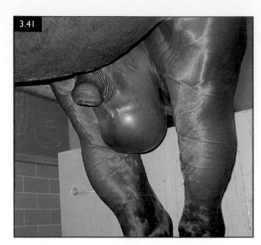

FIG. 3.41 A stallion affected with a severe left scrotal hernia.

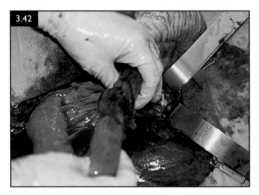

FIG. 3.42 Intraoperative view of strangulated small intestine in the stallion pictured in 3.41.

Differential diagnosis

- scrotal distension in foals:
  - uroperitoneum, trauma, or abscessation.
- distension in adults:
  - testicular torsion, orchitis, and hydrocoele.

Diagnosis

Congenital hernia in the foal

- physical examination.
- ultrasonography of the inguinal region demonstrates presence of normal motile small intestinal loops in the vaginal tunic:
  - tip of caecum or pelvic flexure may be herniated less frequently.

Acquired hernia in the adult

- palpation of the scrotum and testicular region will identify an abnormality.

- definitive diagnosis on per rectum palpation:
  - two loops of small intestine detected passing into the internal inguinal ring.
  - other distended loops of small intestine may be palpable within the abdomen.
- ultrasonography of the distended scrotum helps differentiate testicular torsion from scrotal hernia:
  - transabdominal ultrasonography may reveal distended loops of small intestine.

Management

Congenital hernia in the foal

- most resolve spontaneously by 3–4 months of age.
- daily manual reduction is recommended.
- local bandage following manual reduction can be applied:
  - formation of pressures sores is possible.
- surgery with bilateral closed castration is indicated if:
  - hernia becomes incarcerated.
  - it is very large.
  - not spontaneously resolved by 6 months of age.

Acquired hernia in the adult

- supportive therapy is imperative as cases are often systemically compromised.
- reduce herniation by careful traction on bowel per rectum and/or external manipulations:
  - reducible hernias occur infrequently.
  - stallion sedated plus epidural anaesthesia or GA.
  - rectal tear is a potential complication.
- if manual reduction not possible, immediate surgical correction is required:
  - inguinal approach +/– laparotomy.
  - intestinal resection is often necessary.
  - unilateral or bilateral castration to prevent future herniation.
  - closure of the vaginal tunic and the superficial ring.

Prognosis

- excellent in foals.
- condition is diagnosed rapidly, and resection avoided, the prognosis is good.
- strangulation has occurred, the prognosis is fair to poor.

DISORDERS OF THE CAECUM

Caecal rupture

Definition/overview

- rare and invariably fatal condition because of rapid onset of septic peritonitis.

Aetiology/pathophysiology

- rupture:
  - due to marked distension or devitalisation of the caecal wall.
  - occur secondary to caecal tympany, impaction, or infarction.
- idiopathic caecal rupture can occur in:
  - mares following parturition (see page 39, Book 2):
  - hospitalised horses treated with NSAIDs.
  - absence of any history of disease.
  - suggested that severe tapeworm infection may be associated with rupture.
- can occur without any prodromal signs.
- gross contamination of the abdomen results in rapid onset of severe septic peritonitis.

Clinical presentation

- following caecal rupture may be a short period when the horse appears to have improved because of the immediate relief of severe distension.
- rapidly progressive signs of depression, colic, toxaemia, dehydration, cardiovascular compromise, sweating, and shaking:

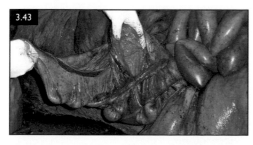

FIG. 3.43 A post-mortem view of a large caecal rupture secondary to a long-term caecal impaction. Note the very severe acute peritonitis and serosal inflammation.

- heart rate increases markedly.
- mucous membranes may be dark red, purple, or blue.
- CRT may be markedly prolonged.
- borborygmi will be decreased or absent.

Differential diagnosis

- septic peritonitis from other causes.
- severe enterocolitis, septicaemia, and pleuritis.

Diagnosis

- haematology may be normal shortly after rupture:
  - rapidly neutropenia with left shift and degenerative neutrophil changes.
- total plasma protein levels decrease as peritonitis progresses, while PCV increases.
- abdominal ultrasonography:
  - excessive flocculent peritoneal fluid.
  - fibrin may be apparent.
- abdominocentesis often reveals dark, foul-smelling peritoneal fluid.
- gritty feel to serosal surfaces may be detected per rectum.
- all above unable to differentiate caecal rupture from rupture of another intestinal viscus.
- definitive diagnosis at surgery or necropsy.

Management

- no viable treatment options.

Prognosis

- invariably fatal (Fig. 3.43).

Caecal infarction

Definition/overview

- uncommon cause of colic.

Aetiology/pathophysiology

- prior to avermectin anthelmintics, *Strongylus vulgaris* infestation was the most likely cause.

- cyathostominosis may also be associated with caecal infarction.
- disseminated intravascular coagulation (DIC) can result in thrombus development in blood vessels, including major vessels in the caecum.
- pathophysiology is dependent on the inciting cause:
  - extensive collateral circulation in the caecum.
  - large thrombi are required to lodge in certain locations.
  - caecal blood supply compromised and ischaemic necrosis ensues.

Clinical presentation

- most affected horses present initially with mild to moderate abdominal pain.
- tachycardia consistent with degree of pain and underlying disease.
- signs of any concurrent disease, particularly if DIC, may obscure signs of infarction.
- caecal rupture leads to signs as described in the previous section.

Differential diagnosis

- variety of causes of colic must be considered.
- must be differentiated from the underlying condition if associated with DIC.

Diagnosis

- clinical examination and palpation per rectum findings are non-specific.
- thickened caecal wall on ultrasonographic examination (difficult to interpret).
- firm mass palpable in the right caudal abdomen (not pathognomonic).
- peritoneal fluid WBC count and protein level will be increased:
  - colour abnormal and worsens with time.
- definitive diagnosis made at surgery or necropsy.

Management

- surgical resection of all infarcted tissue is required:
  - not always possible, depending on the extent of the infarction.
- underlying cause must be addressed:

- if parasitism, farm management should be evaluated.

Prognosis

- fair if infarction is resectable.
- prompt intervention will avoid the onset of peritonitis.

Caecal torsion

Definition/overview

- rare condition.

Aetiology/pathophysiology

- aetiology is unknown in most cases.
- anatomical abnormalities of the caecocolic fold or multiple mesenteric defects are recorded.
- Large colon volvulus may predispose to caecal displacement or volvulus:
  - axis of rotation involves the dorsal mesenteric attachment of the caecum.

Clinical presentation

- accompanied by severe, acute pain and metabolic derangements consistent with strangulation of a large organ.
- characteristic signs of acute colic.

Differential diagnosis

- any strangulating intestinal accident, particularly large colon volvulus.

Diagnosis

- physical examination findings consistent with colic, but not specific for caecal torsion.
- caecal tympany may occur with caecal torsion as outflow obstruction develops:
  - distension and tympany of the right flank may be noted.
- gaseous distension of the caecum often palpable per rectum but not specific
- haematology and abdominocentesis results vary with the degree of caecal compromise.
- definitive diagnosis is made at exploratory laparotomy.

Management

- surgery is required:

- o typhlotomy and decompression.
- o devitalised caecum can be removed by partial typhlectomy.
- o significant ischaemic damage cases may be subjected to intraoperative euthanasia.

Prognosis

- dependent on viability of tissues at the time of surgery:
  - o good if corrected early in the course of the disease.
- recurrence is uncommon except where a congenital defect is present.

Caecal impaction

Definition/overview

- relatively uncommon, but most common cause of caecal disease in the horse.
- Arabian, Morgan, and Appaloosa horses, and horses >15 years of age, may be at higher risk.

Aetiology/pathophysiology

- variety of risk factors have been identified or suggested:
  - o general anaesthesia, pain, and hospitalisation.
  - o poor dentition, poor-quality feed, and parasitic infestation.
  - o role of tapeworms is controversial.
  - o caecal base hypertrophy may cause chronic or recurrent caecal impaction.
- pathophysiology is unclear, but likely involves decreased or abnormal caecal motility.
- allows retention of ingesta in the caecum, particularly at the apex.
- blind-ended nature of the caecum may facilitate impaction formation.

Clinical presentation

- signs of colic ranging from mild and intermittent to severe and protracted:
  - o often mild and slowly progressive.
- no fever.
- heart rate variably elevated.
- GI sounds may be normal or decreased:
  - o typically, decreased or absent borborygmi over right dorsal paralumbar fossa.

- signs of cardiovascular compromise should not be evident.

Differential diagnoses

- colic due to a variety of other causes can present in a similar manner.

Diagnosis

- physical examination and haematology findings are non-specific.
- palpation per rectum is diagnostic:
  - o impacted caecum typically feels firm and doughy.
  - o impaction may not be palpable if present at the caecal apex:
    - ♦ medial caecal band tight and difficult to move.
- caecal impaction can occur concurrently with impaction of the large colon or other abnormalities.

Management

- can be frustrating to treat:
  - o tend to take longer to resolve than large colon impactions.
  - o no clear guidelines for management or when to intervene surgically.
- medical treatment usually attempted initially:
  - o feed restriction.
  - o intravenous fluid therapy in adequate volumes is useful and may speed resolution.
  - o enteral fluid therapy is used but less aggressively than in large colon impaction.
  - o mineral oil, DSS, or osmotic cathartics (e.g. sodium sulphate) are used:
    - ♦ efficacy is unclear.
  - o analgesics administered as required.
  - o usefulness of prokinetics is currently unclear.
- surgery is recommended when:
  - o poor response to medical therapy.
  - o significant caecal distension or abdominal pain.
  - o potential for rupture exists even with apparently small impactions:
    - ♦ some clinicians recommend early surgical intervention.
    - ♦ typhlotomy to remove the impaction.

Prognosis

- most caecal impactions resolve with medical therapy but may require prolonged treatment.
- caecal rupture is a concern and can occur without warning:
  - suspected in any horse with caecal impaction that deteriorates suddenly.
  - grave prognosis.
- recurrence of caecal impaction is common in some animals:
  - underlying problems in intestinal motility.
  - intestinal wall damage from initial impaction.
  - continued presence of predisposing factors.
  - surgical bypass may be indicated in recurrent cases.

Caecal tympany

Definition/overview

- gaseous distension of the caecum.

Aetiology/pathophysiology

- primary caecal tympany occurs in the absence of an outflow obstruction:
  - arises via excessive caecal gas production and/or a reduction in caecal motility.
  - dietary changes, lush pasture, and high-grain diets may be predisposing factors.
- secondary caecal tympany occurs as a result of a caecal outflow obstruction:
  - large colon displacement, impaction, or volvulus.

Clinical presentation

- non-specific signs of colic of varying severity.
- heart rate elevated consistent with the degree of pain:
  - very high rates and severe pain can be present in severe tympany or due to an underlying process such as large colon volvulus.
- abdominal distension and especially bloating of the right paralumbar fossa.
- area of resonant tympany usually present over the right flank.

- borborygmi may be decreased on the right side.
- signs of toxaemia or cardiovascular compromise are not present with primary caecal tympany.
- tachypnoea if significant abdominal distension and pressure on the thoracic cavity.

TABLE 3.8 Protocol for caecal trocarisation
1 Tympanic area over the right paralumbar fossa should be clipped, surgically prepared, and blocked with local anaesthetic
2 14G catheter or trocar set should be used. The catheter or trocar should be inserted perpendicular to the skin surface, until gas escapes. Suction can be used to expedite decompression
3 May be beneficial to inject 10 ml of sterile saline through the catheter prior to removal to lessen contamination of the body wall as the catheter is removed. Some degree of local peritonitis is expected, and severe peritonitis may develop secondary to laceration of a viscus or leakage from the site of intestinal puncture although this is rare
4 Single dose of broad-spectrum antimicrobial prophylaxis (e.g. sodium/potassium penicillin 20,000–40,000 IU/kg i/v and gentamicin 6.6–8.8 mg/kg i/v) is indicated

Differential diagnosis

- other causes of colic, particularly those resulting in gaseous distension of the large colon.

Diagnosis

- per rectum palpation of a large, gas-distended caecum in the right side of the abdomen:
  - marked distension may lead to the base of the caecum protruding into the pelvic canal.
  - sometimes difficult to differentiate caecum from large colon.
- other diagnostic tests are unlikely to differentiate the caecum from the large colon.

Management

- approach to tympany depends on severity of signs and whether primary or secondary.
- secondary tympany:
  - inciting cause must be addressed.
- most cases of primary caecal tympany respond to withholding of feed, walking, and analgesics.
- intravenous fluid therapy is indicated in dehydrated horses (may be useful in all cases).
- marked caecal distension, either with primary or secondary tympany:
  - caecal trocharisation may be required (Table 3.8).
- caecal rupture can occur, mainly with severe and/or chronic distension:
  - exploratory coeliotomy and caecal decompression or typhlotomy may be required.
- management (particularly diet) should be evaluated:
  - access to lush pasture should be restricted.
  - high-grain diets should be avoided, and dietary changes made gradually.

Prognosis

- very good for primary caecal tympany.
- recurrence usually the result of ongoing management issues rather than a primary caecal abnormality.
- secondary caecal tympany depends on the primary cause.

Tapeworm infection

Definition/overview

- common worldwide.
- usually, benign.
- infestation with *Anoplocephala perfoliata* can be associated with colic, particularly if large numbers are present.

Aetiology/pathophysiology

- *A. perfoliata*, *A. magna*, and *Paranoplocephala mamillana* are tapeworms found in horses.
- *A. magna* and *P. mamillana* are not typically considered to be pathogenic.
- prevalence of tapeworm infestation can be very high (up to 80%) in some areas:

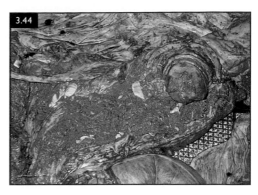

FIG. 3.44 Ileocaecal intussusception. Note the numerous tapeworms.

  - usually in temperate climates as compared with hot and arid areas.
- tapeworms have an indirect life cycle:
  - horses are infected by ingestion of oribatid mites, the intermediate host.
  - adult tapeworms found in the intestinal tract 1–2 months following ingestion:
    - *A. perfoliata* is commonly found around the ileocaecal junction.
- mucosal congestion, focal ulceration, and mucosal thickening may develop at the site of *A. perfoliata* attachment:
  - most cases, no clinical signs result.
  - inflammation at the site is thought to predispose to ileocaecal intussusceptions (Fig. 3.44).
  - may also be associated with spasmodic colic and ileal impaction, and possibly an increased incidence of colic overall.
  - risk proportional to the tapeworm burden.
  - tapeworm-associated colic more common in horses 5 years of age or younger.

Clinical presentation

- most horses display no clinical abnormalities.
- tapeworm infestation itself not thought to produce signs of ill-thrift, weight loss, or diarrhoea.
- ill-thrift to severe colic may be observed because of intussusception, spasmodic colic, or ileal impaction secondary to tapeworm infestation.

Differential diagnosis

- variety of causes of colic should be considered.

Diagnosis

- Faecal flotation commonly used:
  - sensitivity can be poor depending on the testing methodology.
  - some solutions effective for flotation testing of other parasite eggs are not effective.
  - saturated sucrose solution (450 g in 350 ml water) reported to be more effective.
  - *A. perfoliata* eggs are D-shaped with a thick shell.
- serological assays more useful for population studies than diagnosis of individual animals.
- saliva-based tapeworm test is available.
- adult tapeworms are uncommonly found in faeces and, if present, might suggest a high burden.

Management

- most routinely used anthelmintics are not effective against tapeworms.
- may be overlooked in deworming programmes.
- pyrantel pamoate can be effective, used at twice the nematocidal dose.
- praziquantel (1.0–1.5 mg/kg p/o) is effective against tapeworms:
  - products containing a combination of ivermectin (0.2 mg/kg) or moxidectin (0.4 mg/kg) and praziquantel (1.0–1.5 mg/kg) are available in many countries.
- annual deworming for tapeworms is recommended.

Prognosis

- simple infestation with tapeworms carries an excellent prognosis due to ease of treatment and limited clinical signs.
- poorer prognosis if a tapeworm-associated intestinal accident has occurred.

DISORDERS OF THE LARGE COLON

Colitis

Definition/overview

- acute colitis is a potentially life-threatening disease characterised by:
  - diarrhoea.
  - varying degrees of depression, dehydration, toxaemia, abdominal distension, and abdominal pain.

Aetiology/pathophysiology

- variety of pathogenic organisms may be involved, including:
  - *C. difficile, C. perfringens, Salmonella* spp.
  - *Neorickettsia risticii* (Potomac horse fever [PHF]).
  - equine coronavirus (equine enteric coronavirus [ECoV]).
- identification of the aetiological agent can be difficult because of limitations of available tests and incomplete understanding of the GI microflora.
- majority of cases are idiopathic in most parts of the world.
- outbreaks can occur, particularly in equine hospitals and on breeding farms.

Salmonellosis

- Salmonellosis occurs when the appropriate combination of host (immune status, GI microflora, pain), bacterial (pathogenicity, dose), and environmental (stressors) factors is present.
- faecal–oral inoculation or proliferation of small numbers of *Salmonella* organisms already in the GI tract may occur.
- large numbers are typically required to cause disease in normal animals.
- compromised animals (young, concurrently ill, antimicrobial treated, hospitalised) may be infected with much lower doses.
- certain *Salmonella* strains may be able to cause disease with lower numbers (Fig. 3.45).

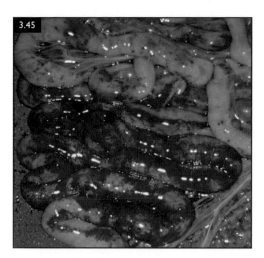

FIG. 3.45 Marked hyperaemia of the serosal surface of the small intestine of a foal with fatal salmonellosis.

Clostridium difficile infection

- *C. difficile* is a spore-forming bacterium found in a small percentage of normal horses, particularly young horses and those treated with antimicrobials.
- can proliferate and produce toxins in certain situations:
  - *C. difficile* infection (CDI) can develop following ingestion of toxigenic strains.
  - overgrowth of *C. difficile* residing in low levels in the GI tract.
- antimicrobial therapy is a risk factor for the development of CDI:
  - absence of this history does not rule out CDI.

Clostridium perfringens-associated diarrhoea

- *C. perfringens* is a Gram-positive spore-forming anaerobic bacterium that can produce a wide variety of toxins (Table 3.9):
  - clinical relevance of some strains is unclear.
  - normal inhabitant of the GI tract in a large percentage of normal horses and foals.
- *C. perfringens* can overgrow and produce a variety of toxins in some situations:
  - antimicrobial therapy.
  - dietary changes.
  - stress and transportation.
  - concurrent disease.
- *C. perfringens* enterotoxin and beta-2 toxin associated with diarrhoea in adults and foals.
- type C strains have been implicated in severe enterocolitis in foals.

Potomac horse fever

- *N. risticii* (formerly *Ehrlichia risticii*) is an obligate intracellular bacterium that has an affinity for monocytes.
- most cases occur during summer and early autumn.
- cases often have a proximity to freshwater.
- variety of aquatic invertebrates may be involved in natural transmission of the disease.
- mechanism by which *N. risticii* causes diarrhoea and other clinical signs is unclear:
  - interference with intestinal sodium and chloride absorption may be involved.
- cause of the laminitis, which frequently develops concurrently, is not known.

Equine enteric coronavirus

- equine coronavirus (ECoV) is a beta coronavirus that manifests as an enteric disease:

TABLE 3 Toxin production by different *Clostridium perfringens* types

Type	<TCH> Alpha	Beta	Epsilon	TOXINS Iota	Beta-2	Enterotoxin
A	√				±	±
B	√	√	√		±	±
C	√	√			±	±
D	√		√		±	±
E	√			√	±	±

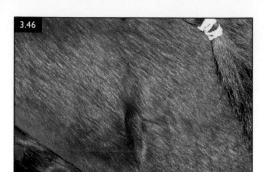

FIG. 3.46 Prolonged skin tent in the neck of a horse estimated to be 10–12% dehydrated.

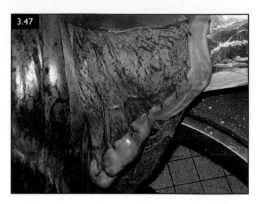

FIG. 3.47 Small intestine and mesentery of a horse with DIC secondary to colitis.

- ○ considered an emerging disease in the United States, Europe, and Japan.
- ECoV is closely related to bovine coronavirus.
- transmission via the faecal–oral route.
- more common in the cold weather months.
- virus is highly contagious between horses.
- currently no evidence that ECoV is infectious to humans:
  - ○ **basic biosecurity protocols are recommended.**
- pathophysiology is currently not well understood.

Idiopathic colitis

- syndrome involving a variety of different bacterial organisms and mechanisms of disease.
- disruption of the normal microflora probably allows for the proliferation of pathogenic organisms.
- antimicrobial therapy, concurrent disease, transportation, diet changes, and high-grain diet are potential risk factors.

Antimicrobial-associated diarrhoea

- not a specific disease but refers to cases of acute diarrhoea that are temporally associated with antimicrobial administration.
- administration of any antimicrobial via any route can predispose horses to diarrhoea:
  - ○ certain antimicrobials, including macrolides, are considered higher risk.
- geographical differences also appear to be present.

- variety of infectious agents such as *C. difficile*, *C. perfringens*, and *Salmonella* spp. can be involved.
- presumed that antimicrobials disrupt the normal protective bacterial microflora in the intestinal tract, permitting overgrowth of pathogenic bacteria.

Clinical presentation
General

- highly variable and depends on a number of factors.
- spectrum of disease can range from soft faeces with no other clinical abnormalities, to peracute, fatal, necrohaemorrhagic enterocolitis.
- diarrhoea is usually present but clinical signs may develop before its onset.
- varying degrees of dehydration (Fig. 3.46), toxaemia, depression, abdominal pain, cardiovascular compromise, and abdominal distension.
- DIC can occur (Fig. 3.47):
  - ○ non-strangulating infarction of the colon from DIC should be considered in horses with colitis that deteriorate suddenly.

Salmonellosis

- 'classical' presentation of salmonellosis includes:
  - ○ fever, depression, diarrhoea, and severe toxaemia.
  - ○ combination occurs in 50% or less of affected horses.
  - ○ fever of unknown origin may be the only presenting sign.

- diarrhoea can be mild, of short duration, or not evident in some cases.
- septicaemia and extraintestinal infection are of most concern in foals.
- sloughing of the intestinal mucosa (Fig. 3.48) may be evident as the passing of casts in the faeces.

Clostridial diarrhoea

- clinical presentation of CDI and *C. perfringens*-associated diarrhoea is highly variable and non-specific.
- range from mild disease with only soft faeces, to peracute necrohaemorrhagic colitis with rapid progression to death.

Potomac horse fever

- fever that can be very high (up to 41.7°C [107°F]).
- usually, there is an initial episode of mild depression, anorexia, and fever.
- moderate to severe diarrhoea may ensue in approximately 60% of cases.
- severe toxaemia and depression may accompany colic.
- laminitis may develop in 25–40% of cases:
  - may be more severe than expected based on the severity of intestinal and systemic disease.
- abortion may occur several months after disease resolution because of fetal infection.

Equine enteric coronavirus

- equine coronavirus commonly presents with anorexia, lethargy, and fever of 38.6–41.1°C (101.5–106.0°F)

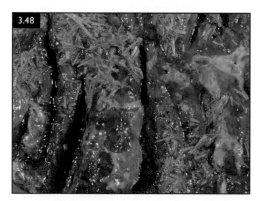

FIG. 3.48 Intestinal mucosa of a horse with salmonellosis. Note the mucosal casts detaching from the mucosal surface.

- soft formed faeces are common and profuse diarrhoea can occur but is less common.
- mild colic signs are common.
- nasogastric reflux associated with enteritis has been reported.
- neurological abnormalities may be seen secondary to hyperammonaemia.

Differential diagnosis

- noninfectious causes of colitis such as right dorsal colitis and sand enteropathy.
- intestinal accident is a differential diagnosis in severe cases.
- cantharidin toxicosis and cyathostominosis should be considered depending on the geographical location, time of year, and clinical presentation.
- rotavirus and *Lawsonia intracellularis* infection should be considered in foals.
- other toxic causes of colitis such as arsenic toxicosis are uncommon but should be considered in some situations.

Diagnosis
General

- clinical signs and haematology are non-specific and not diagnostic:
  - leucopenia, neutropenia, left shift, and neutrophil toxic changes are common.
  - leucocytosis and monocytosis may occur more commonly with PHF.
- urinalysis should be performed, particularly if elevations in urea and creatinine levels are present.
- total plasma protein levels should be evaluated.
- monitoring of plasma electrolyte concentrations is useful to guide treatment.
- tests for specific pathogens are described below:
  - **coinfection can occur, so a broad range of testing is recommended.**

Salmonellosis

- faecal culture is the most common diagnostic tool:
  - intermittent shedding and relatively low sensitivity of testing.
  - single negative culture cannot rule out salmonellosis.
  - 3–5 negative samples are required.

- rectal mucosal biopsy specimens can also be submitted for culture:
  - not commonly performed.
  - useful in cases of chronic colic or fever of unknown origin versus fulminant colitis.
- utility of PCR testing of faeces remains unclear, but it may be a useful screening test.

Clostridium difficile infection

- detection of *C. difficile* toxins in faecal samples is diagnostic for CDI:
  - tested for presence of both *C. difficile* toxins A and B.
  - fresh, refrigerated samples are preferred.
  - *C. difficile* toxins are stable *in vitro*.
- ELISA detection of *C. difficile* toxin A and B in faecal samples is the preferred test:
  - toxins are stable if samples are kept chilled.
- quantitative PCR for *C. difficile* toxin A and B is now widely available:
  - relevance of identification of toxigenic strains in the absence of demonstrable toxin is unclear.
  - ELISA detection of toxins may be more clinically relevant.
  - negative PCR result is helpful for ruling out *C. difficile* as toxins are shed early in the disease and a single sample is thought to be adequate.
- culture is usually reserved for epidemiological purposes.

Clostridium perfringens-associated diarrhoea

- difficult as *C. perfringens* can be isolated from the faeces of a large percentage of normal horses.
- no correlation between numbers of *C. perfringens* or bacterial spores in faeces and diarrhoea has been reported:
  - typing of bacterial isolates or PCR can be useful to determine what toxin genes they possess.
  - relevance of identifying toxigenic strains in the absence of demonstrable toxin is unclear.
  - type C strains are uncommonly identified in normal animals and detection of these strains is highly suggestive of disease.

- identification of genes coding for beta-2 toxin and *C. perfringens* enterotoxin (CPE) production is suggestive.
- significance of identification of type A, the most common strain, in the absence of beta-2 toxin or CPE genes is debatable.
- diagnosis is best based on identification of toxins in faecal samples:
  - detection of CPE is highly suggestive of disease.
  - ability to diagnose this condition will improve as rapid tests to detect other *C. perfringens* toxins become available.

Potomac horse fever

- presumptive diagnosis often made based on appropriate clinical signs at appropriate time of year in endemic areas:
  - not definitive, as other sporadic causes of diarrhoea cannot be differentiated clinically.
- response to empirical treatment with oxytetracycline is suggestive, but not diagnostic.
- serological testing is available:
  - four-fold change in antibody titre between acute and convalescent samples is supportive, but often does not occur.
- PCR testing is now readily available and more useful:
  - early in the disease, blood samples may be PCR positive and faecal samples PCR negative.
  - may be reversed later in the disease:
    - both blood and faecal samples should always be submitted.
  - blood samples should be collected prior to administration of oxytetracycline for increased sensitivity.

Equine enteric coronavirus

- haemogram can be unremarkable:
  - leucopenia secondary to neutropenia or lymphopenia.
  - hypoalbuminaemia may be seen.
- definitive diagnosis via faecal quantitative PCR testing:
  - samples should be kept chilled or frozen.

Antimicrobial-associated diarrhoea

- diagnosis is based on temporal association of antimicrobial administration and onset of clinical signs.
- specific pathogen testing should be performed.

Idiopathic colitis

- diagnosis of exclusion when other known causes of enterocolitis have been ruled out.

Management

- **aggressive supportive therapy, particularly fluid therapy with large volumes of balanced electrolyte solution, is the most important component of treatment.**
- intravenous fluid therapy is required in all but the mildest of cases:
  - intravenous hypertonic saline (4–6 ml/kg of 5–7% NaCl) may be useful in severely dehydrated horses but must be followed by large volumes of isotonic fluids.
  - supplemental potassium, magnesium or calcium may be required:
    - based on monitoring of blood electrolyte levels.
    - ionised calcium should be measured:
      - total calcium levels will decrease if the horse is hypoalbuminaemic, while metabolically active total calcium may be normal.
  - sodium bicarbonate is rarely required, even in severely acidotic animals:
    - aggressive fluid therapy will correct the acid–base status in most cases.
- total protein levels should be monitored because severe hypoproteinaemia can develop.
- endotoxaemia is very common, regardless of the aetiology:
  - flunixin meglumine (1.1 mg/kg i/v) indicated but used judiciously in dehydrated horses.
  - polymyxin B (6000 IU/kg i/v q12h) may be used to bind endotoxin.
- metronidazole (15–25 mg/kg p/o q8–12h) appears to be effective in the treatment of clostridial diarrhoea and many cases of idiopathic colitis:
  - metronidazole-resistant strains of *C. difficile* are rare but have been reported.
- broad-spectrum antimicrobial therapy is controversial:
  - concerns include prolonging shedding of *Salmonella* (if present), development of antimicrobial resistance, and further disruption of the intestinal microflora.
  - parenteral antimicrobial therapy mainly indicated in adults to protect against bacterial translocation and is not necessary in most cases.
  - sodium penicillin/aminoglycoside combination is often indicated in neonates and immunocompromised individuals.
  - parenteral administration in salmonellosis is directed at prevention and treatment of extraintestinal infection.
- oxytetracycline (6.6 mg/kg slowly i/v q12h for 3–5 days) is indicated in cases of diagnosed or highly suspicious PHF:
  - typically, a response is noted within 12 hours.
  - abatement of fever usually the first sign, followed by improvement in attitude and appetite.
  - no response is noted within 24–48 hours, the diagnosis should be reconsidered.
- di-tri-octahedral smectite (1.5 kg/adult horse p/o, followed by 450 g p/o q6–8h) may be useful as an adsorbent.
- *Saccharomyces boulardii* (25–50 g p/o q12h) may be beneficial:
  - other probiotics are widely used.
  - no evidence of efficacy and may cause diarrhoea.
- no specific treatment for equine coronavirus:
  - supportive treatment, including NSAIDs, fluids, electrolytes, and gastrointestinal protectants is recommended as needed.
- horses not displaying signs of abdominal pain should be fed grass hay *ad libitum*.
- small volumes of concentrates may be gradually introduced to horses that require additional caloric intake.
- most horses with moderate to severe colitis will lose significant body condition, regardless of dietary intake.

- parenteral nutrition may be required where feeding is withheld for more than a few days.
- affected horses require intense monitoring to detect changes in clinical condition and development of complications.
- laminitis, the most severe complication, is addressed elsewhere (see page 58, Book 1):
  - all four feet should be iced continuously during the acute inflammatory stage of the disease.
- **all horses with colitis should be assumed to be infectious until proven otherwise:**
  - salmonellosis is transmissible to horses and is zoonotic.
  - *C. difficile* can be transmitted between horses and may also be zoonotic.
  - risk of transmission of *C. perfringens* is probably lower, but precautions should still be taken.
  - coronavirus can be transmitted between horses.
  - PHF is not transmissible by horses.
  - idiopathic cases should be treated as infectious.
- where a transmissible disease is considered possible:
  - precautions should be taken to decrease the risk of transmission to other horses and to humans.
  - affected horses should be completely isolated from other animals.
  - if not feasible, cases should be separated as much as possible from other horses, particularly neonates.
  - barrier precautions, including overboots, gloves, and either disposable gowns or dedicated coveralls, should be used.
  - medical instruments (e.g. thermometers, nasogastric tubes) and other items (buckets, shovels, wheelbarrows) should be used only for affected horses or completely disinfected after each use.
  - area outside the stall should be cordoned off and disinfected frequently.
  - horses with colitis should not be allowed on common pasture.

Prognosis

- variable and should be considered fair in horses with severe, acute colitis.

- death can occur due to:
  - severe toxaemia, necrotising enterocolitis, and intestinal rupture.
  - intestinal infarction from DIC.
  - laminitis.
  - high cost of treatment.
- infarction of intestinal blood vessels (result of severe toxaemia and DIC) can account for sudden deterioration.
- laminitis and catheter site complications may occur in up to 25% of severe cases.
- long-term GI complications are uncommon after recovery:
  - may take weeks to months to return to normal body condition.
- salmonellosis cases that recover may shed the bacteria for weeks to months following resolution of clinical signs:
  - three to five negative faecal cultures obtained before the horse is considered no longer infectious.
- vaccination for PHF appears to reduce the severity of disease.
- vaccines for the prevention of *C. perfringens*-associated disease are available for ruminants:
  - not recommended for use in horses because of limited evidence of efficacy.
  - apparent high incidence of adverse vaccine reactions.
- prognosis for PHF is good if diagnosed early and appropriate therapy is started:
  - worsens if laminitis develops.
- morbidity for equine coronavirus is reported to be 10–83%; mortality is low:
  - death is often due to secondary complications including septicaemia, endotoxaemia, and hyperammonaemia-associated encephalopathy.
- judicious use of antimicrobials, particularly those that tend to be associated with a higher incidence of diarrhoea, is important.

Sand enteropathy

Definition/overview

- uncommon but regionally important cause of diarrhoea.

Aetiology/pathophysiology

- accumulation of sand in the large colon is usually associated with sand impaction; however, sand enteropathy can also result.
- more common in areas with loose sandy soil.
- sand may be ingested while grazing on sandy soil or from ingestion of sand in sandy paddocks, arenas, or stalls.
- horses that are underfed or kept in overstocked, closely grazed pastures may be at greater risk.
- sand accumulation can result in chronic irritation of the colonic mucosa resulting in diarrhoea:
  - reduction of the absorptive surface area.
  - interference with normal intestinal motility.

Clinical presentation

- diarrhoea is the main presenting sign:
  - acute or chronic.
  - usually mild and not associated with severe dehydration, toxaemia, or cardiovascular compromise.
- pyrexia, anorexia, weight loss, and intermittent colic may be present.
- 'sand sounds' may be heard over the ventral abdomen.
- colonic rupture secondary to severe inflammation and irritation is rare but will result in the development of septic peritonitis.

Differential diagnosis

- infectious causes of colitis, including *Salmonella*, *C. difficile*, *C. perfringens*, and *N. risticii* (PHF).

Diagnosis

- history of exposure to sand, or sandy soils, and clinical signs.
- faecal sand content evaluation:
  - suspension of faeces and water allowed to settle out in a rectal sleeve:
    - not recommended.
    - quantity of sand correlates poorly with large colon accumulation.
- palpation per rectum is unremarkable unless there is a concurrent large colon impaction.

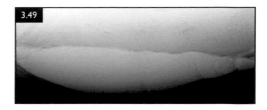

FIG. 3.49 Radiograph demonstrating sand accumulation in the ventral abdomen. (Photo courtesy K Niinistö)

- sand accumulation may be evident radiographically (Fig. 3.49) or ultrasonographically, particularly in the cranioventral abdomen.
- haematology should be unremarkable:
  - changes consistent with the degree of dehydration.
  - mild neutropenia is occasionally present.
- total protein levels do not decrease as compared to enterocolitis.
- peritoneal fluid is usually unremarkable.

Management

- enteral fluid therapy is useful in mild cases.
- psyllium (1.0 g/kg) combined with magnesium sulphate (1.0 g/kg) daily via nasogastric tube has been shown to be effective in the removal of sand accumulations:
  - continued for 3–5 days.
  - followed by repeat radiographic or ultrasonographic examination.
- following resolution, periodic evaluation (every 3–6 months) via abdominal radiography or ultrasonography should be considered:
  - particularly if management changes are not feasible.
- intermittent administration of psyllium may help reduce sand accumulation, but the response is highly variable between individuals:
  - 0.25 kg of psyllium/500 kg once daily for 7 days, performed monthly, has been recommended but is of questionable benefit.
- discussion of management practices with the owner is important.

Prognosis

- excellent overall.
- small proportion of cases, severe colon irritation may result in chronic diarrhoea and ill-thrift.
- management changes are often required to prevent further cases.

Right dorsal colitis

Definition/overview

- uncommon syndrome characterised by ulcerative inflammation of the right dorsal colon.

Aetiology/pathophysiology

- chronic or excessive administration of NSAIDs is the most common risk factor:
  - history of NSAID use is not always present.
  - concurrent dehydration or hypotension increases the risk.
  - phenylbutazone use is most reported:
    - unclear whether this drug is higher risk, or it is used more often.
  - performance horses are most affected because of the increased use of NSAIDs in this group.
- NSAID administration results in decreased prostaglandin levels:
  - prostaglandins are involved in local protection in the colon.
  - high levels and for prolonged periods of time, +/− concurrent dehydration or hypotension:
    - mucosal inflammation and ulceration develop as local protective effects are overwhelmed.
    - inflammatory response generated further damages the intestinal mucosa.
- clinical signs can result from intestinal inflammation, damage to the mucosal barrier with subsequent absorption of bacterial toxins, and exudation of plasma proteins.

Clinical presentation

- two general syndromes are observed:
  - acute form:
    - colic is the predominant clinical sign.
    - often accompanied by fever, depression, lethargy, and signs of endotoxaemia.
    - diarrhoea may also be present.
  - chronic form:
    - weakness, weight loss, depression, lethargy, intermittent colic, and peripheral oedema may be observed.
    - diarrhoea is less common.

Differential diagnosis

- acute form:
  - salmonellosis, clostridial enteritis, PHF, coronavirus, peritonitis, intestinal accident, and sand enteropathy.
- chronic form:
  - inflammatory bowel disease, intestinal neoplasia, cyathostominosis, protein-losing nephropathy, and *Lawsonia intracellularis* infection (weanlings).

Diagnosis

- only definitively diagnosed via surgical biopsies or necropsy.
- clinically, only a presumptive diagnosis.
- complete blood cell count and serum biochemical profile should be submitted:
  - hypoproteinaemia is the main abnormality.
- abdominal ultrasonography:
  - thickened right dorsal colon.
  - difficult to identify.
- urinalysis to rule out renal protein loss.
- abdominocentesis will help identify other differentials.
- presumptive diagnosis is usually made with:
  - appropriate clinical signs and a history of NSAID administration.
  - severe hypoproteinaemia.
  - exclusion of other causes.

Management

- NSAID administration ceased if possible.
- continued analgesia required, alternatives include:
  - transdermal fentanyl.
  - epidural or parenteral opioids.
  - intravenous CRI lidocaine or ketamine.
- acute disease:

- o intravenous fluid therapy with a balanced electrolyte solution.
- o overly aggressive fluid therapy avoided, particularly in hypoproteinaemic animals.
- chronic disease: fluid therapy is usually not indicated.
- acute or chronic disease:
  - o transfusion of plasma or synthetic colloids in severely hypoproteinaemic animals.
  - o sucralfate (20–40 mg/kg p/o q6h) may be useful:
    - ♦ unclear if significant drug levels are achieved in the right dorsal colon.
  - o synthetic prostaglandin misoprostol (5 µg/kg p/o q12h) has been used:
    - ♦ effect is not known, and adverse effects can be encountered.
- diet:
  - o long-stem roughage (hay) withheld.
  - o complete pelleted diet fed until all clinical/haematological abnormalities resolved.
  - o pasture should be avoided.
  - o feed small meals frequently.
  - o body weight cannot be maintained:
    - ♦ dietary fat increased:
      - – additional high-fat concentrate diet.
      - – supplementation with corn oil (250 ml q12h).
- addition of psyllium (50–100 g/500 kg/day, divided into 1–4 doses) could be useful:
  - o hydrolysed to short-chain fatty acids.
  - o important energy source for colonic enterocytes.
- surgical intervention may be indicated in severe, acute presentations or refractory chronic cases.

Prognosis

- guarded overall.
- prognosis for return to normality is better in horses with acute disease and when NSAID cessation is possible.
- poor in horses with severe, chronic hypoproteinaemia.
- gradual but steady elevation in serial blood albumin levels – good prognostic indicator.
- full recovery may take months.
- laminitis is a possible complication, particularly in acute cases.

Cyathostominosis

Definition/overview

- small strongyles (cyathostomes) are important GI parasites worldwide.
- infection can cause a range of signs including inapparent infection, ill-thrift, and severe protein-losing enteropathy and diarrhoea (larval cyathostominosis).
- some geographical regions (e.g. the UK):
  - o larval cyathostominosis considered the most common cause of diarrhoea in adult horses.

Aetiology/pathophysiology

- small strongyle group consists of approximately 50 different species:
  - o differences in prevalence, pathogenicity, and life cycle.
  - o speciation is rarely performed, and multiple species are often present.
- younger horses more likely to be infected with large numbers of small strongyles:
  - o may be more likely to develop clinical disease with lower numbers compared to adults.
- risk factors for infection include:
  - o high stocking density.
  - o inappropriate deworming programmes.
  - o poor manure management.
  - o overgrazing of pastures.
- larval cyathostominosis typically a seasonal problem:
  - o more common during the late winter and spring in most temperate areas.
  - o cases are more common in late fall and winter in some other regions.
  - o horses 1–3 years of age are most affected.
  - o recent anthelmintic treatment is a risk factor:
    - ♦ may trigger disease by removing the negative feedback of adult worms in the intestinal lumen, thereby resulting in excysting of larvae.
- small strongyle eggs are shed in faeces and develop into infective L3 on pasture.
- after ingestion, the L3 enter the mucosa of the large colon and caecum and encyst.
- encysted larvae may remain hypobiotic for up to 2 years.

- at any point, L3 can develop into L4, excyst, and migrate back to the intestinal lumen, where they mature into adults.
- prepatent period varies with different strongyle species (range 5 to 18 weeks).
- encysted larvae may incite a granulomatous reaction:
  - main problem occurs during emergence of hypobiotic larvae.
  - marked inflammatory response:
    - characterised by oedema, ulceration, and protein exudation.
  - nutrient/fluid absorption and intestinal motility can be affected.
  - syndrome is termed 'larval cyathostominosis'.
- encysted larvae are more common in the caecum and ventral colon:
  - represent the majority of small strongyle burden.
  - may vary with geographical region and time of year.
  - ventral colon main site for adult worms, followed by dorsal colon and caecum.
- adult worms in the intestinal lumen may cause disease:
  - lesser importance.
  - pinpoint mucosal ulceration.

Clinical presentation
- infection with adult small strongyles:
  - may produce mild and vague signs, such as weight loss or ill-thrift.
  - increased risk of colic may be present:
    - association with caecocaecal and caecocolic intussusceptions.
  - may be seasonal, recurrent, or sporadic.
  - chronic weight loss and chronic diarrhoea have been reported:
    - clinically may mirror low-grade, undifferentiated inflammatory bowel disease.
- larval cyathostominosis is the most serious clinically:
  - may present with severe diarrhoea, weight loss, depression, and peripheral oedema:
    - **diarrhoea is not present in all cases.**
    - severe hypoproteinaemia is common.

Differential diagnosis
- protein-losing enteropathy, acute infectious colitis of a various aetiologies, and right dorsal colitis.
- various differential diagnoses exist for the mild, general disease caused by adult worms.

Diagnosis
- **difficult for larval cyathostominosis as most findings are non-specific:**
  - faecal egg counts are often low when clinical disease is present:
    - disease is associated with encysted larvae, not egg-producing adults.
    - disease may be triggered by recent anthelmintic therapy:
      - eggs and adult worms less likely to be present.
  - haematology is non-specific:
    - peripheral eosinophilia is uncommon, even in severe cases.
  - hypoalbuminaemia is common:
    - often more severe than expected from severity and duration of the diarrhoea.
  - elevations in alpha-2 and beta-1 globulins have been reported.
  - late L4 larvae occasionally evident on faecal smears or rectal gloves after palpation.
  - abdominal ultrasonography:
    - thickening of the large colon wall may be evident.
  - identification of large numbers of encysted and/or emerging larvae in the large colon:
    - encysted cyathostomes can sometimes be detected on rectal mucosal biopsy.
    - exploratory laparatomy can be diagnostic:
      - affected animals are often poor surgical candidates.
  - definitive diagnosis often achieved at necropsy:
    - oedema and thickening of the intestinal wall.
    - encysted cyathostomes may be evident grossly in the intestinal mucosa (Fig. 3.50).

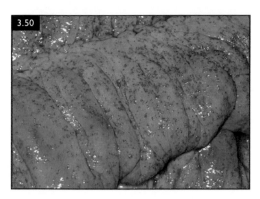

FIG. 3.50 Mucosal surface of the large colon from a foal with severe cyathostominosis. Note the numerous small larvae in the mucosal wall.

Management

- two aspects to management.
- treatment of overt enteric disease (diarrhoea and/or hypoproteinaemia):
  ○ largely supportive.
  ○ correction of fluid and electrolyte imbalances with intravenous fluid therapy.
  ○ plasma or synthetic colloids in severely hypoproteinaemic animals.
- reduction of parasite burdens (Table 3.10):
  ○ different treatment regimens have been proposed to reduce the parasite burden.
  ○ moxidectin (0.4 mg/kg p/o once):
    ♦ good efficacy against encysted larvae.
    ♦ considered treatment of choice as elicits less inflammatory response than fenbendazole and resistance is less of a concern.

○ other regimens include:
  ♦ fenbendazole (10 mg/kg) on days 1–5, 16–20, and 31–35, with ivermectin on days 6, 21, and 36).
  ♦ single course of fenbendazole (10 mg/kg p/o q24h for 5 days).
○ concurrent administration of anti-inflammatories may be useful:
  ♦ inflammatory response associated with the emergence or death of larvae.
  ♦ corticosteroids (e.g. prednisolone, 1 mg/kg p/o q24h).
○ **routine preventive control is critical:**
  ♦ few drugs are effective against encysted larvae.
  ♦ optimal deworming programmes vary between premises based on a variety of factors.
  ♦ period of highest risk for infection should be considered when designing a deworming programme:
    – more likely to be exposed in spring and fall in temperate climates.
    – winter in subtropical climates.
  ♦ annual or biannual deworming may suffice on farms with a reasonable stocking density and good manure management.
  ♦ other farms may require more frequent deworming.
  ♦ multiple-anthelmintic-resistant small strongyles are a serious concern.
- management factors such as stocking density, manure management, and pasture rotation need to be assessed:

TABLE 3.10 Anthelmintic treatment options for cyathostominosis

DRUG	DOSE	FREQUENCY	COMMENTS
Ivermectin	0.2 mg/kg p/o	Once	Effective against adults
Moxidectin	0.4 mg/kg p/o	Once	Effective against adults and encysted larvae
Fenbendazole	50 mg/kg p/o 10 mg/kg p/o	Once q24h for 5 days	Effective against adults; resistance is a concern
Oxfendazole	10 mg/kg p/o	Once	Effective against adults; resistance is a concern
Pyrantel tartrate	2.2 mg/kg p/o	Daily	Effective against ingested larvae; resistance is a concern

- o manure should be removed from pastures twice weekly to prevent accumulation of infective larvae.
- o harrowing of pastures may be effective in hot/dry weather as infective larvae are susceptible to desiccation.
- o ruminants are resistant to small strongyles, so pasture rotation with these species is useful.

Prognosis

- approximately 40% of horses with larval cyathostominosis will survive if given appropriate treatment.
- some cases will die within 2–4 weeks of initial clinical signs:
  - o complicated by difficulty in diagnosing cases.
- prolonged recovery period may be required depending on degree of mucosal damage.
- prognosis is poorer if clinical signs have been present for more than 3 weeks.

Chronic diarrhoea

Definition/overview

- continuous or intermittent passage of soft or watery faeces for prolonged period.
- animals of all ages can be affected.
- relatively common and often frustrating problem.

Aetiology/pathophysiology

- variety of possible causes and most cases are idiopathic:
  - o inflammatory, infectious, neoplastic, and nutritional causes are all possible.
- pathophysiology is variable, depending on the specific aetiology:
  - o net result is intermittent or continuous passage of soft faeces.
  - o due to disruption of normal fluid homeostasis mechanisms in the large colon.
  - o small intestinal disease may be present concurrently.
- note small intestinal disease alone should not produce diarrhoea in an adult horse.

Clinical presentation

- intermittent or continuous passage of soft faeces often only clinical complaint.

- other clinical abnormalities, include:
  - o weight loss, ill-thrift, anorexia, peripheral oedema, depression, and fever.
  - o may suggest more severe underlying disease.

Differential diagnosis

- variety of infectious, inflammatory, neoplastic, and nutritional causes exist:
  - o see specific diseases covered elsewhere.
- occasionally, non-intestinal diseases may cause chronic diarrhoea:
  - o liver disease, Cushing's disease, and hyperlipidaemia.

Diagnosis

- thorough history should be obtained:
  - o characterise the changes in faecal consistency.
  - o try to make an association between diarrhoea and certain management areas:
    - ♦ feeding, exercise, travel, or drug therapy.
- variety of diagnostic tests can be performed to identify the aetiology (Table 3.11).
- investigation of undifferentiated inflammatory bowel disease is warranted in cases refractory to dietary management and non-specific therapy.

TABLE 3.11 Diagnostic options for chronic diarrhoea

Haematology
- complete blood cell count
- serum biochemical profile
- plasma fibrinogen
- serum amyloid A

Faecal analysis
- *Salmonella* culture
- *Clostridium difficile* toxin A/B ELISA
- *Clostridium perfringens enterotoxin* ELISA
- Faecal float and smear

Abdominal radiography

Abdominal ultrasonographic examination

Rectal mucosal biopsy
- culture
- histology

Carbohydrate absorption tests

Exploratory laparotomy/laparoscopy with biopsies

Management

- absence of a specific diagnosis – variety of treatments can be tried:
  - diet change and nutritional analysis is recommended.
  - diet consisting of mainly, or exclusively, hay or pasture grass can be beneficial.
  - **note some horses will respond to provision of a hay-free diet.**
- moxidectin (0.4 mg/kg p/o once) is often prescribed.
- metronidazole (25 mg/kg p/o q8–12h for 5 days) is often used but is questionable.
- probiotics are widely used, but no beneficial effect has yet been demonstrated:
  - yogurt is unlikely to be effective:
    - contains low viable bacteria numbers.
    - does not contain organisms with any known benefit in horses.
- treatment for sand enteropathy may be useful in known problem areas.
- corticosteroids are often used after other treatments have failed:
  - dexamethasone (5–10 mg/450 kg i/m q24h for 21 days, then tapering).
  - prednisolone (1 mg/kg p/o q24h, for 3 weeks).

Prognosis

- generally fair, if diarrhoea is accompanied by other clinical abnormalities such as weight loss or hypoproteinaemia.
- good for survival and normal function if the diarrhoea is the only complaint but the problem may persist.

Colonic tympany (gas colic)

Definition/overview

- intestinal tympany, also known as gas colic, is a common cause of colic.

Aetiology/pathophysiology

- variety of risk factors have been suggested including:
  - diet change.
  - feeding of highly fermentable substrates (grain, lush grass, wilted grass).
  - rapid eating.
  - electrolyte abnormalities.
  - dental abnormalities.
- excessive production of intestinal gas and/or alterations in colonic motility may result in colonic tympany (rate of gas production exceeds the rate of elimination).
- intestine distends with gas and signs of pain may develop.
- colonic tympany secondary to obstructive lesions is covered under the specific obstruction.
- caecal tympany is often present concurrently.

Clinical presentation

- signs of abdominal pain will vary with the degree of abdominal distension:
  - rolling, pawing, flank-watching, stretching, recumbency, and anorexia.
  - pain can range from mild and intermittent to continuous and severe.
- heart rate usually elevated, consistent with the degree of pain.
- gross abdominal distension may be present:
  - usually bilateral (as opposed to caecal tympany).
  - marked distension may result in tachypnoea via pressure on the diaphragm.
- mucous membranes are usually normal unless severe distension is present.
- borborygmi may be normal, increased, or decreased:
  - high-pitched tympanic sounds may be heard during simultaneous auscultation and percussion of the abdomen.

Differential diagnosis

- variety of types of colic must be considered, particularly spasmodic, large colon impaction, and large colon displacement.

Diagnosis

- important to rule out the presence of surgical disorders such as large colon volvulus or displacement.
- distension of the large colon may be palpable per rectum:

  - o **thorough examination required to identify a causal lesion.**
- gaseous distension of the stomach may be present concurrently on nasogastric intubation.
- abdominal ultrasonographic examination is unremarkable.
- peritoneal fluid analysis and haematology should be unremarkable.

Management

- analgesic administration is usually required:
  - o drugs affecting intestinal motility should be used judiciously.
- mineral oil (4 litres via nasogastric tube) may coat fermentable substrates, but efficacy is unclear.
- feed should be withheld.
- frequent walking may be useful to simulate intestinal motility.
- short periods of trotting on a lunge line may be useful, particularly in more severe cases.
- severe abdominal distension also involving the caecum:
  - o caecal trocharisation may be required (see Caecal tympany, page 233).
- surgical intervention may be required in:
  - o severe, uncontrollable pain.
  - o severe abdominal distension.
  - o progression of clinical signs.
  - o decompress the intestine and rule out the presence of a concurrent surgical lesion.

Prognosis

- most cases respond well to conservative therapy.
- clinical condition deteriorates or there is a poor response to treatment:
  - o re-evaluate horse to ensure that another problem is not present.
- large colon displacement or volvulus can occur secondary to gaseous distension of the large colon.
- management reviewed to identify and address any risk factors that are present.

Colonic volvulus

Definition/overview

- relatively common cause of severe, life-threatening colic.

- both non-strangulated and strangulated volvulus may occur (latter is more frequent).
- strangulated large colon volvulus (LCV) rapidly induces hypovolaemic and endotoxaemic shock and affected horses require emergency surgical treatment.
- prognosis for survival with strangulated LCV is guarded to poor.

Aetiology/pathophysiology

- precise cause of LCV in horses is not currently known.
- broodmares just before or after parturition appear at increased risk:
  - o changes in digestion and/or visceral positioning during pregnancy may predispose mares.
- change in large colon motility may predispose any horse to the development of LCV.
- equine large colon has only two fixed attachment points:
  - o caecocolic ligament.
  - o transverse colon.
- most cases of LCV, the right ventral colon displaces dorsomedially (viewed from behind) (clockwise rotation).
- pathophysiology of LCV depends on the degree of rotation of the colon:
  - o rotation <270°:
    - ♦ blood supply to the large colon is usually not compromised.
    - ♦ only colonic lumen is obstructed to normal passage of gas and ingesta.
  - o rotation >270°:
    - ♦ blood supply (venous or arterial and venous) is compromised.
    - ♦ lumen of the large colon is obstructed.
    - ♦ **strangulating lesion.**
    - ♦ most cases, venous occlusion and haemorrhagic strangulating obstruction:
      - – sequestration of blood in the strangulated portions of the colon.
      - – ischaemic lesions of the mucosa:
        - ◊ dies within a few hours and intraluminal leakage of plasmatic fluids and absorption of endotoxin occur.

◊ rapid development of hypovolaemic and endotoxaemic shock.

Clinical presentation

- clinical signs vary with the degree of colonic rotation.
- non-strangulated LCV (rotation <270°) display clinical signs similar to those associated with large colon impaction or non-strangulating displacements.
- strangulated LCV have peracute colic and severe, intractable abdominal pain:
  ○ moderate to severe abdominal distension causing respiratory compromise.
  ○ signs of toxaemia and cardiovascular compromise may be present and severe.

Differential diagnosis

- non-strangulated LCV includes:
  ○ large colon impaction.
  ○ large colon displacement both right and left dorsal.
- strangulated LCV induces the most acute and violent signs of colic:
  ○ incarcerated internal hernia:
    ♦ diaphragmatic hernia.
    ♦ epiploic foramen entrapment.
    ♦ incarceration in the gastrosplenic ligament.
    ♦ strangulated inguinal hernia.

Diagnosis

- history of imminent or recent parturition or previous management changes is typical.
- severe colic with abdominal distension unresponsive to analgesics is characteristic of strangulated LCV.
- rectal palpation may identify large colon distension with tight taeniae:
  ○ strangulated volvulus, oedema of the large colon wall is occasionally palpable.

Management

- non-strangulated volvulus will rarely respond to conservative medical treatment:
  ○ most horses require surgical treatment.
- **strangulated volvulus is a surgical emergency.**

- about 5% of nonbreeding mares and males have a LCV recurrence.
- broodmares are at a higher risk:
  ○ after one episode, 15% chance of developing a second LCV.
  ○ after two episodes, the risk is increased to 80%.
  ○ colopexy or large colon resection indicated to prevent recurrence after two episodes of LCV.

Prognosis

- non-strangulated LCV is guarded to good.
- strangulated volvulus is associated with fatality rates of approximately 70%.
- time from development of volvulus to surgical intervention is critical:
  ○ strangulating lesions corrected within 4 hours of onset of signs have a better prognosis.

Strongyloides westeri infection

Definition/overview

- *Strongyloides westeri* ('threadworm'), is a common parasite in foals, but is usually of minimal clinical significance.

Aetiology/pathophysiology

- *Strongyloides* are capable of both a parasitic and a free-living reproductive cycle.
- only female worms are involved in the parasitic cycle, living in the small intestine and producing eggs via parthenogenesis.
- after hatching, larvae usually mature into free-living adult worms.
- under certain conditions the L3 can infect horses via skin penetration or ingestion:
  ○ develop into adult worms in the small intestine.
  ○ foals may also be infected from larvae present in the tissues of mares:
    ♦ larvae mobilise from arrested states in tissues of the abdominal wall.
    ♦ subsequently excreted in milk.
- infections peak within 4–6 weeks of age and are eliminated naturally by 20–25 weeks.

Clinical presentation

- infection is usually inapparent.
- disease is characterised by acute diarrhoea in foals in first few weeks of life.

Differential diagnosis

- other causes of neonatal diarrhoea including:
  - foal heat, clostridia, salmonellosis, and rotavirus.

Diagnosis

- eggs may be evident on faecal flotation:
  - use fresh faeces to avoid confusion with larvated strongyle-type eggs.
  - identification of eggs not diagnostic by itself because of high counts present in healthy foals.

Management

- specific treatment is rarely indicated because rarely a cause of disease.
- transmission of *S. westeri* from mares to foals markedly reduced by treatment of mares with ivermectin (0.2 mg/kg p/o) within 24 hours of parturition.
- treatment of foals with ivermectin at 1–2 weeks of age can hasten the elimination of *S. westeri*.

Prognosis

- excellent.

Large strongyle infestation

Definition/overview

- large strongyles are significant where routine deworming is not performed.
- prior to the widespread use of ivermectin, they were a common cause of severe colic.

Aetiology/pathophysiology

- *Strongylus vulgaris*, *S. edentatus*, and *S. equinus* may be involved:
  - *S. vulgaris* is the most clinically important.
- adult strongyles live in the large intestine and caecum:
  - reddish, thick, and up to 4 cm in length.
- eggs passed in faeces and infective L3 develop in the environment.

- following ingestion, *S. vulgaris* L3 penetrate the intestinal mucosa and moult to L4 in the submucosa:
  - invade small arteries/arterioles and migrate to cranial mesenteric artery and branches:
    - inflammation of the arteries can develop in response to the larvae.
    - thrombosis can cause ischaemia in areas of the intestinal tract.
    - thromboemboli may develop and cause ischaemic necrosis of other areas of the intestinal tract.
    - intestinal aneurysms are less common.
  - after several months, moult and L5 migrate to the intestinal wall:
    - nodules form around them and subsequently rupture into intestinal lumen.
    - releases young adults.
- after ingestion, *S. edentatus* penetrates the intestinal mucosa and reaches the liver via the portal circulation:
  - further liver migration occurs, and then the larvae travel under the peritoneum and eventually reach the intestinal lumen.
- migratory route of *S. equinus* is less well understood:
  - L4 larvae form in the intestinal wall, enter the peritoneal cavity, migrate into the liver, then moult in the pancreas and return to the large intestine.
- strongyle migration has been suggested to be the cause of haemomelasma ilei, a typically benign condition (Fig. 3.51).

Clinical presentation

- few clinical signs are produced by the presence of adult worms in the GI tract:
  - mild diarrhoea, ill-thrift, and anaemia are possible with chronic, severe burdens.
- migration of *S. edentatus* and *S. equinus* larvae can produce:
  - haemorrhagic tracts in the liver.
  - nodule formation in the gut wall or peritoneum.
  - subsequent clinical signs are rare.
  - pancreatitis is rare or rarely identified.
- intestinal infarction is more serious:
  - clinical presentation varies, depending on:

- ◆ degree of intestinal ischaemia, duration of disease, and location of the lesion.
- ◆ pain may be mild to severe.
- ◆ heart rate is elevated (can exceed 100 bpm).
- ◆ respiratory rate may also be elevated.
- ◆ may sweat profusely and appear anxious.
- ◆ with significant intestinal ischaemia or septic peritonitis:
  - – mucous membranes congested and hyperaemic, with prolonged CRT.
- ◆ borborygmi are decreased to absent.

Differential diagnosis

- strangulating intestinal infarction, severe enterocolitis, and peritonitis.

Diagnosis

- eggs are usually readily identifiable on a faecal flotation test:
  - ○ small and large strongyle eggs cannot be differentiated ('strongyle-type' eggs).
  - ○ absence of identifiable eggs does not rule out infection.
- impossible to definitively identify a non-strangulating infarction without surgery or necropsy.

Management

- Large strongyles are generally susceptible to:
  - ○ ivermectin (0.2 mg/kg p/o).
  - ○ moxidectin (0.4 mg/kg p/o).
  - ○ fenbendazole (10 mg/kg p/o q24h for 5 days, or 60 mg/kg single dose).
- resistance to pyrantel has been reported.

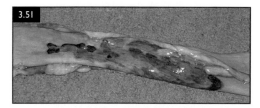

FIG. 3.51 Characteristic appearance of haemomelasma ilei, a benign condition.

- pasture management is important:
  - ○ provision of adequate stocking density.
  - ○ routine (twice weekly) removal of faeces.
  - ○ pasture rotation.
- intestinal infarction is present:
  - ○ prompt surgical intervention is required.
  - ○ affected intestine must be resected.
  - ○ resection of all the damaged intestine is often not possible, leading to euthanasia.

Prognosis

- excellent unless intestinal infarction is present.
- infarction present:
  - ○ guarded with surgical intervention and hopeless if surgery is not an option.

Displacement of the large colon

Definition/overview

- large colon movement is only restricted by its attachment to the caecum and transverse colon, and it is therefore relatively mobile.
- variety of displacements can occur and result in abdominal distension and pain.

Aetiology/pathophysiology

- aetiology is unknown and likely to be variable.
- reported risk factors for displacements include:
  - ○ advancing age (>7 years).
  - ○ Warmblood breed.
  - ○ large body size.
  - ○ foaling.
  - ○ diet changes.
- anything resulting in excessive production or accumulation of gas within the large colon could predispose to development of a displacement.
- two common displacements are:
  - ○ nephrosplenic entrapment (left dorsal displacement).
  - ○ right dorsal displacement.
- gaseous distension is often associated with a mild–moderate large colon impaction.
- right dorsal displacements can occur in two directions:

- clockwise:
  - more common.
  - pelvic flexure is displaced between the caecum and body wall in a cranial-to-caudal direction.
- counterclockwise:
  - pelvic flexure travels in a caudal-to-cranial direction.
- once the colon is displaced, the normal flow of ingesta and/or gas may be restricted:
  - abdominal distension and pain.
  - colon vascular supply is minimally affected.

Clinical presentation

- signs of mild to severe abdominal pain may be evident, depending on the degree of abdominal distension:
  - continuous or intermittent.
  - heart rate elevated according to the degree of pain.
- presentation may be acute or chronic.
- moderate to severe abdominal tympany may be present.
- signs of toxaemia or cardiovascular compromise should not be evident.
- occasionally, horses with a nephrosplenic entrapment may appear to be in pain:
  - but heart rate is not correspondingly elevated, presumably due to vagal effects.

Differential diagnosis

- any condition causing colic, particularly with gaseous distension of the large colon.

Diagnosis

- may be difficult to diagnose and to differentiate from large colon impaction or volvulus.
- should be suspected when there is progressive gaseous distension with a large colon impaction.
- palpation per rectum is useful for a presumptive diagnosis of right dorsal displacement:
  - typically, distended colon palpable on the right side of the abdomen.
  - caecum is not palpable.
  - colon may be palpable between the caecum and body wall.
  - large colon impaction may be palpable concurrently.

- diagnosis of a nephrosplenic entrapment can be difficult on rectal palpation:
  - nephrosplenic space can be difficult to palpate in large horses.
  - nephrosplenic entrapment may be suspected based on medial displacement of the spleen.
  - not unusual to detect loops of small colon in the nephrosplenic space:
    - often incidental and must be differentiated from entrapped large colon.
- transabdominal ultrasonography useful to rule out a nephrospenic entrapment:
  - left kidney and spleen visualised in direct apposition, then entrapment is unlikely.
  - gas-filled viscus obliterating the view of the dorsal border of the spleen suggests a nephrosplenic entrapment.
  - inability to visualise the left kidney is not, in itself, diagnostic.
  - displaced colon not gas filled, a displacement may not be identified.
- nasogastric reflux is not typically present.
- abdominocentesis is useful when deciding whether surgical intervention is required:
  - peritoneal fluid is usually normal in an uncomplicated displacement.

Management

- medical therapy will often be successful:
  - feed should be withheld until the displacement resolves.
  - fluid therapy is useful:
    - soften an impaction, if present.
    - stimulate intestinal motility.
    - intravenous fluid therapy is preferred.
    - oral therapy (up to 8–10 litres q30min) can be useful in milder cases.
    - horses may experience more pain after fluid therapy has started because of increased colonic distension.
  - analgesics provided as required.
- re-examined frequently to ensure that a more severe intestinal accident such as a LCV has not developed.
- some cases may have severe, progressive abdominal distension and intractable pain:
  - surgery is indicated in these cases.

- displacement is unlikely to correct spontaneously if marked tympany is present:
  - trocharisation of the distended bowel may temporarily relieve intestinal tympany where surgery is not an option.
- horses occasionally improve clinically:
  - gaseous distension abates.
  - impaction (if present) resolves.
  - yet the colon will remain displaced after a few days of medical therapy:
    - very conservative feeding may stimulate intestinal motility and resolve the displacement.
    - if unresponsive, surgical correction will be required.
- left dorsal displacement of the colon lateral to the spleen but without entrapment in the nephrosplenic space will often correct with conservative therapy.
- nephrosplenic entrapment requires specific measures:
  - phenylephrine (3–5 μg/kg/minute for 15 minutes), followed by 15–20 minutes of lunging or jogging is sometimes effective at correcting the displacement:
    - causes splenic contraction, making it easier for the entrapped colon to return to its normal position.
    - effects are short-term and administration can be repeated.
  - rolling under general anaesthesia:
    - successful in >90% of cases but lower in horses with marked gas distension.
  - surgery may be required in:
    - severely painful cases.
    - those not responding to medical treatment.
    - where rolling has been unsuccessful.

Prognosis

- very good, with the majority of cases responding to medical treatment.
- uncommonly some horses develop repeated displacements:
  - underlying causes should be sought and addressed where possible.
  - ablation of the nephrosplenic space, colopexy or large colon resection can be considered in recurrent displacements requiring surgical correction.

Large colon impaction

Definition/overview

- impaction with ingesta is a common cause of colic.

Aetiology/pathophysiology

- impactions occur from accumulation of dehydrated and densely packed ingesta:
  - often at a site where the large colon narrows.
  - most commonly pelvic flexure.
  - right dorsal colon impactions are not uncommon (Fig. 3.52).
- factors affecting hydration of the colonic contents and intestinal motility may predispose to the development of impactions and include:
  - ingestion of highly fibrous grass or hay.
  - poor diet.
  - decreased water intake:
    - restricted access, excessively cold water, change in water source.
  - management changes including sudden exercise restriction.
  - transportation.
  - pain.
  - sand enteropathy.
  - EGUS.
- many cases occur in the absence of these factors.

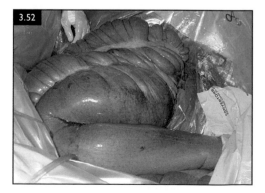

FIG. 3.52 Severe impaction of the right dorsal colon that required surgical intervention.

- firm ingesta accumulates in the affected area leading to colonic distension from ingesta and altered movement of intestinal gas causing variable signs of pain.

Clinical presentation

- non-specific signs of abdominal pain including:
  - anorexia.
  - flank-watching, pawing, rolling, and tail-swishing.
  - straining to defaecate, and sweating.
  - intermittent pain over a few days may be reported.
  - pain can range from mild and intermittent (over days) to severe and continuous.
  - heart rate is correspondingly elevated.
- borborygmi are often decreased.
- signs of systemic compromise or toxaemia should not be evident.
- dehydration may be present, depending on the duration of signs.
- intestinal tympany may be present.
- decrease in faecal production.
- passage of firm, dry faeces sometimes reported.
- faeces may be covered in mucus, indicating delayed intestinal transit.

Differential diagnosis

- other causes of mild to moderate colic without intestinal compromise:
  - spasmodic colic, intestinal tympany, sand impaction, enteroliths, and large colon displacement.
- extraintestinal diseases such as laminitis, pleuritis, peritonitis, urinary obstruction, exertional rhabdomyolysis, and reproductive tract lesions.

Diagnosis

- most impactions of the large colon are palpable per rectum:
  - identification of a section of ingesta-filled and distended large colon.
  - pelvic flexure impactions are most obvious and may extend into the pelvic canal.
  - size and texture of the impaction should be noted.
  - occasionally, an impaction may lie beyond reach of the examiner.

- gastric reflux is unusual, but can occur:
  - small intestinal compression by distended large colon.
  - pain-induced ileus.
- transabdominal ultrasonography is useful in horses too small for per rectum palpation.
- abdominocentesis should be performed with care to avoid penetrating a markedly distended, friable large colon:
  - peritoneal fluid is normal in most cases.
  - should be performed in horses that deteriorate acutely to determine whether colonic rupture may have occurred.

Management

- feed should be withheld:
  - restricted from otherwise healthy adult horses for a week without adverse consequences in most cases:
    - ♦ take care in obese animals to avoid inducing hypertriglyceridaemia.
- analgesics will usually be required.
- treatment via nasogastric tube may be useful in horses without gastric reflux:
  - mineral oil (4 litres) has traditionally been used but efficacy has not been proven:
    - ♦ can pass around dense impactions without any beneficial effect.
    - ♦ more useful in mild impactions.
  - DSS can be administered orally (beneficial effect has not been demonstrated):
    - ♦ repeated administration avoided as irritation and toxicity can develop.
  - osmotic cathartics can be useful:
    - ♦ magnesium sulphate (1 g/kg q24h) most used.
    - ♦ do not use high doses of cathartics when very large, firm, and potentially obstructive impactions are present:
      - – potential for development of marked colonic distension.
      - – preferable to soften the impaction with fluid therapy prior to administration of cathartics.
  - administration of water via a nasogastric tube is cost-effective and successful:

♦ tube can be left in place and water (8 litres up to q30min–2h) administered.
♦ repeated monitoring of correct placement.
♦ excessive quantities of water (>30 l/day) associated with hyponatraemia.
♦ use of balanced electrolyte solutions will control this problem:
 – simple, cheap, balanced electrolyte solution can be made with 45 ml NaCl and 15 ml KCl (30 ml table salt and 30 ml 'Lite' salt) per 8 l water.
 ○ fluids stopped until the horse is re-evaluated if signs of colic progress or if gastric reflux develops.
• intravenous fluid therapy may be required for more severe cases, or those that are refractory to oral therapy:
 ○ less effective than repeated enteral fluid administration.
• most impactions resolve with medical treatment.
• surgery is warranted:
 ○ very large impactions that do not respond to medical treatment.
 ○ cases with severe intractable pain.
• following resolution of the impaction, important that feeding is reintroduced gradually:
 ○ small volumes of hay, hay cube slurries, grass, or bran mashes used initially.
 ○ small volumes offered every few hours.
 ○ volume increasing over time, so a normal hay or grass ration is offered by 24–48 hours.
 ○ underlying disease and risk factors for impaction, including management and dental disease, should be evaluated to help prevent recurrence.

Prognosis

• very good in general, but worse if surgery is required.
• severe and/or long-standing impactions may damage stretch receptors in the intestinal wall, predisposing to recurrence.
• rupture of the large colon during exteriorisation is a concern if surgical correction is needed.
• large colon rupture is invariably fatal.

Sand impaction

Definition/overview

• accumulation of large volumes of sand in the large colon is a common cause of colic in some geographical areas.

Aetiology/pathophysiology

• sand may be ingested while:
 ○ grazing on sandy soil.
 ○ kept in sandy paddocks, arenas, or stalls.
 ○ greater risk if underfed or kept in overstocked, closely grazed pastures.
 ○ some horses, particularly foals, may intentionally ingest sand (pica).
• post-ingestion, sand can settle in the large colon:
 ○ continued ingestion may lead to partial or complete obstruction, and signs of colic.
• right dorsal colon is the most common site of sand accumulation:
 ○ impactions can develop anywhere in the large colon, and at multiple sites.

Clinical presentation

• mild to severe colic may be observed:
 ○ signs can be intermittent or continuous.
• accompanied by varying degrees of anorexia, depression, and abdominal distension.
• faecal production may be decreased, and soft faeces may be present.
• concurrent large colon displacement or volvulus may affect the presentation.

Differential diagnosis

• other causes of mild to moderate colic including:
 ○ large colon impaction or displacement.
 ○ intestinal tympany, EGUS, and enterolithiasis.

Diagnosis

• history of potential exposure to sand is usually present.
• sand impaction can be difficult to differentiate from other causes of colic.
• abdominal auscultation:
 ○ characteristic 'sand sounds' heard, particularly over the ventral abdomen.

- o similar to friction rubs or movement of sand in a paper bag.
- o relatively sensitive and specific indicator of sand accumulation.
- haematological changes are uncommon, non-specific, and not diagnostic.
- per rectum palpation:
  - o difficult to detect sand impactions as they are often located cranially.
  - o gaseous distension of the large colon and caecum is often palpable:
    - ♦ may also indicate a large colon displacement or volvulus.
- abdominocentesis should only be performed if essential:
  - o undertaken with care because of concerns about lacerating the distended colon.
  - o enterocentesis yields sand – sand impaction is invariably present.
- sand accumulation may be evident radiographically (Fig. 3.49), particularly in the cranioventral abdomen.
- sand evident ultrasonographically within the large colon in the cranioventral abdomen.
- sand sedimentation test has a poor correlation with the presence of sand in the large colon and is not advised.

Management

- enteral fluid therapy is useful in most cases.
- removal of impacted ingesta as per a typical large colon impaction should be performed prior to attempting to remove accumulated sand.
- once the animal is comfortable and passing normal faeces:
  - o specific therapy targeted at removing sand should be commenced:
    - ♦ psyllium (1.0 g/kg) combined with magnesium sulphate (1.0 g/kg) daily via nasogastric tube is effective in the removal of sand accumulations.
    - ♦ continued for 3–5 days followed by repeat radiographic or ultrasonographic examination.
- following resolution periodic evaluation (every 3–6 months):
  - o via abdominal radiography or ultrasonography.
  - o particularly if management changes are not feasible.

- intermittent administration of psyllium may help reduce sand accumulation but the response between individuals is highly variable.
- medical treatment is usually effective, but surgical intervention may be required in:
  - o horses with intractable pain.
  - o poor response to medical therapy.
  - o deteriorating cardiovascular status.
- feed should be gradually reintroduced after the impaction has resolved.
- management practices should be changed to avoid further sand impactions.

Prognosis

- good but compared with ingesta impactions, sand impactions tend to be:
  - o more difficult to treat.
  - o more likely to require surgery.
  - o have a higher mortality rate.
- rupture of the large colon during exteriorisation of the large colon during surgery is not uncommon.

Intramural lesions of the large colon (ILLC)

Definition/overview

- intramural lesions (lesions within the wall) of the large colon are uncommon and usually lead to mild to moderate intermittent colic.
- treatment is surgical, and the prognosis varies with the aetiology of the lesions.

Aetiology/pathophysiology

- multicentric and intestinal lymphosarcoma and adenocarcinoma reported in a limited number of cases of ILLC.
- segmental eosinophilic colitis is an uncommon disease that results in a local thickening and obstructive lesion of the colon in horses:
  - o precise aetiology is not known, but parasite involvement is suspected.
- abdominal abscessation limited to the wall of the large colon can be a rare cause (Fig. 3.53).
- local thickening and obstructive lesions of the colonic wall result in potential partial or complete obstruction of the colonic lumen.

Clinical presentation

- clinical signs are non-specific.
- most common are mild to moderate recurrent colic episodes associated with abdominal distension and pelvic flexure impaction.
- lethargy, weight loss, pyrexia, and diarrhoea may also be observed.

Differential diagnosis

- causes of:
  - simple colon obstruction (food and foreign body impaction).
  - primary large colon tympany.

Diagnosis

- abdominal mass attached to the large colon and/or large colon distension may be palpable per rectum.
- ultrasonographic examination of the large colon may show an increased wall thickness or confirm the presence of an abdominal mass.
- peritoneal fluid:
  - total nucleated cell count and protein concentration are usually increased.
  - exfoliated tumour cells are rarely observed.
- definitive diagnosis is made at exploratory laparotomy (biopsies can be taken).

Management

- usually initially treated in a supportive manner using:
  - restricted diet, analgesics, intravenous and/or enteral fluids, and laxatives.
- clinical signs are temporarily responsive to medical treatment:
  - recur as food is reintroduced or the action of the analgesics abates.

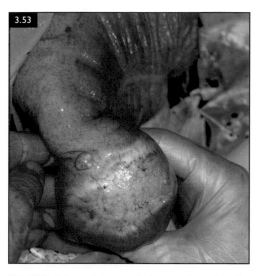

FIG. 3.53 A large intramural abscess found in the large colon of a horse presented for exploratory laparotomy for investigation of chronic abdominal pain.

- eventually managed by exploratory laparotomy and identification of the lesion.

Prognosis

- guarded to poor for intestinal neoplasia as the tumour may extend to other organs.
- retrospective study of 22 cases with segmental eosinophilic colitis treated surgically had a good prognosis for survival.
- abdominal abscesses that require treatment in addition to long-term antimicrobial administration have a poor to guarded prognosis.

DISORDERS OF THE SMALL COLON AND RECTUM

Small colon impaction

Definition/overview

- most common disorder of the small colon:
  - seems to be predisposed to impaction as the lumen of the large colon narrows acutely through the transverse colon into the small colon.

- ponies, American miniature horses, and Arabs develop small colon impactions more frequently than other breeds.

Aetiology/pathophysiology

- aetiology of small colon impaction includes:
  - ingestion of poor-quality roughage.

- poor dentition.
- parasitism dehydration.
- motility disorders.
- older horses are more frequently affected, probably due to deteriorated dentition and decreased small colon motility.
- more frequent during the autumn and winter:
  - access to water may be decreased.
  - consumption of coarse roughage material is increased.
- impaction causes an intraluminal obstruction of the small colon resulting in:
  - ingesta, fluid, and gas accumulation in segments of the GI tract proximal to the impaction.
- horses deteriorate slowly because of the aboral location of the small colon and the large space for the ingesta, fluid, and gas to accumulate orad to the impaction.
- as the impaction persists, the intestinal segments proximal to the obstruction, mainly large colon and caecum, become more and more distended and the affected horse experiences colic.

Clinical presentation

- initially present with only mild signs of colic and reduced faecal output.
- abdominal distension and moderate to severe colic with progression.
- nasogastric reflux is inconsistent.

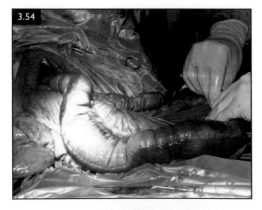

FIG. 3.54 Intraoperative photograph of an impacted small colon in a miniature pony showing a large amount of the small colon distended with firm faecal material.

Differential diagnosis

- any intraluminal obstruction of the large intestine in horses:
  - large colon and caecal impactions.
  - foreign body, enterolith, and faecalith obstructions.

Diagnosis

- based on clinical signs and rectal palpation:
  - usually decreased faecal production and distended abdomen.
  - exhibit moderate to severe signs of colic.
  - one/several firm, tubular, and digesta-filled loops of small colon on palpation:
    - thickness of the wall and palpation of a single, free taenial band helps identify the small colon.

Management

- medical conservative management is often successful in the treatment of mild to moderate impactions:
  - aggressive enteral and/or parenteral fluid therapy is used to:
    - overhydrate the horse.
    - stimulate intestinal secretion production.
    - breakdown the impaction.
  - analgesics to control abdominal pain.
  - exercise is used to stimulate intestinal motility.
  - **administration of an enema in standing horses is not recommended unless:**
    - impaction located in distal portion of small colon near the rectum.
    - horse tolerates them well.
    - can be associated with traumatic rupture of the small colon.
- surgical treatment (Fig. 3.54) is recommended with:
  - severe impactions.
  - when the impaction fails to respond to medical treatment.
- horses with small colon impaction may have a higher incidence of developing salmonellosis in some areas:
  - unclear aetiology but worth noting if diarrhoea develops during treatment.

Prognosis

- good for survival if respond to medical conservative treatment.
- horses undergoing surgery commonly develop postoperative complications such as fever, diarrhoea, salmonellosis, and laminitis leading to a guarded prognosis.

Small colon strangulation

Definition/overview

- obstruction to the vasculature of the small colon and ischaemic damage to the intestinal tissue due to:
  - strangulating lipoma.
  - volvulus (see page 224).
  - entrapment of small colon through a congenital or acquired defect.

Aetiology/pathophysiology

- small colon has a short mesentery compared with the distal small intestine, which accounts for the lower incidence of strangulation.
- small colon can become entrapped in:
  - defects in the gastrosplenic and broad ligaments, and caecocolic fold and mesocolon.
  - through a vaginal tear.
  - inguinal and umbilical herniation of the small colon have been reported.
- congenital defects including vitelloumbilical anomalies may create abnormal spaces through which the small colon can become incarcerated.
- entrapment leads to obstruction of the small colon vascular supply:
  - tissues become oedematous and turgid.
  - further swelling of the entrapped intestine obstructs arterial supply to the intestine, resulting in ischaemic damage.
- orad distension of the small, transverse and ascending colon occurs due to intraluminal obstruction.

Clinical presentation

- present with signs ranging from mild to moderate abdominal discomfort to acute severe abdominal pain.
- nasogastric reflux is an inconsistent finding.

Differential diagnosis

- any strangulating obstruction of the intestine including:
  - strangulating lipomas, inguinal and other hernias, volvulus, epiploic foramen entrapment, and entrapment of bowel in mesenteric or ligamentous rents.
  - small intestinal strangulations tend to occur more acutely and with a more rapid deterioration in clinical signs and haematological parameters.

Diagnosis

- rectal palpation:
  - variable location of the strangulation can lead to inconclusive rectal findings.
  - common finding is impaction within the cranial small colon and, in chronic cases, colonic distension.
  - transrectal ultrasound is useful for diagnosing small colon impactions.
- peritoneal fluid often serosanguineous with elevated protein concentration and WBC.
- elevated blood lactate level may demonstrate tissue ischaemia.
- transabdominal ultrasonography findings include:
  - distended, non-motile small colon with a thickened wall (>3–4 mm).
  - normal colon and SI wall thickness help localise the lesion to the small colon.

Management

- surgical management is critical.

Prognosis

- approximately 50% of these cases survive.

Small colon obstruction

Definition/overview

- obstruction can be intraluminal or extraluminal in origin.
- causes for intraluminal obstructions include:
  - impaction, foreign bodies, enteroliths, faecaliths, and bezoars (Fig. 3.55).
- causes for extraluminal obstruction include:

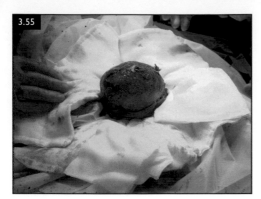

FIG. 3.55 A large trichobezoar is being removed from the small colon at exploratory laparotomy via a flank incision. Note the careful draping around the colon to minimise contamination of the abdomen.

    ○ intramural haematoma and, rarely, neoplasms such as leiomyomas.

Aetiology/pathophysiology

- foreign bodies involved are usually nylon, plastic, or rubber material from halters, hay nets, bale twines, synthetic fencing material, and plastic trash can liners.
- after ingestion, foreign bodies reach the large colon (particularly the right dorsal colon) where they can remain for extended periods of time.
- covered with mineral precipitate, which increases their bulk:
  ○ usually an irregular shape, often containing sharp projections.
  ○ sharp projections may cause pressure necrosis of the intestinal wall.
- eventually pass into the transverse/small colon and cause obstructions.
- foreign body obstructions occur mostly in horses less than 3 years of age:
  ○ not as discriminative as older horses in their eating habits.
- intramural haematomas are caused by haemorrhage between the small colon mucosa and muscularis layers:
  ○ unknown aetiology but mainly observed in older horses.
  ○ haemorrhage occludes the intestinal lumen.
  ○ dissects along the intestine and produces intestinal necrosis.

Clinical presentation

- signs of moderate to severe colic.
- mild to moderate abdominal distension.
- reduced or lack of faecal production.

Differential diagnosis

- any obstructive conditions of the large intestine such as:
  ○ faecal impaction of the caecum and large and small colon.
  ○ foreign bodies, enteroliths, and faecaliths.
- small colon foreign body obstruction tends to occur more acutely, with a more rapid deterioration in clinical signs, than small colon faecal impaction.

Diagnosis

- clinical signs and rectal palpation but often difficult to diagnose.
- rectal palpation:
  ○ one or several firm, tubular, and digesta-filled loops of small colon.
  ○ foreign body is rarely palpable.
- definitive diagnosis made during exploratory coeliotomy.

Management

- surgical treatment is recommended for complete obstruction of the small colon.

Prognosis

- guarded for small colon obstruction due to a foreign body or an intramural hematoma.
- postoperative complications include diarrhoea, laminitis, and anastomosis leakage.

Small colon segmental ischaemic necrosis

Definition/overview

- Segmental ischaemic necrosis of the small colon is a rare condition usually observed in broodmares.

Aetiology/pathophysiology

- mesocolon rupture is main cause of disruption of the mesocolonic vasculature and of small colon segmental ischaemic necrosis in horses.

- ○ occurs during parturition when the small colon may become trapped between the uterus and the body wall.
- ○ type 3 or 4 rectal prolapses:
  - ♦ mesocolon vasculature disrupted if >30 cm of distal small colon and rectum prolapse.
- rupture of the vasculature results in infarction, causing segmental ischaemic necrosis and functional obstruction of the small colon.
- signs of colic and septic peritonitis occur subsequently.

Clinical presentation

- mild signs of colic occur within 24 hours of parturition in broodmares.
- affected horses fail to pass faeces.
- cardiovascular status slowly deteriorates, and signs of septic peritonitis and shock develop.

Differential diagnosis

- early signs need to be differentiated from the mild abdominal pain associated with uterine contractions.
- other differentials include conditions associated with small colon obstruction, septic peritonitis, and parturition-associated reproductive tract disease.

Diagnosis

- history of recent parturition or rectal prolapse with reduced or lack of faecal production with mild signs of colic.

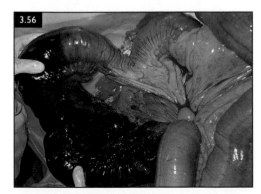

FIG. 3.56 Typical post-mortem appearance of an infarct lesion of the peritoneal rectum and distal small colon. The lesion in this broodmare resulted from a rupture of the mesocolon, which had occurred during parturition.

- rectal palpation may not be initially diagnostic, but as the condition progresses:
  - ○ one/several firm, tubular, and digesta-filled loops of small colon palpated.
- abdominocentesis initially reveals abdominal haemorrhage:
  - ○ increased WBC count and protein level as the condition progresses.
- exploratory laparotomy or necropsy for definitive diagnosis (Fig. 3.56).

Management

- surgical treatment with exploratory laparotomy, resection/anastomosis of the ischaemic segment or end colostomy.

Prognosis

- directly correlated with the location of the lesion:
  - ○ orad enough for resection/anastomosis, fair.
  - ○ too aborad for an anastomosis to be performed, the prognosis is grave.

Rectal tears

Definition/overview

- rectal tear occurs when at least one of the rectal wall layers is disrupted.
- most rectal tears occur during transrectal palpation:
  - ○ generally located 20–30 cm from the anus, in the dorsal portion of the rectum.
  - ○ have a longitudinal direction.
- young horses, males, and Arabian horses are more frequently affected.

Aetiology/pathophysiology

- most commonly iatrogenic in origin and the aetiology includes:
  - ○ transrectal palpation and enema administration.
  - ○ reproductive complications such as dystocia and breeding injury.
- spontaneous tears are rare but have been described.
- pathophysiology varies with the location and the degree of severity of the tears.
- rectum is approximately 30 cm long in a 450 kg horse:
  - ○ oral half in the peritoneal cavity.

- ○ aboral portion retroperitoneal.
- ○ most tears are 20–30 cm from the anus and are within the peritoneal cavity.
- classification reflecting degree of severity has been established:
  - ○ *Grade 1 tears:* only the rectal mucosa and submucosa are torn.
  - ○ *Grade 2 tears:* rectal muscularis layer is torn, causing the mucosa and submucosa to form a diverticulum as they protrude through the defect.
  - ○ *Grade 3 tears:*
    - ♦ grade 3a tears: all layers are affected except the serosa.
    - ♦ grade 3b tears: all layers are affected except the mesorectum.
  - ○ *Grade 4 tears:* complete tears involving all the rectal wall layers.
- Grade 1 tears are usually not associated with complications.
- Grade 2 and 3 tears:
  - ○ faecal material becomes impacted in the defect.
  - ○ development of a perirectal or retroperitoneal abscess, dissecting cellulitis, or rectal wall necrosis that can eventually result in abdominal faecal contamination.
- Grade 4 tears:
  - ○ usually massive faecal contamination of the abdominal cavity.
  - ○ leads to septic peritonitis, septic shock, and ultimately death (Fig. 3.57).

Clinical presentation

- presence of whole fresh blood on the rectal examination sleeve or sudden relaxation of the rectum during examination is suggestive of a serious rectal injury.
- clinical signs may not be present in the short term even after serious tears.
- tenesmus, abdominal pain, tachycardia, pyrexia, and ileus may develop within hours after the injury.
- grade 4 rectal tears develop septic shock and peritonitis very shortly after the injury.

Diagnosis

- evaluate horses with rectal tears immediately to determine location, size, and depth of the tear.
- performed after the horse is well sedated and epidural anaesthesia has been administered.
- rectum should be carefully evacuated.
- digital palpation with a bare hand is the most effective procedure for assessing the tear.
- endoscopic evaluation of the rectum is also useful for assessment of the tear (Fig. 3.58):
  - ○ prevent excessive insufflation of the rectum during the procedure to reduce the risk of further tearing of the defect.
- abdominocentesis should be performed if a grade 4 tear is suspected.

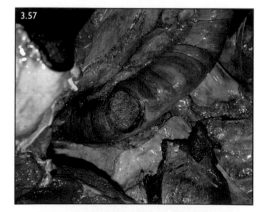

FIG. 3.57 Typical post-mortem appearance of an iatrogenic grade 4 rectal tear. Note the obvious faecal contamination of the peritoneal cavity.

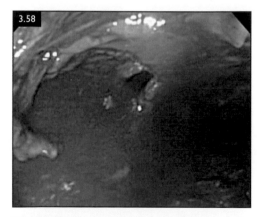

FIG. 3.58 Endoscopic image of a mare with a grade 4 rectal tear that occurred following palpation for routine reproductive evaluation.

Management

- management varies with the grade of tear.
- grade 2 tears are treated conservatively:
  - administration of systemic broad-spectrum antimicrobials, NSAIDs, and laxatives.
  - grade 1 tears are treated similarly except antibiotics are not necessary.
- **grade 3 and 4 tears should be referred to a hospital facility for further evaluation and treatment after the following first aid treatment:**
  - prevent faecal contamination of the abdomen with a well-lubricated stockinet packed with cotton inserted into the rectum to a level approximately 10 cm cranial to the tear:
    - ♦ soaking the cotton in povidone–iodine prior to insertion is recommended.
  - close the anus using towel clamps or a purse-string suture.
  - intravenous systemic broad-spectrum antibiotics and NSAIDs should be given.

Prognosis

- good for survival with a grade 1 rectal tear. Grade 3 tears warrant a poor prognosis and grade 4 tears a grave prognosis.

Rectal prolapse

Definition/overview

- occurs when rectal tissue evaginates and protrudes through the anus.
- rare in horses.

Aetiology/pathophysiology

- any condition causing tenesmus may lead to rectal prolapse in horses:
  - diarrhoea, constipation, intestinal parasitism, proctatitis, colic, and rectal foreign body/tumours.
  - type 4 prolapse usually occurs in mares during foaling or dystocia.
- anal sphincter applies pressure on the protruded rectal tissue and impinges on the venous return.
- protruded tissue eventually becomes oedematous and necrotic making it prone to irritation and trauma.

Clinical presentation

- four types of rectal prolapse have been described in the equine:
  - Type 1: only the rectal mucosa (or part of it) protrudes through the anus (Fig. 3.59).
  - Type 2: occurs when there is an eversion of the entire ampula recti (Fig. 3.60).
  - Type 3: complete eversion of the ampula recti, complicated by an intussusception of the peritoneal portion of the rectum.
  - Type 4: intussusception of the peritoneal rectum and a variable length of the small colon, both protruding through the anus (Fig. 3.61).

Diagnosis

- initial diagnosis is made by observation of an abnormal mass of tissue protruding beyond the anus:
  - tissue is usually inflamed and cyanotic.

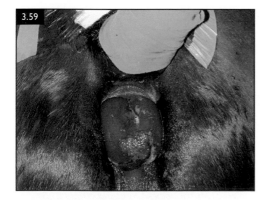

FIG. 3.59 Type 1 rectal prolapse.

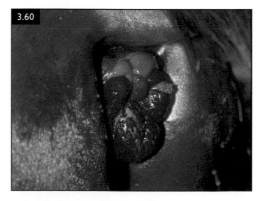

FIG. 3.60 Type 2 rectal prolapse.

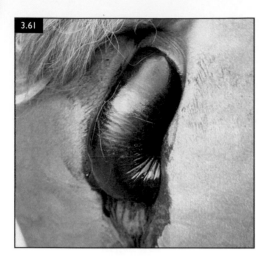

FIG. 3.61 Type 4 rectal prolapse.

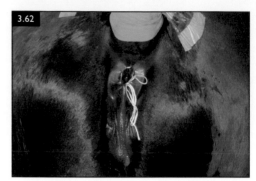

FIG. 3.62 Purse-string suture correction of a type 1 rectal prolapse.

- degree of trauma and necrosis is variable.
- rectal palpation help differentiate between types 2 and 3 cases.
- type 3 or 4 cases may develop septic peritonitis:
  - abdominocentesis should be performed in these cases.

Management

- acute and circumscribed types 1 and 2 cases should be treated conservatively:
  - topical application of lidocaine jelly onto the protruded tissue.
  - repeated administration of epidural anaesthesia to reduce straining.
  - placement of a purse-string suture for 48–72 hours:
    - made of a double strand of 6 mm (1/4 inch) umbilical tape applied 1–2 cm lateral to the anus with four wide bites (Fig. 3.62).
    - open the suture every 2–4 hours to manually remove rectal faeces.
  - mineral oil by nasogastric tube and fasted for 24 hours.
  - laxative diet fed for 10 days following purse-string removal.
  - **treat the primary cause of straining.**
- long-standing or recurring types 1 and 2 rectal prolapses should be treated surgically.
- type 3 and 4 rectal prolapses should be manually reduced immediately after they occur:

- usually associated with severe vascular injury to the rectum and/or distal small colon.
- exploratory laparotomy is recommended:
  - resection/anastomosis or permanent end colostomy may be necessary.

Prognosis

- good for types 1 and 2 prolapses.
- poor to grave for types 3 and 4 prolapses as usually associated with severe injuries to the vascular supply and mesentery disruption.

Anorectal lymphadenopathy/ perirectal abscess

Definition/overview

- uncommon condition that affects mostly young horses and results in extraluminal obstruction of the rectum.
- treatment involves systemic antimicrobials and anti-inflammatories, prevention of rectal impaction, and drainage of the abscess when present.

Aetiology/pathophysiology

- most cases the cause is unknown, but may develop following:
  - rectal or vaginal puncture or trauma.
  - secondary to gravitation of a gluteal abscess following an intramuscular injection.
  - *Streptococcus zooepidemicus* and *Escherichia coli* are most implicated.

- Anorectal lymph nodes are located dorsally in the retroperitoneal tissue surrounding the rectum.
- sepsis causes these nodes to enlarge, which may result in an extraluminal obstruction of the rectum.
- rarely, infection progresses into the abdominal cavity and induces a septic peritonitis.

Clinical presentation

- signs of mild abdominal pain, depression, anorexia, reduced faecal output, tenesmus, and fever.

Differential diagnosis

- perirectal abscesses need to be differentiated from neoplasms that develop in perirectal tissue:
  - extensive perineal melanoma and melanosarcoma may produce similar clinical signs.

Diagnosis

- based on palpation of a firm perianal mass per rectum.
- transrectal ultrasonography reveals enlargement of the anorectal lymph nodes or the presence of a mature abscess.

- cytological examination and bacteriological culture of aspirates collected percutaneously or through the rectal wall confirm sepsis of the anorectal lymph nodes.

Management

- management of anorectal lymphadenopathy aims to:
  - treat the anorectal lymph node infection.
  - decrease perirectal swelling and pain.
  - preventing rectal obstruction.
  - NSAIDs, a prolonged course of antimicrobials, and oral laxatives administered.
- perirectal abscesses drained based on their location, either rectally or perianally:
  - performed under epidural anaesthesia with the horse standing.
  - postoperatively, drained abscesses are flushed twice daily with antiseptic solution.

Prognosis

- good to excellent unless there is extension of the septic process into the abdominal cavity.

DISORDERS OF THE PERITONEUM

Haemoperitoneum

Definition/overview

- blood loss into the abdominal cavity is an uncommon but potentially life-threatening problem.
- most common in multiparous mares over 11 years of age.

Aetiology/pathophysiology

- occurs in broodmares:
  - mainly because of ruptured uterine vessels during or after parturition.
  - other causes (Fig. 3.63) include:
    - rupture of ovarian granulosa cell tumours or ovarian follicular haematomas.
    - uterine leiomyomas, or leiomyosarcomas.

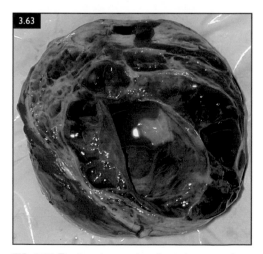

FIG. 3.63 Ruptured capsule of ovarian granulosa cell tumours can be the source of abdominal haemorrhage.

- less frequently, intra-abdominal haemorrhage originates from the GI tract:
  - entrapment of the small intestine within the epiploic foramen and subsequent rupture of the caudal vena cava.
  - rupture of mesenteric arteries secondary to *Strongylus vulgaris* larval migration.
- splenic rupture secondary to blunt trauma or neoplasia.
- haemorrhage secondary to a coagulopathy is uncommon.

Clinical presentation

- clinical manifestations are frequently non-specific.
- initial clinical signs include:
  - depression, lethargy, partial or complete anorexia, and colic.
- anaemia and hypovolaemia intensify:
  - signs of hypovolaemic shock:
    - tachycardia, tachypnoea, weak peripheral pulses, pale mucous membranes.
- ileus and abdominal distension may occur if a large volume of blood accumulates.

Differential diagnosis

- all conditions resulting in colic.
- broodmares:
  - uterine torsion, uterine rupture, and dystocia.

Diagnosis

- abdominal fluid accumulation, abdominal masses, or reproductive tract abnormalities may be palpable per rectum.
- transabdominal ultrasonography reveals:
  - presence of hyperechoic fluid within the abdomen:
    - typically, with a characteristic swirling pattern.
  - origin of haemorrhage is rarely identified.
- abdominocentesis definitively diagnoses haemoperitoneum:
  - **be careful to ensure that iatrogenic haemorrhage during abdominocentesis or centesis of the spleen is not misinterpreted.**

- erythrocyte count:
  - early stages, generally less than or equal to peripheral blood erythrocyte count.
  - chronically, usually equal to or greater than the peripheral blood erythrocyte count, due to protein and fluid resorption.
- cytological examination:
  - platelets not typically present unless the haemorrhage is peracute.
  - evidence of erythrophagocytosis suggests haemorrhage is subacute or chronic.
  - chronic haemorrhage:
    - hypersegmented pyknotic neutrophils and haemosiderophages observed.
- haematological abnormalities associated with acute blood loss after the initial 24 hours:
  - anaemia and decreased total plasma protein.
- hypoproteinaemia usually observed prior to the decline in haematocrit:
  - most common following initiation of intravenous fluid therapy.
- no obvious explanation for haemorrhage:
  - coagulation profile assessed to rule out coagulopathy.
  - thrombocytopenia is common and usually secondary to blood loss.
  - immune-mediated thrombocytopenia (IMTP) can occur.

Management

- initial treatment directed towards treating hypovolaemic shock:
  - intravenous fluid therapy (isotonic crystalloid solution) increases vascular volume:
    - fluid rate varies depending on cardiovascular status and volume of blood loss.
    - three times estimated volume of blood loss replaced with crystalloids.
- replacement of intravascular volume also accomplished with hypertonic saline (4–6 ml/kg of 5.0–7.5% NaCl), followed by administration of isotonic fluids:
  - contraindicated if blood loss is not controlled.

- haematocrit 0.15 l/l (15%) or lower or when the haemoglobin concentration is <50 g/l (5 g/dl):
  - whole blood transfusion usually required, especially in acute cases:
  - chronic blood loss, horses may better tolerate a low haematocrit.
  - clinical signs and blood lactate concentrations should be taken into consideration when deciding whether transfusion is required.
  - volume of blood transfused will depend on rate and quantity of blood loss.
- abdominal surgery may be required to control haemorrhage from tumours, rupture of a viscus, or leaking GI vessels.
- opioid antagonist naloxone (one treatment of 8 mg i/v) or 10% buffered neutral formalin (10–30 ml added to 500 ml of 0.09% NaCl) anecdotally reported as being used:
  - objective evaluation of efficacy is unavailable.

Prognosis

- variable but often poor and depends on the cause of haemorrhage.

Penetrating abdominal wounds

Definition/overview

- wound that breaches the abdominal skin, musculature, and peritoneum:
  - potentially causing damage to the underlying abdominal organs.
- behaviour of horses makes penetrating wounds more common than in other species.

Aetiology/pathophysiology

- impalement on a sharp object (fence post or part of a tree branch) is a common cause.
- occasionally, sustained when landing on an object over which it is jumping.
- reports of shotgun and crossbow wounds to the abdomen.
- pathophysiology will vary depending on:
  - extent of damage to the underlying abdominal organs.

- whether the inciting object has left debris or is still contained within the wound.
  - skin wound may be relatively insignificant:
    - larger amount of damage to the underlying organs is present.
- most of the damage created by deep penetrating wounds affects the spleen and GI tract:
  - splenic damage usually associated with marked haemorrhage and cardiovascular compromise.
  - potential for intestinal perforation and leakage with subsequent peritonitis.
  - large rent in the abdominal wall may lead to evisceration.
  - contaminated penetrating objects mean there is a high probability of infection, both acutely, and chronically during the healing process:
    - wounds may have persistent infection, draining sinuses or abscess formation.

Clinical presentation

- usually, obvious signs of an open abdominal wound:
  - severity of clinical signs may not correspond with the size of the external wound.
  - may be abdominal contents visible or palpable through the wound.
- damage to major abdominal organs is usually accompanied by signs of shock.
- cases with severe internal damage such as intestinal perforation, may not initially appear significantly compromised.
- signs of hypovolaemic shock, endotoxaemia, sepsis, or peritonitis may develop hours after the incident.

Differential diagnosis

- may be confused with deep wounds to the abdominal musculature that have failed to penetrate the peritoneum.

Diagnosis

- usually made by physical examination:
  - any wound over the abdominal region should be explored carefully.
- determine whether abdominal penetration has occurred (regardless of wound size).

- ultrasonographic examination of the abdomen may be useful in:
  - determining organ damage that has occurred.
  - whether there is haemoperitoneum or peritonitis present.
- abdominocentesis is important to determine whether intestinal leakage or haemoperitoneum has occurred.

Management

- acutely injured cases need any cardiovascular compensation stabilised, especially if splenic trauma has occurred (see Haemoperitoneum page 269).
- broad-spectrum antimicrobials should be administered immediately:
  - sodium/potassium penicillin 20,000–40,000 IU/kg i/v q6h or procaine penicillin 20,000 IU/kg i/m q12h and gentamicin 6.6–8.8 mg/kg i/v q24h
  - continued until after the abdominal wound has closed.
- tetanus prophylaxis should be considered.
- exploratory laparotomy may be necessary to determine the presence/extent of intestinal damage:
  - abdominal lavage can be performed during surgery.
- peritoneal lavage can be performed in the standing horse through indwelling drains although these often quickly become blocked.

Prognosis

- varies according to the extent of damage to the underlying organs:

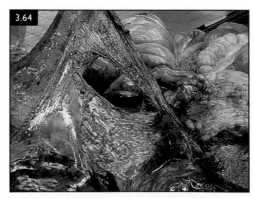

FIG. 3.64 Post-mortem view of the thoracic surface of an equine diaphragm. Note the very large defect in the ligamentous portion of this diaphragm.

- splenic trauma may have a fair–guarded prognosis if the haemorrhage and infection are controlled.
  - perforation of the bowel or evisceration have a grave prognosis.
- injury without trauma to the abdominal organs, the prognosis is improved:
  - wounds in the abdominal wall usually heal well.
  - high risk of infection, abscess formation, and peritonitis during the healing stages.

Diaphragmatic hernia

Definition/overview

- herniation of abdominal viscera into the thoracic cavity through a diaphragmatic defect (Fig. 3.64).

Aetiology/pathophysiology

- herniation through a diaphragmatic defect:
  - congenital:
    - ◆ incomplete fusion of the pleuroperitoneal folds, causing an enlarged oesophageal hiatus.
  - acquired:
    - ◆ increase in intrathoracic or intra-abdominal pressure creates a defect.
    - ◆ external trauma, strenuous exercise, GI distension, or pregnancy.
- herniated viscera decrease thoracic volume and induce thoracic pain, often resulting in hypoventilation.
- herniation may result in simple or strangulating intestinal obstruction.

Clinical presentation

- most frequent in mature horses with a history of trauma, strenuous exercise, breeding, or parturition.
- clinical signs are frequently non-specific and may include:
  - colic, exercise intolerance, and dyspnoea.

Differential diagnosis

- all disorders resulting in acute abdominal pain in the horse.

- diaphragmatic hernia may lead to exercise intolerance and should be included in this differential.
- pneumonia and pleuritis should be included in the differential diagnosis.

Diagnosis

- diagnosis can be difficult:
  - sometimes only made at surgery or necropsy.
- careful thoracic auscultation and percussion:
  - areas of thoracic dullness or reduced cardiac sounds may be identified.
  - referred GI sounds are frequently heard over the caudoventral thorax in normal horses and thus cannot be used for definitive diagnosis.
- perception of an empty caudal abdomen during palpation per rectum.
- standing lateral thoracic radiographs are useful and radiographic signs include:
  - gas-filled intestinal loops in the thoracic cavity.
  - increased ventral thoracic density.
  - absence of the cardiac shadow.
  - loss of part of the diaphragmatic shadow is most consistent finding.
- thoracic ultrasonography may show the presence of pleural fluid and abdominal viscera in the thoracic cavity.
- hypercapnoea due to hypoventilation, may be present:
  - respiratory acidosis or uncompensated metabolic acidosis is usually observed.
  - most common acid–base derangement in horses with colic is metabolic acidosis with respiratory compensation.
- abdominocentesis is usually normal:
  - haemorrhagic fluid may be obtained with an acute acquired diaphragm defect.
  - serosanguineous, turbid fluid if intestinal strangulation has occurred.

Management

- cases with intractable abdominal pain or respiratory distress require an emergency exploratory coeliotomy with assisted positive-pressure ventilation.
- **be careful in sedating suspected diaphragmatic hernia cases as sudden collapse, following the administration of alpha-2 agonists, is not uncommon.**
- acute diaphragmatic defects secondary to trauma may have surgery delayed if the animal's condition is stable:
  - allows for the edges of the defect to fibrose and easier surgical closure.

Prognosis

- poor to guarded prognosis for survival.

Abdominal hernia and prepubic tendon rupture

Definition/overview

- abdominal viscera can herniate through:
  - an anatomical opening.
  - defect in the abdominal wall.
- abdominal herniation includes:
  - ventral hernias.
  - incisional hernias.
  - acquired inguinal/scrotal hernias.
- defects in the abdominal wall in pregnant mares (see pages 30–32, Book 2), may result from:
  - stretching/tearing of the abdominal wall muscles:
    - rectus abdominus, oblique abdominal, and transverse abdominus muscles.
    - prepubic tendon.

Aetiology/pathophysiology

- aetiology of abdominal wall rupture in adult horses:
  - increased intra-abdominal pressure.
  - degenerative changes in the body wall.
  - delayed, or failure of, linea alba healing.
- pregnant mares can suffer ventral hernias and/or prepubic tendon ruptures:
  - associated with degenerative change in the body wall in old broodmares.
  - twin gestation.
  - hydroallantois.
  - and/or trauma.
- incisional herniation is a complication of ventral coeliotomy:
  - reported to occur in 0.7–15% of horses that undergo this procedure.
  - no breed or sex predilection exists.
  - dehiscence (acute incisional disruption) usually develops within 8 days after surgery.

- o incisional herniation can develop up to 3 months after ventral coeliotomy.
- o incisional hernia risk factors include:
  - ◆ postoperative incisional infection and swelling.
  - ◆ postoperative endotoxaemia and pain.
  - ◆ repeated coeliotomy.
  - ◆ use of chromic gut sutures to close the abdominal wall.
- • herniation through body wall defects may result in simple or strangulated intestinal obstruction.

Clinical presentation

- • ventral herniation or prepubic tendon rupture cases display:
  - o severe ventral abdominal swelling/oedema and are reluctant to walk.
  - o often lie down and are distressed with increased heart and respiratory rates.
  - o signs of abdominal pain may be present if the herniated contents are compromised.
- • incisional herniation presents as:
  - o ventral swelling developing over the abdominal incision site.
  - o prior to dehiscence commonly:
    - ◆ brown serosanguineous discharge from the incision.
    - ◆ progressive increase in drainage of peritoneal fluid.

Differential diagnosis

- • ventral herniation should be differentiated from prepubic tendon rupture:
  - o generally, the latter is not correctable surgically.
  - o mares with ventral herniation:
    - ◆ orientation of pelvis and mammary gland is normal.
  - o prepubic tendon rupture:
    - ◆ pelvis rotates cranioventrally as the prepubic tendon tension is lost from the cranial aspect of the pelvis.
    - ◆ lordosis may also be noticed because the pelvis and vertebral column cannot maintain normal alignment.
    - ◆ cranioventral displacement of the udder resulting from the tipping of the pelvis can lead to rupture of the blood supply:

- – blood may be observed in the milk of mares with rupture.
- • postoperative wound infection, severe peri-incisional oedema, seroma, and sinus formation are easily differentiated from incisional hernias, with the abdominal wall being intact on palpation.

Diagnosis

- • external palpation:
  - o ventral and incisional herniation:
    - ◆ define the hernia ring and hernia contents.
    - ◆ may be difficult if there is extensive abdominal oedema.
    - ◆ commonly, mares with ventral hernias resent deep palpation of affected area.
- • rectal palpation:
  - o may help to differentiate ventral hernia from prepubic tendon rupture.
  - o palpation of the abdominal wall defect can be difficult depending on:
    - ◆ defect's location.
    - ◆ size of the fetus.
    - ◆ distended loops of intestine and abdominal pain warrants an immediate exploratory laparotomy.
- • transcutaneous ultrasonographic examination:
  - o 3.5 or 5 MHz transducer.
  - o helpful to rule in herniation.
  - o evaluate extent of the abdominal wall defect (see page 30–32, Book 2).

Management
Ventral hernia

- • surgical herniorrhaphy is advocated:
  - o close to term mare (at least 330 days pregnant):
    - ◆ parturition induced prior to surgery.
    - ◆ delivery assisted as abdominal contractions are often insufficient.
  - o acute herniation without evidence of intestinal obstruction:
    - ◆ delay surgery to allow formation of fibrosis within the hernia ring.
    - ◆ interim management:
      - – application of an abdominal support bandage (see page 32, Book 2).

- – anti-inflammatory drugs to decrease swelling.
  - – feed a low-residue pelleted ration to decrease intestinal bulk volume.
  - ○ evidence of intestinal obstruction:
    - ♦ surgery should be performed without delay.
  - ○ suture or mesh herniorrhaphy depending on the diameter of the hernial ring.

Prepubic tendon rupture

- usually, cannot be surgically corrected.
- conservative treatment may be attempted:
  - ○ parturition induced if the mare is close to term.
  - ○ mare rested in a box stall for several months.
  - ○ abdominal support should be applied.
  - ○ severe oedema initially warrants anti-inflammatory medications.
  - ○ low-bulk pelleted food offered to decrease the volume of digesta.

Incisional hernia

- surgical herniorrhaphy is generally postponed for 4–6 months:
  - ○ allows for resolution of any infection.
  - ○ development of hernial ring fibrosis.
  - ○ many hernias resolve or markedly decrease in size:
    - ♦ no further therapy may be necessary.
- initially, an abdominal support bandage is applied.
- antimicrobials are administered based on wound culture and sensitivity.
- ventral drainage is established.
- infected wound lavaged with diluted antiseptic solution.
- suture or mesh herniorrhaphy is performed when incisional infection has resolved.

Prognosis

- guarded for successful correction of a ventral hernia.
- incisional herniations warrant a favourable prognosis.
- 3–5 months of rest are required after surgical correction of both ventral and incisional hernias.

- prognosis for prepubic tendon rupture is poor.

Septic peritonitis

Definition/overview

- peritonitis is inflammation of the mesothelial lining of the peritoneal cavity.
- any inflammatory stimulus can cause peritonitis.
- septic peritonitis is the most common in horses.

Aetiology/pathophysiology

- leakage or translocation of intestinal bacteria is the most common cause:
  - ○ gastric or intestinal rupture.
  - ○ rectal tear.
  - ○ bacterial translocation in cases of severe enterocolitis.
  - ○ abdominal perforation by foreign bodies.
  - ○ breeding injury in mares.
- rupture of an abdominal abscess.
- small percentage of horses develop peritonitis after colic surgery.
- idiopathic primary peritonitis has been described.

Clinical presentation

- clinical signs are variable and depend on disease duration and degree of contamination.
- signs with acute colonic rupture and gross contamination of the abdomen usually progress rapidly.
- clinical progression may be more gradual with:
  - ○ slowly leaking intestinal viscera.
  - ○ lower level of contamination from bacterial translocation or haematogenous spread.
- intestinal rupture with developing septic peritonitis:
  - ○ affected animals may appear to improve initially as signs of colic abate.
- fever and depression may be present initially.
- condition typically progresses rapidly as septic shock develops.
- body temperature may be elevated, normal, or decreased.

- heart rate is invariably elevated and can be very high (>100 bpm).
- respiratory rate is usually elevated.
- mucous membranes progress from normal to hyperaemic to cyanotic.
- GI sounds decrease.
- dehydration develops as fluid is sequestered in the abdomen.
- variable degree of colic may be evident.
- sweating and anxiety are common.
- idiopathic primary peritonitis typically has milder clinical signs consistent with non-specific colic, although fever is not uncommon.

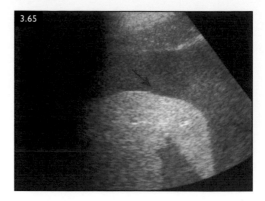

FIG. 3.65 Excessive hyperechoic free abdominal fluid (arrowed) is evident in this horse with septic peritonitis.

Differential diagnosis

- colitis, pleuritis, strangulating intestinal lesions, and other causes of sepsis or endotoxaemia may appear similar.

Diagnosis

- haematology:
  - neutropenia with toxic changes in neutrophils often present but is non-specific.
  - total protein levels tend to decrease rapidly.
  - haematological changes consistent with dehydration and metabolic acidosis may be present.
- rectal palpation:
  - occasionally, the intestinal viscera feel 'gritty'.
  - sometimes, the abdomen feels abnormally empty following intestinal rupture.
- transabdominal ultrasonography:
  - large volume of hyperechoic abdominal fluid usually evident (Fig. 3.65).
- abdominocentesis is invaluable:
  - should be performed in colic cases with an unexplained fever to rule out peritonitis.
  - fluid may range from serosanguineous and turbid to brownish with the presence of ingesta.
  - typically, marked increases in cell count ($15-800 \times 10^9$/l) with degenerative changes in neutrophils and an increased total protein level:
    - intracellular bacteria often evident cytologically.
  - bacterial culture is particularly useful if a ruptured abdominal abscess is suspected.
  - occasionally, normal abdominal fluid is obtained because of pocketing of fluid:
    - particularly early in the disease.
    - abdominocentesis should be repeated if clinical signs progress.
- idiopathic primary peritonitis typically:
  - less marked haematological changes.
  - abdominal fluid varies from mild to markedly increased nucleated cell counts and protein.
  - accumulation of large amounts of free fluid is rare.

Management

- prognosis for severe septic peritonitis is grave and attempts at treatment may not be justified.
- inciting cause should be identified and addressed whenever possible.
- exploratory laparotomy is often indicated (Fig. 3.66).
  - allows for identification of the inciting cause.
  - thorough abdominal lavage and placement of abdominal drains.
- intravenous fluid therapy is often required:
  - high fluid rates often necessary early in the disease because of dehydration and cardiovascular compromise.
  - plasma transfusion may be required.

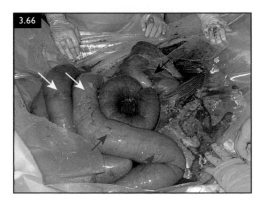

FIG. 3.66 Distended small intestine (white arrows) and caecum (black arrow) with patches of fibrin (red arrows) in a horse with septic peritonitis.

- broad-spectrum antimicrobial therapy, including adequate anaerobic coverage:
  - sodium/potassium penicillin 20,000–40,000 IU/kg i/v q6h.
  - gentamicin 6.6–8.8 mg/kg i/v q24h.
  - metronidazole (25 mg/kg p/o q8–12h).
  - treatment changed as necessary based on culture and sensitivity results.
- flunixin meglumine is typically used (1.1 mg/kg i/v q12h).
- abdominal lavage is essential with severe septic peritonitis:
  - rarely indicated in idiopathic primary peritonitis.
  - lavage via a single ventral drain or combination of dorsal ingress and ventral egress drains.
    - placed in standing sedated horses, ideally with ultrasonographic guidance.
    - horses stabilised before drainage with intravenous fluid therapy to compensate for any fluid shifts that may occur.
    - 10–20 litres of balanced electrolyte solution infused in the adult horse:
      - clamp drain(s) and horse walked for 10–20 minutes to distribute the fluid.
      - drain is then opened.
      - further walking can facilitate drainage.
- intraperitoneal administration of antimicrobials is not usually indicated.
- infusion of other substances (heparin to decrease adhesion formation):
  - efficacy not been proven.

Prognosis

- depends on the cause of the peritonitis and the severity of the disease.
- prognosis is grave where the cause cannot be identified and promptly corrected.
- peritonitis caused by intestinal rupture is almost invariably fatal.
- complications are common and include intestinal adhesions and laminitis.
- treatment can be prolonged and expensive.
- idiopathic primary peritonitis carries a better prognosis with survival in >90% of cases:
  - long-term complications are rare.

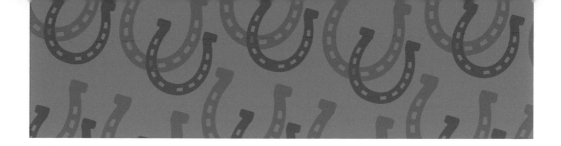

Index